CONTENTS

T0091782

Public health is about creating the conditions for population health. This conceptualization is memorized by all public health students but misunderstood by them and everyone else. Why? Because true comprehension necessitates action and risks upending the arrangement of power in our world. These power structures are the very ones that create the maldistribution of deleterious health outcomes through, for example, environmental catastrophes, economic inequalities, and approaches to globalization.

As an academic who is highly engaged in public health practice, devoting a career to working in public health trenches throughout the world, I have witnessed firsthand the circumvention of important structural issues in favor of protecting power and wealth – whether communities, corporations, countries, or regions. In my work, this happened with HIV and other bloodborne infections, and opioid overdose.

Talking about these issues within the public health community and writing words such as these in public health textbooks are futile endeavors because, as shown during the COVID pandemic, the public health profession is subjugated by the power structures and cannot activate the levers of change. I was reminded of this when I had to admit my surprise that we could not use the podium given to public health to advocate for systemic change during the initial COVID period (2020–2021). Public health remains anemic in effecting climate change, drought, or water scarcity – topics that, strangely, are viewed as being out of public health's "lane." This is likely because public health is speaking to itself.

Our lives and the continuation of our species and our world depend on our collective ability to address root causes of the conditions affecting population health. To do this, we must become an educated electorate. This means fighting for enfranchisement from Gulfport, Mississippi USA to Yangon, Myanmar. This means understanding how law and policy affect the structures and behaviors of systems impacting health outcomes at the population level. This is not about healthcare or pharmaceutical access, although they too are products of the maldistribution of power. This means getting involved in the politics of our communities, states, and countries.

A central lesson is that those who own the framing of a problem (problem definition) determine the playing field for problem solving, the solution options, the actors who have standing for involvement, and the distribution of resulting benefits and burdens. If, for example, the water crisis in the western United States is just a matter of individual water use, then the range of interventions to increase the supply is at the individual or family/household level. But if water scarcity is a function of unbridled development, factory farming, and the inability of the U.S. national government to facilitate solutions with corporations and state and tribal governments, then the options for interventions are quite different.

Let's be honest. Public health colleges, schools, and programs do not prepare students for this level of work. Policy curricula have only been required to accredit U.S. schools of public health in the last 10 years. Public health's professional penchant for individual-level behavioral interventions blinds us to the real fact that it is on the structural level that we must focus, because our lives depend on it.

In this book, Dr. Crosby opens a vital window to our future with a focus on upstream approaches to population health. Readers will recognize critical issues such as COVID, chronic disease, and water scarcity. They will learn (or perhaps recall) civics lessons about the policies and political processes that determine the structure and functioning of government: policies and systems that, for example, facilitate gun violence by precluding meaningful action. Timing is of the essence because as I write this, the United States has experienced its 609th mass shooting *yet* this year, and Haiti and Mexico reel under gun violence fueled by U.S. gun manufacturers.

The take-home message of this book is that public health is centrally political because it addresses the structures that create the conditions for health. Public health is about restoration, justice, and reparation. It is about righting the boat so that we can, together, weather the stormy seas. It is proactive, preventive, population-wide, and courageous. It is about changing our world so that we can, as present and future populations, thrive.

So as you encounter this book and the concepts within, make a promise to yourself that you will take action. You will become a change agent. You will embrace the fact that *we the people* make the policy – but only if we get involved and fix our broken systems. The days of intense focus on individual-level information campaigns have yielded to a new generation of efforts leveraging public support and engagement for the protection of a basic human right: to live healthy and long lives!

Beth Meyerson, MDiv., PhD
Professor of Medicine
Department of Family and Community Medicine
College of Medicine
University of Arizona

When the term **civics** is used in the context of education, most students and teachers in the United States think about the process of learning about the Constitution, the Bill of Rights, co-equal branches of the federal government, and the relationship of state governments to the larger functioning of the nation. Often, however, the approach to civics is less than applied, and the lessons may come across as irrelevant to students. It frequently is not apparent that governments – at all levels – are very much involved in one aspect of our daily lives: promoting and protecting the health of the public. With the year 2020 ushering a global pandemic into the lives of Americans, the term **public health** quickly became used in everyday language, the media, and the offices and meeting rooms of state and federal elected representatives. For most Americans, this was the first time in their lives that public health was not taken for granted.

The COVID-19 pandemic is just one small example of the threats and corresponding public health challenges that can best be met through the collective action of our society. In contrast, 50 years ago, the approach to public health was tightly focused on personal behavior change. This approach originates in medical care and thus is limited to personal actions tied to the ongoing process of monitoring people for the development of chronic diseases and vaccinating people against infectious diseases. The "consult your doctor" advice is all too often a catchphrase used under the rubric of prevention. As the nation has evolved, so has our ability to transcend the limits of medical care and truly embrace the concept of **health for all** (including those without medical care). Decades of funded research have taught the lesson of health being an outgrowth of how we live our lives rather than a product paid for through medical bills.

At this time in history, our nation has an advanced capacity to be proactive about preventing both infectious and chronic diseases at the level of the entire nation (known as **population health**). The approach to population health transcends the personal level and places the responsibility to prevent disease on communities, industries, employers, local and state governments, and the U.S. federal government. This proactive approach functions at a population level as a consequence of an informed and educated electorate – meaning that "we the people" collectively help to shape and maintain the conditions that promote health for all people. This is necessary because the most urgent threats to the health of the public – many of which are results of climate change – demand large-scale adaptations, including immediate actions to reduce the looming health disparities that have plagued America for too long.

As a professor of public health for several decades now, I have carefully selected only the most urgent issues for your attention in this textbook. You will find that each chapter is written with an emphasis on the present and the future as opposed to dwelling on the past. The chapters form a type of unfolding story that begins with how public health has skyrocketed to the center of attention and continues through the issues most in need of – and most amenable to – a prevention-oriented solution, as opposed to the high price of waiting for a clinical disease to develop before intervention occurs. An underlying theme of this textbook is that America must lessen its dependence on medical intervention and become increasingly vigilant about keeping all people from developing risks that lead to premature morbidity and mortality. The last four chapters are particularly novel and important because each is cast as a type of blueprint to design public health responses to events that have yet to become fully catastrophic. We must act now to protect global health in the future!

CHAPTER 1

THE COVID-19 PANDEMIC: A PORTRAIT OF AN EPIDEMIC

The following is an excerpt taken from a speech delivered by President Barack Obama, in the White House, to an assembly of global health leaders. The excerpt begins by referring to recent global pandemics such as Ebola, H1N1, and SARS.

> Each time, it's been harder than it should be to share information and to contain the outbreak. As a result, diseases have spread faster and farther than they should have – which means lives are lost that could have been saved.
>
> —*President Barack Obama, September 26, 2014*

Overview

The last case of smallpox was diagnosed in 1977. The disease caused an estimated 300 million deaths over at least a thousand years, so this final diagnosis represents a milestone in public health practice. The milestone was achieved through one of public health's greatest assets: vaccination! So, it would seem that vaccines will solve everything related to global pandemics. If only this were true! The sobering reality is that Edward Jenner's pioneering work on the smallpox vaccine occurred more than 200 years before the disease was eradicated. The lesson that should have been learned from the globally coordinated smallpox vaccination campaign was that people – and even entire governments – are bound to resist vaccination, regardless of the potential consequences. The **World Health Organization** (a global entity that is widely recognized for being the world authority on the prevention and control of infectious disease) ultimately mobilized health workers to enter even the most remote and culturally unique areas of the planet to convince people to take the vaccine being offered to them at no cost. Sadly, this global smallpox vaccine campaign lasted more than 11 years and was fraught with conflict at the local level in nation after nation.

Now, let's fast-forward to 2021, when healthcare workers around the world were assigned the task of entering remote and culturally unique areas of the planet to convince people to take the vaccine being offered to them at no cost. This time, it was a vaccine against COVID-19. Sadly, populations were not universally glad to have this vaccine; millions of people refused it, despite ample evidence that death from COVID-19 was approximately 11 times more likely among the unvaccinated than the fully vaccinated. This level of refusal was, of course, history repeating itself. But stark differences existed between smallpox vaccination campaigns and vaccination campaigns against **SARS-Cov-2** (i.e., COVID-19). With COVID-19,

Understanding the Science and Practice of Public Health, First Edition. Richard Crosby.
© 2023 John Wiley & Sons, Inc. Published 2023 by John Wiley & Sons, Inc.

LEARNING OBJECTIVES

1. Appreciate and explain the history of the COVID-19 pandemic.

2. Understand disease transmission and the **chain of infection** and how this can be altered to protect the public.

3. Explain basic principles of infection and disease transmission.

4. Describe the function of vaccines.

5. Explain how self-interests in government can hinder public health efforts to control the spread of infectious diseases.

6. Describe examples of corporate interests that overshadowed public health efforts to control COVID-19.

7. Using COVID-19 as an example, articulate how epidemics magnify racial and ethnic disparities in nations such as the United States.

the very same discussions healthcare workers were having with people in isolated tribal villages in Sierra Leone, for example, were also occurring in most U.S. states! Despite an overwhelming level of access to education, COVID-19 vaccine information, and published evidence of the vaccine's safety records, millions of U.S. residents were asking questions such as, "Why should I trust the contents of this vaccine?" and "How do I know this will not give me COVID?" In short, massive uptake of the vaccine did not happen.

As the Delta variant of COVID-19 emerged, it had a huge advantage: many unvaccinated people also were not wearing masks. Due to behavioral factors that were not rectifiable, these two very simple public health measures (vaccination and mask wearing) failed to protect the public. Consequently, hospitals continued to be overwhelmed with COVID patients, workforce productivity was slowed, supply chains were crippled, and economies worldwide slowly imploded under the constant strain of a pandemic that could have ended in record time.

This chapter is not about the history of COVID-19, nor is it about the host of blunders and mistakes made in terms of public health response. Instead, it uses COVID-19 as an example of how public health practice can successfully control the spread of infectious diseases. As the only chapter in this textbook devoted to infectious disease, this topic comes first because controlling epidemics and pandemics is the very origin of public health practice.

As you study this chapter, you will learn basic principles pertaining to the spread and control of infectious diseases. To keep the discussion relevant and timely, each example will be applied to COVID-19. You will also learn a bit about mutation and why, for example, the flu vaccine must be remade and redistributed annually. As the chapter continues, you will come to understand that COVID-19 is not a "once in a lifetime" disaster. Rather, COVID-19 should be viewed as a warning to all humans that our species exists in a fragile balance within a complex web of tiny microorganisms that ultimately can cause massive levels of death and turmoil. Learning to respect this balance and protect it through carefully planned standards of public health practice is an urgent priority for all of us.

All too often public health is taken for granted. The exception is when a nation or the entire world is in the midst of an epidemic or pandemic. Thus, a top priority of public health is the control of infectious disease. If you visualize public health practice as a pyramid, the base is first and foremost the control of rapidly spreading infectious diseases. Indeed, this goal is the origin of public health (see **Chapter 2**). This book also begins with this chapter because COVID-19 teaches a lesson that should greatly inspire all of us: that "we the people" must have an advanced understanding of what may arguably be the most vital function of local, state, and even federal government: protecting the health of the people. Finally, as this is the only chapter in this textbook devoted to infectious disease, you will learn about the overall principles of disease transmission and control. These principles are more important than COVID-19 per se because it is highly likely that many other life-threatening infectious diseases will emerge in the coming decades (Beeler, 2021).

Basic Terminology

Before you read any further in this chapter, it is vital to understand the implied meaning of several terms related to public health practice. The first, of course, is the word **pandemic**. COVID-19 is correctly referred to as a pandemic because it is a global occurrence – thus, pandemics affect multiple nations and continents. When, however, referring to just one nation (such as Britain, China, or the U.S), it is appropriate to use the term **epidemic**. Epidemics are local, whereas pandemics are global. Although you may not be used to thinking about the United States as "local," from a global perspective this is very much the case. Because of significant differences between governments, cultures, and the health status of people, it is

---

two very simple public health measures (vaccination and mask wearing) failed

"we the people" must have an advanced understanding of what may arguably be the most vital function of local, state, and even federal government: protecting the health of the people.

useful to think about how, for example, one nation differs from another in terms of progress in controlling its local version of any given pandemic. A third term in this regard is **endemic**. History shows that most nations can eventually reduce the severity of an epidemic to a low and stable level of annual new cases. At that point, the disease causing that epidemic is correctly referred to as an **endemic**. Sadly, some epidemics reach an endemic level only after several years, or even decades, of public health intervention.

For now, three other terms are vital for you to understand. The first denotes any microorganism having the ability to invade the human body and trigger a disease process: this is a **pathogen**. A pathogen may or may not be a living cell in its own right. COVID-19 is caused by a virus. A virus is not a living cell. Instead, it is a set of genetic instructions looking for cells to invade so it can carry out these instructions. The next term is **immunity**. Without immunity to pathogens, humans would quickly perish. Immunity is typically acquired based on the invasion of a given pathogen followed by a successful immune response. It is very much the case, by the way, that your immune system is your lifeline to survival. Immunity to a specific pathogen can also be acquired through the artificial means of vaccination. When a pathogen invades the immune system (or, in the case of vaccines, when the properties of the vaccine enter the body) and the immune system functions properly, the result is the development of **antibodies**. Depending on the pathogen and the immune system, antibodies may last for a lifetime, several years, or even less than one year. Antibodies maintain a person's health in the near-constant presence of pathogens in daily life.

A Brief History of the COVID-19 Pandemic

In December 2019, stray – and very brief – snippets of the news described a new virus affecting the respiratory systems of people in China. The news was not particularly disturbing or by any means alarming to most people in the United States. In less than two short months, however, all that changed. The virus was quickly gaining traction worldwide, and the United States was far from exempt (as it had been for so many other pandemics that were quickly controlled and soon extinguished). By March 2020, news programs were heavily invested in covering what was then widely known as the COVID-19 pandemic. For the first time in the lives of most Americans, a well-deserved fear penetrated daily life, and it was clear that an era of isolation, mask wearing, and hopes for a vaccine or cure had begun. Stores, restaurants, and business establishments posted signs such as "Temporarily closed." People employed in careers that allowed online work shifted their job site to their living room or den, while those without this ability became unemployed or risked exposure to the new virus on a regular basis. Many others lost their jobs due to shutdowns in the service industries (restaurants, hair salons, retail stores, and so on). Food kitchens and homeless shelters were both overwhelmed and unprepared to meet the rush in demand in ways that were "COVID-safe." The world had dramatically changed in just a few short months.

The world had dramatically changed in just a few short months.

By the end of 2021, it was clear that the U.S. death toll for COVID-19 would soon surpass the milestone 1 one million people. The worldwide myth – emanating from developed nations such as the United States – that any infectious disease could be controlled had been shattered by COVID-19. As **public health** became an everyday term, the public health system became exposed as a tattered web of loosely arranged puzzle pieces that would not fit together in any meaningful way. The public health response was largely a failure. This is not to imply that great measures were ignored; indeed, thousands of institutions – from universities to Fortune 500 companies such as Google and Microsoft – created highly protective policies. University students and their professors, for example, became accustomed to classrooms characterized

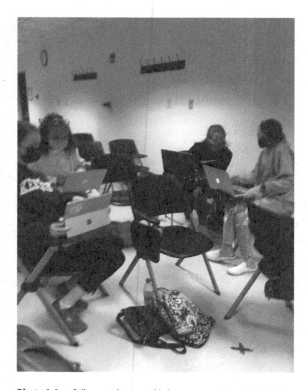

Photo 1.1   College students quickly became accustomed to the idea of mandatory mask use during all classes that were held in person as opposed to online.

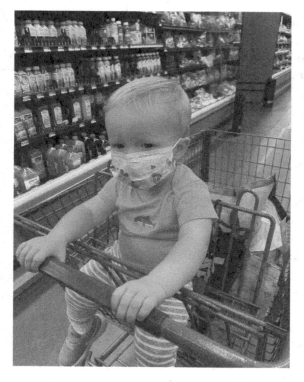

Photo 1.2   People who took the time to understand that even small children could carry and thus transmit the virus were quick to insist that their own children (or grandchildren) must "mask up."

by mandatory mask rules (see **Photo 1.1**). Even when some of the mandates were removed, millions of Americans erred on the side of caution and continued to wear masks in places such as grocery stores (see **Photo 1.2**).

Although most people who lived through the early years of the COVID-19 pandemic probably have their own version of this space in U.S. history (see **Box 1.1**), histories of pandemics are best written by science reporters. For instance, Debora MacKenzie (MacKenzie, 2020) wrote an entire book about why the COVID-19 pandemic "never should have happened." Early in the book, she recounts the events of December 31, 2019. She began the day by reading a report from a prominent organization known as *ProMED (Program for Monitoring Emerging Diseases)*. The report described people with "severe, undiagnosed pneumonia in the central Chinese city of Wuhan, in Hubei province" (MacKenzie, 2020, p. 3). This should have been a wake-up call to the world, but instead it was barely noticed. As it turned out, that day was the unofficial start of what became the largest pandemic since AIDS (a pandemic yet to be fully controlled).

Before COVID-19, scholars and historians frequently referenced a pandemic less recent than AIDS. In 1918, Americans were suddenly in the midst of what became known as the **Spanish flu pandemic**. The flu is a virus; however, unlike COVID-19, it is capable of dramatic shifts in the proteins of its surface structure and DNA. The 1918 flu was a result of an unlikely shift that led to the death (often in just one or two days) of approximately 675,000 Americans in less than 2 years. Prior to COVID-19, this 1918 epidemic was considered the worst in modern U.S. history. Despite warnings from prominent scientists (Garrett, 1995), the world remained largely unprepared for a repeat of the 1918 tragedy. Then, just over 100 years later, the novel coronavirus came along. This was significant because it altered the public illusion that somehow modern medicine would "protect us all."

Unlike COVID-19 (at least for now), Spanish flu was a pandemic of great virulence, with people becoming ill in the morning and dying by nightfall. This rapid destruction of the hosts by the virus led to an equally rapid decline in the pandemic: the virus kept destroying its reservoir (i.e., people) so quickly that infected people had little chance of spreading the disease before they died.

After the Spanish flu pandemic, nations worked together to construct safeguards against future pandemics. But even despite recent warnings from public health experts whose careers were focused on global preparedness against pandemics, the Trump administration (2016–2020) largely dismantled many of the global protections put in place by the previous administration under President Obama (2008–2016). When Americans found themselves in the midst of the COVID-19 pandemic, the broadly ignored global protections were sorely missed. Consequently, variants of COVID-19 such as the

BOX 1.1. ONE SCHOLAR'S PERSPECTIVE ON THE COVID-19 PANDEMIC

While authoring multiple textbooks over two decades, it has always been my practice to avoid writing in the first person. I will violate that rule for only this particular box! As a professor of public health who specialized in the control of HIV, I was immediately struck by the vast similarities between the early years of the HIV pandemic and the first two years of the COVID-19 pandemic. Even before HIV was named, the public experienced a type of mass hysteria, and misinformation spread quickly and rapidly became "fact" in the eyes of people who had a need to embrace beliefs about HIV that best fit their worldview. Homophobic people, for example, were quick to dismiss HIV as a "gay disease." People who viewed drug addiction as a personal choice were quick to view HIV transmitted through the reuse of needles/syringes as an outcome of moral weakness. It wasn't until children became infected by HIV (through blood transfusions or by mother-to-fetus/infant transmission routes) that people could no longer dismiss HIV as being segregated to "bad people." It was soon clear to me that COVID-19 and HIV were strikingly dissimilar because rather than "bad people" dying, the preponderance of people killed by COVID-19 were 70 years of age and older. Yet this dissimilarity created a parallel to the HIV pandemic because young and middle-aged people freely engaged in the belief pattern of "it won't hurt me." This was to me a repeat of all the work I had done in public health since 1983 – people almost always found a way to engage in denial of risk so they would not have to alter their behaviors. Examples include people who smoke, remain obese, and consume high-sodium diets despite knowing that all three of these behaviors are ill-advised from a public health perspective. Denial is easy as long as it works in a person's favor and thus (in this example) lets a person continue the risk behaviors of smoking, eating a diet that causes obesity, and consuming highly processed foods loaded with sodium. It has also been my constant experience that this denial may persist even after, for instance, a mild heart attack occurs. With COVID-19 as the example, denial relative to the value of the vaccine did sometimes (but not always) wane after unvaccinated people were hospitalized with COVID-19 or a family member died of the virus. This is a relatively dim portrait of Americans; however, it played out over and over again as the U.S. epidemic marched onward.

As the global pandemic played out, I was in the process of writing this textbook. I had promised myself I would write this chapter last, hoping that by then at least the U.S. epidemic would be mostly resolved. It did not happen that way: the American epidemic and the global pandemic were constantly "events in motion," as evidenced by emerging variants and the unspoken but always present fear among experts in infectious disease that a variant might come along and evade any immunity provided by the vaccines created in 2021. This very real prospect was terrifying to the point that it was difficult to even imagine the public health consequences. I soon resolved that this chapter would never be finished in terms of summarizing the start and finish of COVID-19. Instead, it became clear to me that all this chapter can do is convey to you a sense of what life was like – from a public health perspective – during what I will refer to as the "early years of COVID-19."

The early years were punctuated by a lack of understanding of the basic disease transmission routes of COVID-19 and the contents of the vaccine against moderate to severe illness (the vaccine was never meant to be one that averted illness entirely). However, this lack of understanding was no surprise, as it had existed in the past for diseases such as influenza. The problem was that the public soon grew weary with the task of learning about COVID-19 and thus gravitated toward creating "local truths" via friendship groups and social media. Masks worn based on mandates were often worn below the nose. Makeshift masks – such as bandanas – were used, despite their complete lack of protective value. Business establishments paid more attention to sanitizing surfaces than enforcing the correct and consistent use of properly fitting and highly protective masks. Even worse, anti-vaccine groups used Facebook, Instagram, Twitter, and other popular forms of social media to finally have their time in the spotlight, sowing doubt about the billions of dollars' worth of carefully conducted research and development that had successfully led to a vaccine in a historically rapid time after the virus was discovered. Our public health system was not robust enough to avoid this near-constant level of information decay.

But information decay was only one problem. The other was that people were used to books, movies, and so on portraying disease outbreaks as time-limited. Business and industry leaders were particularly quick to impose a time frame on the virus and predict dates when life (and work) would "return to normal." Simply stated, none of this rises above the level of wishful thinking. History shows that viral pandemics can last for decades or even centuries. The virus has become part of modern life, and it will run through the human race on a schedule largely determined by its random mutations. As a teacher, I make it a habit to use metaphors when explaining complex phenomena. In that spirit, let me suggest that the public response to the COVID-19 epidemic in the United States was much like people being trapped at the exit of a grocery store by the rapid onset of heavy rain with no end in sight. At first, people gathered by the door, saying, "It won't last long." As time crawled by, some people said "F--- this; I'm going out." As the rain began to subside, others said things like "It's good enough now – I'm out of here." Eventually, others were forced to leave due to obligations beyond their control – they had to leave despite the continuous downpour. Roughly speaking, the vast majority of Americans soon chose to "brave the rain" because they were exhausted from social isolation or decided that this was the new normal. Millions of others fell in the metaphoric category of being "forced to leave due to obligations": their work and/or family life (particularly when schools reopened) allowed no choice except a return to places of employment such as restaurants and bars, where mask wearing was not practical or practiced.

Ultimately, as the third year of the pandemic began, I was humbled about having spent my career as a professor of public health. That title had seemed somehow noble to me, as though we were protecting the public from harm. The reality was that public health was an untested entity in the 21st century, at least until COVID-19 appeared and showed that the public health system was not yet ready for such challenges. There is indeed much to be done, and much of it has to be done differently to be effective in the presence of the next pandemic!

Delta variant and the **Omicron variant** were able to spread rapidly through the world. A variant is nothing more than a random mutation of viral replication, one that successfully creates new properties of a virus that can then propagate.

As the Delta variant quickly dominated the U.S. COVID-19 epidemic, virologists and other scientists feared this could be the new normal. Even prior to Delta, this fear was apparent in the writings of experts; it finally also penetrated the psyche of most Americans. For the first time in their lives, millions of Americans began to realize that something as tiny as a virus could bring industry, business, and the global economy to a near standstill. In the middle of the 2021 holiday season, the WHO warned the world about the even greater dangers of the Omicron variant. By this time, it was clear that humans would have to adapt or face an ever-increasing escalation of daily death tolls.

In early October 2021, the U.S. death toll from COVID-19 surpassed the 700,000 mark. The worldwide myth – emanating from developed nations such as the United States – that any infectious disease could be controlled had been completely shattered by COVID-19. The failed public health system was magnified by Centers for Disease Control (CDC) Director Robert Redfield, who played down the severity of the virus and often altered the findings and conclusions of scientists to create a much less harmful public image of the potential for COVID-19 to destroy lives and greatly diminish the quality of Americans' daily existence.

In contrast to the United States, other developed nations were far more proactive. For example, on December 19, 2020, Britain Prime Minister Boris Johnson delivered a national broadcast to citizens that was essentially a message to please stay home for the holidays and that – despite efforts to the contrary – he was forced to "cancel Christmas." His message was one of protecting Britain from a new and more contagious strain of the novel coronavirus by instructing Brits via a set of nationally established rules pertaining to closures, prohibitions on travel, rules against inter-mingling between households, and the use of safety precautions such as masks and social distancing. His tone and words conveyed a strong sense of urgency, tempered by clarity and confidence. It was an inspirational moment in British history. Unfortunately, a counterpart moment never occurred in the United States. Instead, the U.S. president (Trump) took a nearly opposite approach to the pandemic, engaging the nation in a series of tweets, press statements, and speeches that dismissed the problem as largely inconsequential. As case numbers climbed throughout the spring of 2020 and the death tolls crept into the six-figure range, the White House and the president continued to dismiss the advice of infectious disease experts and appointed largely unqualified people to lead U.S. efforts to curb the spread of the disease. As 2020 was an election year for this president, it was clear that suppressing the severity of the U.S. COVID-19 morbidity and mortality figures was an important priority. The CDC director (Redfield) subsequently admitted to softening the previously drafted directive language used by the CDC to provide guidelines designed to control the spread of the virus in high-risk settings such as meatpacking plants and schools.

As it turned out, the U.S. COVID-19 epidemic was the first time in American history when the disease became a political dividing line between Republicans and Democrats. Even after 2 years of claiming lives and destroying local economies, people took preventive action largely predicted by party affiliation. For instance, Democrats were generally about twice as likely to be fully vaccinated as their Republican counterparts. Even entire states such as Florida and Texas fought mask-wearing mandates, with Florida going so far as to pass legislation against such mandates. Having put mandates into place regarding mask wearing, Governor Gretchen Whitmer of Michigan subsequently became a target of hostile people strongly opposed to this well-established protective action. The hostility elevated to the level of death threats and intruders on her home property. This type of division in the nation set COVID-19 apart from any other national epidemic in U.S. history.

At a time when the people needed most to be united, they were more divided than ever before. Most tragic in this lack of unity was that COVID-19 had disproportionately infected (and killed) people of color – a point that was consistently made by Democrats and seemingly ignored by Republicans. The United States is home to what has consistently been a glaring cascade of **health disparities** that are not unique to COVID-19 and that all favor white, non-Hispanics over people of color (as you progress through this book, you will learn just how insipid and devastating these racial/ethnic disparities are in terms of health and disease).

Just prior to Thanksgiving 2021, the Johns Hopkins system of tracking COVID-19 deaths was used to report that the death toll could be compared to entire states! Using this data, the *Washington Post* reported, "If the Americans who've died of Covid made up a state, it would rank 47th in the country, more populous than Alaska, Vermont, or Wyoming" (Fisher, Royza, & Ruble, 2021).

During the holiday season in 2021, it was widely apparent to all Americans that supplies of merchandise, including big-ticket items such as cars and trucks, were critically low. Further, inflation was at one of the highest points in recent history, and people were leaving their jobs in record numbers. These occurrences are best thought of as ripple effects of COVID-19. Americans who were willing to read credible news sources soon learned that deadly epidemics take a huge toll on the lives of everyone – not just the victims who die from the actual disease. Although heroic efforts in America's intensive care units (ICUs) saved thousands of lives, subsequent studies found that a majority of ICU survivors suffered physical and mental disorders lasting for at least a year; this became known as **post-intensive care syndrome** (Bernstein & Keating, 2021). The overall lesson is identical to the basic lesson of all public health. Specifically, every sector of society – from big industry to hospitals, families, nursing homes, the housing market, and even down to the level of local cafés – will inevitably experience severe and ongoing negative impacts from epidemics of the magnitude reached by COVID-19. This lesson is precisely why our nation and its people must build and constantly reinforce a public health system that is highly functional and immune to political alterations.

our nation and its people must build and constantly reinforce a public health system that is highly functional

Understanding Disease Transmission the Chain of Infection

To begin this discussion, it is important to understand the relationship between what is known as the **host** (i.e., the person potentially acquiring the infection) and the **agent** (i.e., the pathogen). This relationship is greatly influenced by environmental conditions such as being indoors versus outdoors (as was very clear from the start of the COVID-19 pandemic). **Figure 1.1** provides a visual depiction of how the agent, host, and environmental conditions interact to determine the rate of disease transmission in any given population.

The model works much like a children's seesaw found on most playgrounds. If you have been on a seesaw, you know that the heavier person has control over the lighter person. This is because the fulcrum is in the exact middle. In the top half of the figure, you see that the agent is favored (i.e., has control) over the host. Translated to the example of COVID-19, this equates with illness and thus a great potential for person-to-person transmission of the virus. Magnified to a population level, in this scenario the virus has the ability to reproduce at a rate greater than one new infection for every one existing infection. This is known as a **reproductive rate** greater than 1.0.

Now let's look at the bottom half of the figure. Notice that the host is now favored (i.e., has control) over the agent. Translated to COVID-19, this equates with the virus being far less capable of causing illness. Magnified to a population level, the virus no longer has the ability to reproduce at a rate greater than one new infection for every one existing infection. This is known as a reproductive rate of less than 1.0. Once the reproductive rate drops below 1.0, an epidemic will slowly come to an end simply because the agent can no longer populate itself even to the level of replacement.

At this point, if you are following closely, the question becomes, "How can a shift occur to favor the host over the agent?" The answer, of course, involves the environment as well as factors about the host. Early in the U.S. COVID-19 epidemic, for example, a near-national lockdown based on **shelter-in-place** orders changed the crowded environments that previously favored the agent. The closing of schools, restaurants, retail stores, public transportation systems, places of worship, venues for sporting events, and office buildings created a shift in the fulcrum of the seesaw that crippled the agent. As these establishments reopened, mandates for mask wearing and social distancing further moved the fulcrum in favor of the host and also crippled the agent. Subsequently, as the COVID-19 vaccines were administered, millions of potential hosts for the agent were fortified against moderate to severe illness, meaning that

> Once the reproductive rate drops below 1.0, an epidemic will slowly come to an end

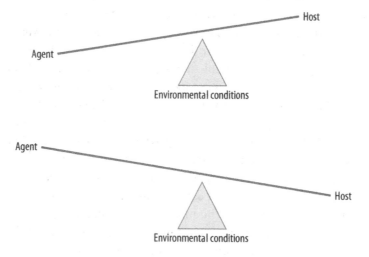

Figure 1.1   How agents, hosts, and environments interact

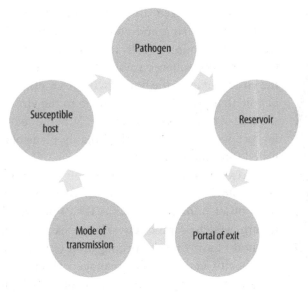

Figure 1.2   The cycle of propagated disease

infections among most of those vaccinated would be short-lived. This, once again, crippled the agent.

The model portrayed in **Figure 1.1** has been used by epidemiologists for decades. Any infectious disease can be thought of in terms of this model, with the challenge being how to alter any one of the three components (i.e., agent, host, environment) to drive down the reproductive rate of the pathogen. From a public health perspective, the environment most often serves as the target to change. This is precisely why public health practice is heavily reliant on the ability to influence policies such as the sanitation of water, the control of rats, and even the practices of food companies relative to keeping their products free of pathogens.

Now that you understand a few basic principles of controlling the transmission of disease, let's move into what is known as the **chain of infection**. This chain applies only to **propagated diseases** rather than diseases that stem from a source such as water-borne illness or food contamination. **Figure 1.2** portrays the chain of infection using a circular model that flows clockwise.

Starting around 12:00 (if you consider the figure like a clock), let's begin with the pathogen of COVID-19. As you know, it is a virus. As a non-living entity, a virus cannot be destroyed with drugs (at best, drugs for a virus greatly slow viral replication). Instead, viral infections are cleared by the body's immune system (but not always completely, as is the case with diseases such as genital herpes and HIV). This is why people with compromised immune systems – such as those living with HIV, pregnant women, people on chemotherapy, and the elderly – are more susceptible to severe cases of COVID-19. Understanding the pathogen is therefore an initial step in understanding the chain of infection.

Now, let's move clockwise to the **reservoir**. With COVID-19, the primary reservoir for the virus is humans. In other words, the virus exists in the world only because humans give it a home. This is why the virus will not just magically disappear, as President Trump claimed in the spring of 2020. As long as at least one human is infected, the virus can always propagate to another person, and another, and so on.

Next up is the **portal of exit**. The word *portal*, in this case, is simply the point at which the virus leaves the body of a person and thus has the potential to infect others. Some infections exit the body via feces, while others exit via secretions such as saliva, semen, and vaginal fluids. With COVID-19, the exit is simply expired air. When humans exhale, a virus can be part of the

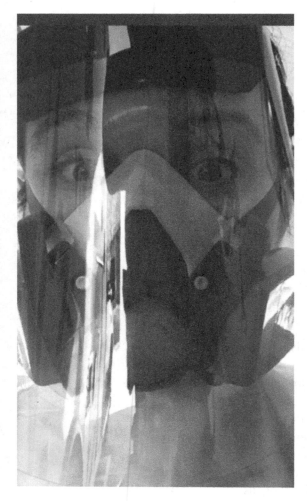

Photo 1.3   Personal protective equipment takes the concept of masking to its highest level.

resulting aerosolized droplets: visible droplets when air is exhaled (including sneezing and coughing) through the mouth and mixed with small amounts of saliva. An overlooked but very common addition is exhaled tobacco smoke. Exhaled smoke provides a free ride to the virus as it exits the body, giving it a method of transport to nearby people that provides an advantage to the virus and greatly enhances the rate of transmission in public. Whether exhaled smoke from vaping produces a similar risk is highly plausible but yet to be established (Sharma & Zeki, 2021).

Breaking the chain of infection at this juncture is possible by either blocking the portal of exit or quarantining the person away from other humans. The COVID-19 portal of exit is the nose and mouth, which is precisely why wearing a mask is the single best method of averting the propagation of COVID-19. It is noteworthy that health care workers managed to stay relatively COVID-free throughout the epidemic because of their high regard for personal protective equipment (**Photo 1.3**).

A properly constructed and correctly worn mask averts the exit of the virus from the body and thus interrupts the chain of transmission. Yet even in states, cities, and other locales that mandated mask wearing to break the cycle of COVID-19 transmission, policies regarding the type of masks and wearing them correctly were not apparent. Sadly, public health has missed a tremendous opportunity to save countless lives through simple mandates. Moreover, the public at large remained mostly uninformed about the concept of mask wearing to avert the transmission of COVID-19 and thus break its cycle of survival.

At this juncture, it becomes important for you to understand the concept of **viral shedding** (see **Box 1.2**). Once you understand shedding, you will be less likely to make the all-too-common assumption made by millions of Americans during the COVID-19 epidemic. That assumption is best characterized by statements such as these:

- "I have already had COVID, so I do not need a mask."

- "COVID-19 doesn't scare me – I am not afraid to get this disease."

- "If I get COVID, I will be okay – it's no big deal for me."

- "Taking chances is part of life – that includes taking a chance on getting COVID by not wearing a mask. Masks are overly safe."

In each statement, the underlying thought is focused on the person perhaps being infected by COVID-19 instead of an assumption that they may be actively transmitting the virus. The difference comes down to self-protection versus a more complex intention to be part of the public health solution to a historic threat to human life. Self-protection was *not* why CDC and other public health authorities recommended mask wearing. Instead, it was recommended as part of a larger effort to interrupt the chain of transmission for the virus, thereby slowing its rate of propagation.

Moving clockwise again in **Figure 1.2**, the next link in the chain is the **mode of transmission**. This link in the chain also includes the target of the transmission, known as the **portal of entry**. Of course, the portal of entry is the point at which the pathogen completes its move

BOX 1.2. THE HUMAN SIDE: WHAT IS VIRAL SHEDDING?

A good way to learn about the concept of viral shedding is to consider a long-standing endemic virus: genital herpes. Given that about 30% of all U.S. people over the age of 12 have been infected by genital herpes, the chances are good that you, too, may have experienced this infection. It begins with a primary infection. This is when the virus initially enters the body and creates visible symptoms. As the immune system responds and thus produces antibodies, these symptoms dissipate and soon disappear. But is the virus really gone?

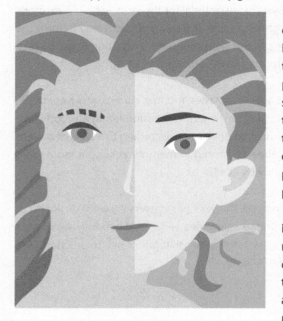

The harsh reality of genital herpes is that it lasts a lifetime. This doesn't mean a person will always have symptoms. Indeed, the opposite is typically true: symptoms of any kind are unusual after the initial infection occurs. The reason this virus is so successful in spreading from person to person has to do with what is now understood as nearly constant levels of very low **viral shedding**. In this example, *shedding* refers to the virus exiting the body through the same general area of genital tissue where the primary infection occurred. As the virus accumulates on the surface of this skin, it becomes a source of contagion for a sex partner. Transmission from one person to the next may therefore happen without either sex partner having any inkling as to what has occurred.

Similar to genital herpes, the virus that causes AIDS – the human immunodeficiency virus – also sheds from the body for a lifetime. Until medications were developed to repress the replication of HIV, the level of shedding was typically great enough to transfer the virus from person to person. Not all viruses last a lifetime, and not all shed for long periods after the initial infection. Although all viruses are different, the one commonality is that they shed for at least several days after noticeable symptoms of the disease are absent. From the perspective of viral success, the longer shedding occurs in otherwise healthy people, the greater the rate of viral transmission from one person to the next.

While it is easy for us as humans to make assumptions about a person's safety against transmitting a recent (or past) virus to somebody else, these assumptions are often made without an understanding of asymptomatic, post-infection viral shedding. So, we believe what we can see, and our eyes tell us that everything is fine. This aspect of human nature – seeing is believing – has the unfortunate consequence of leading people to make unfounded judgements about who is "safe" in terms of whether they may be transmitting (i.e., shedding) the COVID-19 virus. As rational beings, humans will someday have to learn that what can't be seen can still be dangerous.

from one person to the next. Because COVID-19 is capable of riding the airwaves (in aerosolized form) and thus being inhaled (the nose or the mouth therefore being the portal of entry), it is a relatively easy infection to acquire. Note that the word *acquire* in this case means to become a host to a pathogen. Acquisition is the counterpart to transmission, with *transmission* meaning the pathogen is passed onto another person. Thus, the portal of exit refers to transmission, whereas the portal of entry refers to acquisition. It is also noteworthy that COVID-19 can be transmitted by direct contact through a highly vulnerable area of the face: the eyes and eyelids. Because people often touch their eyes with their fingers, it is easy for a pathogen surviving on a finger to be transported into the body through this portal of entry. This is why public health messaging about sanitizing surfaces had great value, despite the messaging not being constructed in a way that made the reasons clear to the public. A more simplistic message might have been something like "Touching your eyes can introduce

Acquisition is the counterpart to transmission, with *transmission* meaning the pathogen is passed onto another person.

BOX 1.3. COMMON MYTHS AND MISCONCEPTIONS ABOUT COVID-19

1. Food spreads the virus.

The coronavirus enters the body through the nose, mouth, or eyes. When it enters through the mouth, it must be inhaled (in droplet form) rather than swallowed and thus sent to the high-acid environment of the stomach. The acids of the stomach will quickly destroy the COVID-19 virus.

2. A mask offers full protection.

The virus can enter the host three ways: (a) the nose and the nasal system are optimal for the virus – this warm, moist environment helps the virus thrive; (b) air inhaled into the lungs through the mouth is also an efficient way in from the perspective of viral spreading; and (c) the virus, like many other pathogens, can enter through the eyes. Thus, finger-to-face contact must be avoided to avert droplets on surfaces from being introduced into this third portal of entry.

3. Vaccines offer complete protection.

Some vaccines do offer complete protection, including the vaccines against measles, mumps, rubella, and hepatitis B. The COVID-19 vaccine, however, does not work this way. Instead, it works like most vaccines by stimulating antibody production ahead of a true episode of COVID-19 acquisition. The antibodies must be developed according to a type of pattern (genetic code). After these vaccine-induced patterns have been made, they are stored in memory cells so a more rapid immune response can occur in the event of an actual invasion into the body by COVID-19.

4. Vaccinated people cannot carry or spread the virus.

None of the COVID-19 vaccines were produced to avert infection. Instead, the vaccines universally were designed to prevent moderate or severe illness from infection with COVID-19, including its numerous variants. When fully vaccinated people proudly insist that they are free not to wear masks, they are missing the larger point that public health practice relies on all potential carriers (symptomatic or not) to not openly exhale COVID-19-laden air.

COVID-19 into your body. This habit should be avoided entirely." Again, in the absence of a massive and constant public health campaign to inform people about the transmission and acquisition of COVID-19, an outbreak of misconceptions occurred (see **Box 1.3**).

Finally, moving clockwise one last time in **Figure 1.2**, the cycle relies on a **susceptible host**. That a pathogen enters the body is one thing; it must also be able to successfully reproduce before it can cause disease. To begin reproducing, it must first attach itself to the cells of its host. In the case of viruses, this attachment is where the genetic codes of the pathogen can be integrated into the cellular machinery of the body, soon making millions of copies via altered cells. Blocking this attachment is one of the many strategies used in the public health practice of preventing HIV transmission.

To begin reproducing, it must first attach itself to the cells of its host.

In cases where a pathogen attaches successfully to host cells, the chain of infection can still be altered by greatly slowing its reproduction rate. Antibiotics, for example, work against bacterial pathogens by weakening their cell walls, thereby creating a fragile and short-lived invasion of the pathogen. In the case of viral infections, progression can be slowed by interrupting the synthesis of proteins needed for replication. For pandemic viruses such as HIV and COVID-19, a host of antiretroviral medications were developed and approved for use; these significantly slow viral replication, and the success was especially phenomenal against HIV. However, the most valuable public health strategy for limiting the reproduction of pathogens that have invaded the body is vaccination, which now becomes the focal point of this chapter.

the most valuable public health strategy for limiting the reproduction of pathogens that have invaded the body is vaccination

How Do Vaccines Work?

To the surprise of much of the world, when the COVID-19 vaccines became available, there was no overwhelming and universal response. Instead, the term **vaccine hesitancy** suddenly entered into everyday public health vocabularies. In the United States, this translated into just under two-thirds of the eligible public being fully vaccinated as the winter months of 2021 rolled around (the vaccine first became available in February of that year). Although a great deal of speculation has occurred – and will continue to occur – regarding the reasons for vaccine hesitancy, a primary cause was certainly a lack of clarity and thus understanding about how vaccines work (**Photo 1.4**).

As noted in **Box 1.3**, most vaccines work by simulating the invasion of a pathogen. It is also true that some vaccines use weakened versions of a virus (the polio vaccine is a good example), rather than simulating the virus with surface proteins. An easy way to think about this simulation is to visualize pieces of a picture puzzle that fit together only one way. Most vaccines are for viral infections, so let's go with the term *virus* here rather than the larger term *pathogen*. The invading virus has a distinct shape determined by protruding structures, attachment sites, and so on. The immune system has the

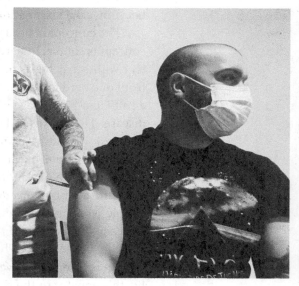

Photo 1.4   Vaccine hesitancy became a new term for Americans as a result of the COVID-19 pandemic.

ability – among other defenses – to create a second and complementary shape that attaches itself to the virus and thus renders it changed and harmless. This second and complementary shape is known as an **antibody**. Like all cellular structures, antibodies are created through a set of genetic instructions. For most viral invasions, the immune system requires several days, or in some cases weeks, to create this specific set of genetic instructions. During this time, the virus is successfully replicating in the body and creating cellular havoc that presents as physical disease. A shorter period between entry into the body and the development of the genetic instructions for the specific antibody leads to a shorter course of – and less severe – disease. This is where things become interesting, because that set of genetic instructions can be made by the simulated invasion mentioned previously. As long as some **memory cells** (dormant antibodies) remain in the body, any actual invasion can be attacked and blocked (with the complementary second shape) in a comparatively short time. Inducing this simulated response typically involves using a vaccine with surface protein structures that simulate the virus. The key word in all of this is *simulated*. Like most vaccines, the COVID-19 vaccine does *not* introduce living virus into the body. It is simply not possible to get COVID from the COVID vaccine, as many Americans falsely believed and echoed through various social media platforms. The vaccines against COVID-19 are very safe. This is not to dismiss isolated cases of issues such as blood clots, as seen during the development of the Johnson & Johnson vaccine. From a population health perspective, the incidence of death or long-term disability from these rare occurrences is minuscule in contrast to the mortality and morbidity imposed at the population level by COVID-19. This type of math – calculated at the population level – fully justifies vaccine mandates.

However, the overarching philosophy of population-level math runs counter to the medical approach to health, which is very much based at the individual level with providers and patients considering only what is best in each person's case of risk and benefit. Had this same individual-level approach been dominant during the global effort to vaccinate every living human against smallpox, humans might have already perished as a species. It became ever

However, the overarching philosophy of population-level math runs counter to the medical approach

Had this same individual-level approach been dominant during the global effort to vaccinate every living human against smallpox, humans might have already perished as a species.

clearer during the early years of COVID-19 that the idea of a collective and unified public response to the epidemic was undermining the single best tool available to public health practice: universal vaccination, which would create **herd immunity**.

The concept of herd immunity stems from the agricultural practice of raising animals. The concept is simple. In herds of animals that are not self-contained – meaning the herd is in contact with other herds of the same species – the potential for an infectious disease to spread from one herd to another is very high. However, this potential can be reduced to nearly zero if a sufficient percentage of the herd yet to be exposed has been vaccinated against the pending disease. The entire herd does not need to be vaccinated because any infectious agent entering the herd will not have an efficient chain of animal-to-animal transmission. The same concept applies to people, but it is not similar to animal herds because people may intermingle (even randomly) with one another in a way that is not like two herds of animals coming into contact. Thus the threshold needed to confer a slower progression of disease spread is much higher in people compared to animals. With COVID-19, this threshold is estimated to fall somewhere between 70 and 80% of any given population. For instance, if 80% of all the people living and working in the city of Philadelphia were immunized against COVID-19, the disease would be subject to a reproductive rate of far less than 1.0. In terms understandable to the general public, this equates to the chain of transmission being broken, thereby crippling the ability of the virus to spread from host to host. When a case turned up occasionally, it would garner the full attention of public health authorities in the region to conduct thorough **contact tracing**. The idea behind contact tracing is simply that anyone who may have been exposed to the new case must be quickly located and tested. A period of isolation from others (i.e., quarantine) is imposed on any contacts who test positive, for the safety of the community.

Now that you understand herd immunity, you are better equipped to appreciate why vaccination for infectious diseases (not just COVID-19) must be widespread and therefore mandatory. Mandating vaccination (see **Box 1.4**) is a key intervention point for public health because it is how vaccines can ultimately lead to the eradication of a disease, as was the case with smallpox.

the threshold needed to confer a slower progression of disease spread is much higher in people compared to animals.

BOX 1.4. MANDATING VACCINES, AND OTHER PUBLIC HEALTH SAFETY MEASURES

The famous singer and songwriter Eric Clapton, who may be a musical icon for your parents' generation, became a focal point of controversy in late 2021. This was because he recorded and released a song that served as a protest to mask mandates. Some of the more notable lyrics are as follows:

Do you wanna be a free man, or do you wanna be a slave? Do you wanna wear these chains until you're lying in the grave?

Eric Clapton was inducted into the Rock and Roll Hall of Fame three times. He was idolized by millions of fans and admired by his singer/songwriter colleagues. However, his 2021 anti-mask and anti-vaccination songs, interviews, and photos (such as one taken with Governor Greg Abbott of Texas, an avid critic of mask and vaccine mandates) caused him to lose much of his acquired status as well as long-standing fans.

Ultimately, the story of Eric Clapton speaking out against COVID-protection mandates became the story of the entire United States. Unlike our Asian counterparts, for example, the United States has a history of individualism as opposed to one characterized by the term *collectivism*. The concept of collectivism implies that people work together for the common good of society as a whole, deferring personal gain and individual goals into a subservient position. For instance, in China and Japan, mask wearing has always been a custom among people suffering from an illness as mild as a common cold. The ethic in this example is that part of being a good citizen is to engage in public health practices that serve other people. Sadly, this ethic was all-too-often absent in America during the first years of the U.S. COVID-19 epidemic. Thus, mandates became the alternative – they were not the first thing suggested by state and local governments. But millions of Americans cried out that these mandates were an infringement on their rights and freedoms.

What was lost to the Americans who were opposed to COVID-protection mandates is that public health has historically played a heavy role, including vaccine mandates, in efforts to protect people against the spread of infectious diseases. Examples include an entire series of vaccinations that you as a student were most likely required to have to be admitted to the college or university you are attending. In 2021, 30 U.S. states had active laws making sexual intercourse a crime for people living with HIV. Upon being hired, restaurant workers and food handlers in all 50 states are required to show proof of not having an active case of tuberculosis. Legal quarantine of people with active cases of tuberculosis is still common in the United States. None of these mandates have ever been an issue for the American public – they are generally viewed as an important form of protecting the public. So the question that must be posed to people such as Eric Clapton becomes, "How are COVID-related mandates any different from dozens of other public health mandates that have been enforced for decades?"

Vaccines confer **acquired immunity**. Immunity can be acquired by (a) having the disease or (b) having a weak version of the disease, as is the case with immunization (in the case of COVID-19, this immunity appears to be even stronger than the naturally acquired immunity triggered by having the actual virus enter the body and cause disease). If the host has acquired immunity to the virus, the virus will still enter the body, but it will not be able to copy itself in large enough numbers to survive and be efficiently transmitted to other humans. This point is important to herd immunity; however, in the case of highly efficient viruses –such as the Delta variant of COVID-19 – evidence suggests that vaccinated people can still carry enough active virus to spread the disease to others, particularly those who are not vaccinated.

in the case of highly efficient viruses –such as the Delta variant of COVID-19 – evidence suggests that vaccinated people can still carry enough active virus to spread the disease

In the absence of ambitious and omnipresent public health campaigns teaching the public these basics facts regarding how vaccines work, misinformation flourished. This was evident time after time, with examples from vaccinated parents unwilling to allow their children to be vaccinated to members of the Air Force refusing a federal mandate to comply with the policy requirement that service members must be fully vaccinated by November 1, 2021. Of all the concerns expressed by people unwilling to be vaccinated or to vaccinate their children, the one with a small degree of credibility pertained to **Guillain-Barré syndrome**. This syndrome affects the nervous system, and it was first linked to vaccines in the late 1970s when the swine flu vaccine was found to be the culprit behind this chronic disorder. The syndrome was found to occur in persons vaccinated against COVID-19, but at a rate not much greater than would be expected from ordinary influenza vaccines.

Before moving to the next section of this chapter, it is well worth asking, "Can COVID-19 ever be eradicated, as was done with smallpox?" Sadly, the answer to this question is "No." This dismal outlook has to do with the concept of **zoonotic disease**. In November 2021, it became apparent that COVID-19 had a non-human reservoir: white-tailed deer (**Photo 1.5**). As the term implies, a zoonotic

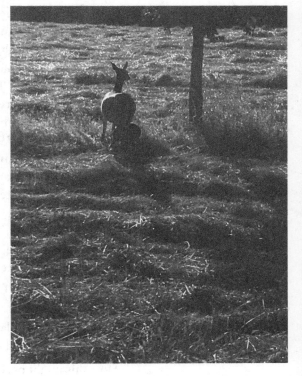

Photo 1.5 White-tailed deer are abundant in many parts of the United States; they may also carry COVID-19.

disease is one with the ability to infect both animals and humans. Given the impracticality of vaccinating wild deer, humans will need to adapt to COVID-19. The best-case scenario for an end game will be fairly low levels of endemic spread.

Self-Interests in Government and Racial Disparities in the Era of COVID-19

During the Trump administration, a key person in the White House was Dr. Deborah Birx, the coronavirus response coordinator. Despite excellent credentials and qualifications in the area of infectious disease control, Dr. Birx frequently stood down regarding the president's ongoing efforts to claim that COVID-19 was quickly resolving. It wasn't until nearly a year after the election of President Joe Biden that Dr. Birx publically stated, to a congressional committee, that President Trump had not accepted advice to ramp up testing, test younger people, or impose stricter mandates on vaccination and mask wearing for federal employees.

By 2022, it was clear that President Trump had deliberately placed his self-interests for re-election far ahead of the ever-pressing needs imposed by the COVID-19 epidemic. In late 2021, a congressional investigation of the Trump administration's handling of the COVID-19 epidemic included testimony from six senior officials directly involved in efforts to minimize the U.S. response. A subsequent news article summed up the investigation nicely: "The Trump administration repeatedly interfered with efforts by the Centers for Disease Control and Prevention last year to issue warnings and guidance about the evolving coronavirus pandemic, six current and former health officials told congressional investigators in recent interviews" (Diamond, 2021). Looking back on the history of failed federal responses to an American epidemic, this example is unrivaled.

One outgrowth of a White House overly involved in a public health response is that the CDC may alter its practices based on presidential directives. This is, of course, nothing less than dangerous. But sitting presidents appoint their own CDC directors, thereby creating a less-than-independent relationship. During the Trump administration, the conflict between politics and public health was especially apparent in what CDC did *not* do. This was painfully obvious in terms of health communication, and it continued into the Biden administration.

For decades, the CDC employed people trained specifically in health communication. Their task was to carefully balance the messaging from the CDC to achieve a desired response from the public that also avoided the hysteria our nation witnessed during the first decade of the HIV crisis (which ranged from sanitation workers refusing to handle routine garbage containers used by hospitals to grade schools expelling students who were living with HIV). Balanced messaging was considered a necessity by the CDC and most other national and international organizations devoted to health promotion. Then, when it mattered the most, the CDC commitment to balanced messaging seemed to come to an end.

A prime example comes from the Biden Administration's CDC Director Rochelle Wolinsky, who has stated that fully vaccinated people may once again safely congregate without wearing masks or practicing social distancing. So, what is wrong with this public health message? Think about

- How this would play out in the real world. Would unvaccinated people be socially and physically screened out of such gatherings?

- How this might become a license to abandon mask wearing and social distancing practices that were costly to business and industry, such as airlines not selling the middle seat in a

sitting presidents appoint their own CDC directors, thereby creating a less-than-independent relationship.

For decades, the CDC employed people trained specifically in health communication.

row of three seats, restaurants serving food only on a to-go basis, or business establishments allowing employed to telecommute.

• What this implies in terms of an end point to the epidemic. How much would it sway public opinion toward a general feeling of "It is almost over"?

• The assumption behind the message in terms of time. The COVID-19 vaccines were not developed with the idea of everlasting immunity; vaccine experts knew that immunity would wane and thus leave fully vaccinated people at varying levels of protection and risk.

In parallel with the federal government's mistakes in responding to the COVID-19 epidemic, it was apparent that racism was –as is usually true with all forms of preventable diseases – playing a strong hand in the epidemic. Counted on the basis of **case rates** (e.g., the number of infected people per 100,000 in a defined population), far more people of color were infected with the virus than white, non-Hispanic persons. Further, on a case-rate basis, far more people of color ultimately died from the disease.

Early in the process of vaccinating the American public against COVID-19, a key issue was rigorously debated by the **Advisory Committee on Immunizations Practices** (ACIP). In a nutshell, it came down to whether essential workers should be prioritized for the vaccine (following health care workers). This debate centered on the point that people of color are vastly overrepresented in jobs such as housekeeping, fast food chains, grocery stores, and so on, meaning that shelter-in-place safeguards against COVID were not equitably available for millions of minority members. In the December 18, 2020 edition of the *Washington Post*, the following was noted: "The focus on essential workers as a way to advance equity has gained support from all 14 members of the independent panel [the ACIP]" (Stanley-Becker & Sun, 2020). This focus on essential workers ultimately served as one example of an effective public health response to the racial and ethnic disparities of the U.S. COVID-19 epidemic.

This focus on essential workers ultimately served as one example of an effective public health response to the racial and ethnic disparities

By September 2021, the CDC reported compelling surveillance data relative to the wide racial and ethnic divide between non-Hispanic white people and persons of four different categories of race/ethnicity. **Figure 1.3** shows this comparison. To understand the figure, read each column as the number of times greater risk. For instance, you can see that both Black/African Americans and Hispanic/Latinx Americans had, at this early stage of the epidemic, a nearly threefold greater risk of being hospitalized with COVID-19 and a twofold greater risk of dying from COVID-19. Using surveillance to count cases, hospitalizations, and deaths is certainly a valuable public health function; however, the real challenge becomes one of rectifying these glaring disparities.

Rate ratios compared to White, Non-Hispanic persons	American Indian or Alaska Native, Non-Hispanic persons	Asian, Non-Hispanic persons	Black or African American, Non-Hispanic persons	Hispanic or Latino persons
Cases	1.7x	0.7x	1.1x	1.9x
Hospitalization	3.5x	1.0x	2.8x	2.8x
Death	2.4x	1.0x	2.0x	2.3x

Figure 1.3   The racial and ethnic divide with COVID-19 hospitalization and death
Source: Centers for Disease Control and Prevention. Risk for COVID-19 infection, hospitalization, and death by race/ethnicity. Updated September 9, 2021. https://www.cdc.gov/coronavirus/2019-ncov/covid-data/investigations-discovery/hospitalization-death-by-race-ethnicity.html.

Corporate Interests and the Spread of COVID-19

COVID-19 was unique in the American experience because it was arguably the first time an epidemic of such large proportions could be said to be largely preventable. Describing the reasons is beyond the scope of this chapter; however, two excellent books give complete accounts of the multiple missteps and outright deceptions marking this time in history (MacKenzie, 2020; Slavitt, 2021). Indeed, throughout much of the early COVID-19 epidemic, it became clear that corporate practices and profit margins were more sacred than human life and the prevention of COVID illness. Delta Airlines personified this in its somewhat thinly veiled messaging to customers — messaging that was focused on the health of passengers and emphasized that federal regulations required all passengers to wear a mask during the entire duration of the flight. In the same e-mail sent to soon-to-be passengers, Delta also featured its snack and beverage service. Apparently the airline either wanted to be sure people were fed and hydrated at the expense of exposing them to COVID-19 or needed the revenue generated by the sales of alcoholic beverages during the flight. People who flew in 2021 were no doubt used to this somewhat bipolar stance on the part of airlines: a strict stand on masks along with permission to remove masks when eating or drinking. So, assuming a planeload of people board and sit while fully masked during their snack time, the finite level of available oxygen in the airplane quickly becomes saturated by the expiration of the virus as people chew and drink. That level of saturation may be zero (if nobody on board is pre-symptomatic, symptomatic, or just recovering from symptoms), or it may be a linear function of the amount of virus being collectively expired by the crew and passengers. All of this, of course, is absolute insanity when it comes to the highly infectious variants of COVID-19 (such as the Delta variant). It is no more logical than the teenage male who uses a condom only part of the time when he engages in sexual intercourse with a partner.

Following the metaphor of condoms, another level of insanity was widely apparent during the days of mandatory mask use in public places. Just as most people who use condoms report having a substantial number of issues using them correctly, the same was true for mask-wearing behaviors. Sadly, many Americans could not understand that COVID-19 enters — and exits — the body through the nose. Thus, mandatory mask wearing became a mere symbolic exercise for people who decided that covering the mouth alone was ample. In the obvious absence of enforcement, mandatory mask wearing was about as effective as continuing to have sexual intercourse after a condom breaks: the intent may have been good, but the protective value was subverted. For example, it was not unusual to read about flight attendants enforcing the use of seatbelts but not the correct wearing of masks.

The insanity was not limited to airlines. School classrooms were another example of how people can bend a guideline to the point of complete ineffectiveness. Elementary teachers, for instance, were found to remove their masks when reading stories out loud to children. Teachers, students, and school staff routinely ignored the entire concept of social distancing. Mask wearing was loosely defined, thereby creating a vast potential for spreading the virus via air expired from countless uncovered nostrils.

At the same time public places were being less than stringent about consistent and correct mask wearing, there was also an emphasis on sanitizing. This emphasis may have made the public feel a bit safer; however, sanitizing surfaces and hands is a preventive measure typically applied to pathogens spread through ingestion rather than inhalation. COVID-19 and its variants are pathogens that enter the body through the **olfactory system** (i.e., the nose and nasal cavities of the head). Thus, while people were dutifully devoting their energies to hand sanitizing, for example, the nation ignored the very real threat of superspreader events such as football games (even outdoor stadiums pose a risk because people are crowded into closed areas

it became clear that corporate practices and profit margins were more sacred than human life

such as restrooms and food courts), basketball games, theatre performances, and religious services (those featuring singing are particularly implicated, as COVID-19 spreads efficiently from the rapid expiration of air that has been in the lungs).

The more ubiquitous insanity in 2021 revolved around state governors. Florida, for instance, banned schools from mandating mask wearing. Soon after the 2021/2022 school year began in Florida, the state experienced a record number of new COVID cases among young people. Other states had similar bans on mask mandates; however, still other states stood on the opposite end of this continuum and fully supported mask mandates for schools. Some cities were even proactive enough to pass and enforce citywide mask mandates. Of course, the problem was the lack of national coordination: where people lived at the time was the critical factor in terms of their risk of acquiring COVID. Most developed nations (including the United States) have historically had stringent government-based controls against the spread of highly infectious diseases, yet this same control was not exercised to a substantial degree in the early years of the U.S. COVID-19 epidemic.

A Few Thoughts About the Future of COVID-19 and Other Emergent Diseases

The future of public health practice will become increasingly focused on controlling emerging epidemics and pandemics, with COVID-19 being a forerunner. This focus will, by necessity, have to occur at structural levels such as federal and state policies and laws designed to foster conditions that lead to the protection of the public against propagated diseases. This future will include steps to avert the spread of any airborne disease. An example of such a step is converting public indoor areas (including office space) to a more open-air concept in terms of building design. For example, in modern public buildings, windows that are made of heavy glass and do not open will be replaced with windows that let air flow freely in and out. This is a great example of how small changes matter in terms of public health. In outdoor air, liquid droplets carrying the virus quickly diminish. Indoors, a goal will be to optimize total **air changes per hour** (ACH). ACH is a measure of the volume of fresh air added (in cubic feet) over 1 hour divided by the total volume of indoor space under consideration (also in cubic feet). With this architecture-based formula in mind, you can imagine how architects may soon become a key part of public health practice.

> small changes matter in terms of public health.

This future will doubtlessly be marked by a competing series of laboratory victories followed by missed opportunities at the level of voluntary vaccination. In many ways, the search for an AIDS vaccine (initiated in the 1990s) laid a strong foundation for the relatively quick development of the COVID-19 vaccines. Our capacity to quickly design and manufacture safe and highly effective vaccines against emergent diseases will continue to increase. Unfortunately, this ability will not automatically translate into increased public uptake of new vaccines. Thus the future may well hold vaccine mandates and vaccine cards that people must carry and present to be admitted to public spaces.

> Our capacity to quickly design and manufacture safe and highly effective vaccines against emergent diseases will continue to increase.

Given the near-daily attention given to controlling COVID-19 by the CDC and other key health agencies in the United States, government-based public health institutions will probably always be well funded. Whether and how these institutions will become politically insulated from the whims or self-interests of elected federal officials – particularly in the executive and legislative branches – is yet to be seen.

Additionally (and this is certainly long overdue), the COVID-19 pandemic may force high-income nations, such as the United States, to begin acting on the fact that microbes left unchecked will only continue to advance deeper into the human species. It is not enough, for example, to use vaccines only to protect people living in wealthy nations, as doing so leaves a fertile playground of humans in middle-income and low-income nations to become incubators for microbial mutations. Yet at the end of 2021, global reports indicated that approximately three-quarters of the people in high-income nations had been vaccinated, compared to less than one-half of people residing in middle-income nations and only about 5% of those living in low-income nations. The public health approach to averting pandemics must always be global and equitable.

A final point to ponder is the extent to which public health laws pertaining to infectious disease can be enforced. Passing health-protective laws is important; however, without strict enforcement, these efforts will fail in their mission to protect the public. With COVID-19, this pertains to mask wearing, vaccination, and social distancing. For example, consider the local mandates that limited the number of restaurant patrons who could be seated at one time. **Box 1.5** provides an example based on an interview with a waitress working in a small New England dinner.

> The public health approach to averting pandemics must always be global and equitable.

BOX 1.5. WHAT GOOD ARE PUBLIC HEALTH LAWS WITHOUT ENFORCEMENT?

The following information is based on an interview that I (the author) conducted with a waitress working in a highly prized New England steakhouse. She had worked at this steakhouse for many years prior to COVID-19. I interviewed her in late 2021. She explained that when the state first mandated COVID-19 restrictions on restaurant capacity, the steakhouse was very compliant. These regulations included provisions such as seating no more than six people at any one table, ensuring that all people at any one table resided in the same household, and keeping tables six feet apart (meaning many tables had to be "closed" by placing reserved signs on them). Thus, seating capacity was greatly reduced, and a burden was placed on restaurant management to ascertain the "same household" rule.

As the interview continued, the waitress explained that other restaurants in the area also adopted these initial regulations; however, they soon became very lax in enforcement. Consequently, the steakhouse where she worked had to also become lax in its enforcement; otherwise, business would go to these nearby competitors. She noted that by Thanksgiving 2020, the steakhouse's owners mostly abandoned earlier attempts to enforce the COVID-19 safety regulations and often served a full house. A small percentage of the clientele protested the lack of enforcement by leaving the restaurant. But her description of the time progression created an overall image of the owners simply letting go of the safety regulations a little more each day. Referring to enforcement of the regulations at the start of the U.S. epidemic, she exclaimed, "It all just went out the window." When I asked her whether any state inspectors attempted to gauge compliance with the safety regulations, she described a one-time inspection that was "a 30-second walkthrough, with no questions asked."

After the interview concluded, I found myself wondering, "What if states enforced highway safety rules this way?" The takeaway is that states may posture about safety regulations against an airborne pathogen such as COVID-19. However, in the absence of at least minimal enforcement (such as issuing speeding tickets to keep traffic flow generally with the speed limits), these public health regulations are only as valuable as the business owners make them. The difference between voluntary regulation and actual regulations should be discernable – state-imposed mandates in the absence of enforcement become little more than voluntary suggestions.

Review and Key Terms

This chapter began by teaching you about the difference between a **pandemic**, an **epidemic**, and the term **endemic**. Pandemics, such as the historic **Spanish flu**, are ultimately handled by the **World Health Organization**, as has recently been the case with **SARS-Cov-2** (i.e.,

COVID-19). As the chapter proceeded, you learned about **immunity** via **antibody** development, which can be stimulated through vaccination. Most importantly, you learned how vaccination can lower the **reproductive rate** of a **pathogen**, thus leading to declines in **case rates**. The **memory cells** in a vaccinated person are capable of mounting a rapid response to an invading pathogen such as COVID-19, thereby limiting the ability of that pathogen to use the **host** as a long-term **reservoir** and thus a source of transmission to other people (i.e., it limits disease **propagation**).

In the absence of vaccination or immunity **acquired** by having the disease, the pathogen will greatly multiply and slowly undergo **shedding** from the host through its **portal of exit** (which differs from pathogen to pathogen). The pathogen can then be transmitted to others via its portal of entry (which, again, differs from pathogen to pathogen). For instance, the most common portal of entry for COVID-19 is the **olfactory system**. Public health interventions that interrupt this **chain of infection** (such as mask wearing) are therefore vital for keeping the reproductive rate of any given pathogen low.

This chapter also taught you about reaching **herd immunity**, a public health goal of every vaccination campaign. Sadly, you learned that reaching herd immunity via vaccination often occurs unevenly in any given nation, thus exacerbating **health disparities**. This type of disparity was particularly apparent in the U.S. COVID-19 epidemic when the **Delta variant** became dominant, and it continued with the **Omicron variant**. Although factors such as **vaccine hesitancy** and various **environmental conditions** (e.g., poverty, overcrowding, lack of health care) favor the **agent** (such as COVID-19), intensified public health efforts to favorably alter these factors are a priority. Rapid approval of vaccines by the **Advisory Committee on Immunization Practices**, as well as nationwide efforts to greatly expand **contact tracing** services, are two hallmarks of the larger public health actions implemented against COVID-19. Education is also important, with the example of helping people understand the exceedingly low risk of **Guillain-Barré syndrome** as a result of the COVID-19 vaccine (and others).

The chapter concluded with a number of talking points about the future of COVID-19. For instance, the concept of public health architecture was presented, with indoor spaces designed for optimal **air changes per hour**. As this pandemic continues, it will be incumbent on public health practice to create ongoing safety guards against disease transmission and to continually strive to reach herd immunity through well-coordinated and highly effective vaccination campaigns. More importantly, the public health lessons learned from COVID-19 can become valuable for application against subsequent epidemics and/or pandemics.

For Practice and Class Discussion

Practice Questions (answers are located in the appendix to this textbook)

1. Which one of the following terms is **not** applicable to understanding how vaccines work?
   a. Memory cells
   b. Antibodies
   c. Neurotransmitters
   d. Surface proteins

2. The most common portal of entry for the COVID-19 virus is:
   a. The olfactory system
   b. The lower eyelids
   c. Ingesting the virus via contaminated foods
   d. The mouth

3. The concept of corporate interests taking precedence over public safety from COVID-19 is **best** illustrated by which example?
    a. Increasing taxes for middle-class Americans
    b. A rush to return to retail sales and dining in indoor restaurants
    c. Mandatory vaccination of all employees

4. Regarding the history of COVID-19, which statement is **true**?
    a. The virus entered the United States almost one year after it first appeared in China.
    b. The Trump administration engaged in prolonged denial about the severity of this virus.
    c. The U.S. Department of Defense quickly vaccinated all members of the military, even before the American public began receiving the vaccines.
    d. The COVID-19 pandemic was inevitable – it could not have been any less devastating in terms of cases or human lives lost.

5. Which part of the chain of infection for COVID-19 pertains to white-tailed deer?
    a. Reservoir
    b. Portal of exit
    c. Acquired immunity
    d. Mutation of the pathogen

6. The difference between an **epidemic** and the term **endemic** is:
    a. All epidemics begin as endemics.
    b. Only endemics occur on a global scale.
    c. Epidemics are not controllable.
    d. Epidemics are characterized by massive case rates; when these fall to a low and stable level, the term endemic applies.

7. Which example **best** illustrates the principles of a propagated disease?
    a. A common source serves as a point of infection for most new cases.
    b. An animal-to-human mode of transmission becomes dominant.
    c. Human-to-human transmission of the pathogen is favored by environmental conditions such as overcrowding.
    d. After several successive mutations, the pathogen develops memory cells.

8. Which statement is **most** applicable to understanding the health disparities of COVID-19?
    a. The protective behavior of sheltering in place was less possible for essential workers.
    b. Black Americans lacked health insurance needed to receive the vaccine.
    c. Latinx Americans were often refused hospital care.

9. Which organization has the **most** influence relative to controlling pandemics?
    a. The U.S. Advisory Committee on Immunization Practices
    b. The World Health Organization
    c. The Centers for Disease Control and Prevention

10. Which statement about COVID-19 is **false**?
    a. Immunity can be acquired by having the disease.
    b. Although the vaccine is extremely safe, there is a very small risk of Guillain-Barré syndrome.
    c. The virus can enter the body through the eyes.
    d. Fully vaccinated people cannot transmit the virus to others.

For Discussion (in class or small groups, or online)

11. As has been true with HIV/AIDS, the COVID-related racial disparities described in this chapter are likely to become worse as the U.S. epidemic moves toward becoming endemic. Given this, go online to locate what you consider to be a highly informative infographic on this topic. At this time in history, what is your best theory as to why these racial disparities are occurring? (Describe this in a post or a tweet for others who may benefit.)

12. This chapter included myths and misconceptions about COVID-19. Other than those, identify at least one other myth or misconception that you know about in your own community. Then, find another person taking this class who has also done this exercise. Taking turns, describe the realities and science that counter the selected myths and misconceptions you each chose.

13. The period between the Spanish flu pandemic and the COVID-19 pandemic was just over 100 years. Most experts in emerging disease epidemiology predict that future pandemics of a similar magnitude will begin to occur far more frequently. Applying what you have learned in this chapter, plus going online to learn about climate change and emerging diseases, compose a one-page position paper that speculates about what pandemic may next occur and how we (as humans) can best respond to this threat.

References

Beeler, B. (2021, October 27). To see climate change in action, just look in your own backyard. *Washington Post.* https://www.washingtonpost.com/opinions/2021/10/27/see-climate-change-action-look-your-own-backyard/

Bernstein, L., & Keating, D. (2021, November 12). For many ICU survivors and their families, life is never the same. *Washington Post.* https://www.washingtonpost.com/health/2021/11/12/covid-icu-intensive-care-syndrome/

Diamond, D. (2021, November 12). Messonnier, Birx detail political interference in last year's coronavirus response. *Washington Post.* https://www.washingtonpost.com/health/2021/11/12/messonnier-birx-coronavirus-response-interference/

Garrett, L. (1995). *The coming plague: Emerging diseases in a world out of balance.* Penguin Books.

Fisher, M., Royza, L., & Ruble, K. (2021, November 3). 750,000 Americans dead as many families feel unity in pain but division in mourning. *Washington Post.*

MacKenzie, D. (2020). COVID-19: *The pandemic that never should have happened and how to stop the next one.* Hachette Books.

Sharma, P., & Zeki, A. A. (2021). Does vaping increase susceptibility to COVID-19? *American Journal of Respiratory and Critical Care Medicine, 202*(7), 1055.

Slavitt, A. (2021). *Preventable: The inside story of how leadership failures, politics, and selfishness doomed the U.S. coronavirus response.* St. Martin's Press.

Stanley-Becker, I., & Sun, L. H. (2020, December 18). COVID-19 is devastating communities of color. Can vaccines counter racial inequity? *Washington Post.* https://www.washingtonpost.com/health/2020/12/18/covid-vaccine-racial-equity/

CHANGING LIVES A "MILLION AT A TIME": PUBLIC HEALTH IS VERY DIFFERENT THAN THE MEDICAL PROFESSION

We the people of the United States, in order to form a more perfect union, establish justice, insure domestic tranquility, provide for the common defense, promote the general welfare . . ."

—*Preamble to the Constitution of the United States*

Overview

Please read the preamble to the Constitution a second time. Now, reflect on these key terms: *justice, domestic tranquility,* and *general welfare.* In each of these three concepts lies the assumption that the public as a whole is basically healthy and protected from the harms of most diseases and other forms of premature death or loss of quality of life. As important, if not more so, is the opening phrase, "We the people." As you learned in Chapter 1, even one disease can have profound negative effects on an entire nation, creating economic and social upheaval as well as loss of life and loss of quality of life among those who do not die from the disease. The essential lesson learned from COVID-19 is that public health is a public responsibility!

This chapter will give you a broad overview of how "we the people" are – whether we know it or not – ultimately in control of what is known casually as public health. Just as "we the people" are in control of our governmental issues (e.g., taxes, public spending, government-based price supports, boosting the economy, and passing laws), we are also tasked with creating conditions that allow for the health and welfare necessary to truly prosper. This daily responsibility is distinctly different from a medical approach to public health because the medical paradigm is based on treatment as opposed to prevention. Treatment is expensive. Treatment also spawns inequalities in terms of which people receive the best care and services. Conversely, prevention is inexpensive, and it can be applied to all people equally.

As you read this chapter, bear in mind that public health is not a profession per se. Instead, it is a shared action of responsible citizens. Although some professions (e.g., agriculture, environmental science, consumer law, biotechnology, pharmacy, and even architecture) are highly relevant to public health, its day-to-day maintenance is a product of an informed public and an active electorate (meaning that voting at local, state, and federal levels is vital). Also, as you read, be open to the

LEARNING OBJECTIVES

1. Understand that public health is a public responsibility rather than a profession per se.

2. Describe how COVID-19 shaped and defined public health practice.

3. Name and describe seven risk conditions that place the public's health in jeopardy.

4. Name and describe seven health-protective conditions that preserve and promote the public's health.

5. Understand basic concepts and terms from the science of epidemiology.

6. Differentiate between three forms of prevention (primary, secondary, and tertiary), and describe the centrality of prevention to public health practice.

7. Describe how population-level health is vastly different from a medical approach to health.

8. Discuss the varied, yet complementary, roles of education, regulatory actions, and a structural-level approach to protecting and improving public health.

9. Understand a sequential model of the available tools to improve public health.

10. Identify the role of public health research in terms of public health practice.

11. Explain the importance of public health from an economic viewpoint.

The essential lesson learned from COVID-19 is that public health is a public responsibility!

Treatment is expensive. Treatment also spawns inequalities in terms of which people receive the best care and services.

idea that public health research has revealed an enormous amount of new information and evidence about how disease and other threats to our welfare can be prevented. This body of prevention science suggests a need for daily actions and massive changes, in contrast to the medical paradigm of using pills and procedures to cure illness after it occurs. Unfortunately, "we the people" have thus far been slow to adopt the more progressive daily approach over the all-too-familiar treatment approach. But this unfortunate reality is changing!

The Need for Organized Public Health Practice

In December 2019, a few spotty news stories described a new and prolonged illness infecting people in parts of China. As you learned in Chapter 1, the disease soon spread globally, and the COVID-19 pandemic dominated the lives of people and economies in every corner of the world. With the exception of the AIDS pandemic, COVID-19 became the first pandemic ever experienced by people in developed nations such as the United Kingdom, the United States, Italy, France, Brazil, and so forth. Suddenly two words became popular: *public health*! As these two words played out in daily actions, people began to see what public health is all about: *creating conditions that control and even reverse the tide and trajectory of any one nation's current epidemics.* They also began to understand that the two words implied a need to rectify the health disparities that so quickly emerged, especially for people of color in nations such as the U.S., who were vastly more likely to acquire, and die from, COVID-19. A new title – "the nation's leading public health expert" – was used daily to refer to the director of the *National Institute of Allergy and Infectious Disease*, Dr. Anthony Fauci.

As 2020 gave way to 2021, people all over the world began learning about variants of the virus and how the different vaccines work to prevent people from having moderate to severe cases of COVID-19. Politicians, economists, corporate executives, and small business owners all became self-taught in the finer points of flattening the curve as well as what US policies were needed to strengthen the public health response (i.e., improve prevention practices) and improve the medical response (i.e., bolster the ability of hospitals to successfully treat people with severe cases). This distinction – between public health and medical care – became an ordinary part of news stories and studies of the pandemic. Suddenly the world seemed to understand that prevention and treatment are two very different things! This difference has always defined how public health rises above medicine in purpose. An effective public health response averts the overwhelming needs of an "after the fact" medical response.

An effective public health response averts the overwhelming needs of an "after the fact" medical response.

Just as public health applies to saving lives, protecting wellbeing, and preserving economies in the era of COVID-19, it also applies to future emerging diseases: diseases that have become endemic (meaning they have leveled off at some stable rate on a year-to-year basis, HIV/AIDS being a prime example) and the all-encompassing chronic diseases (such as heart disease, stroke, and cancers of all kinds) that drain life years from massive numbers of people on a predictable, and often escalating, schedule. Although this virtuous role of public health seems clear, that clarity has not always been the case.

Although this virtuous role of public health seems clear, that clarity has not always been the case.

Even in the new millennium, people claiming to engage in public health practice are actually serving as adjuncts to medical practice. This frequently occurs under the banner of *community health* – a practice often characterized by medical screenings meant to find early signs of chronic disease such as heart disease, breast cancer, and cancer of the colon. This work is valuable and clearly needed, but it occurs with a medical mindset, meaning the work is done one person at a time. The roots of preventing disease at the population level (see **Box 2.1**) and its outgrowth demonstrate that public health greatly differs from community health by taking on intervention approaches that affect massive numbers of people – it is not a one-person-at-a-time endeavor.

public health greatly differs from community health by taking on intervention approaches that affect massive numbers of people – it is not a one-person-at-a-time endeavor.

BOX 2.1. CHOLERA CONTROL IN THE 1800S

Paramount to understanding public health is the concept of *thinking* about health with respect to entire populations rather than specific individuals or even patients. This is the case for *actions* as well. These actions may be relatively simple. Although it may take the equivalent of moving mountains to heal a person with advanced heart disease, for example, the public health actions needed to avert the onset of heart disease may simply consist of governments subsidizing plant-based foods and removing price supports for animal-based foods. To help you with this somewhat abstract notion of simple actions, let's consider an example from history.

To truly appreciate this history-based example, it is important to first understand the disease known as *cholera* (which is still common today). Cholera is a diarrheal disease that most often resulted (and even today still results) in death. The bacterium that causes cholera is well adjusted to modern life, and its evolution has allowed it to survive globally. It is able to encapsulate itself and float in ocean waters for months! This means it still exists in many populated areas of the world. Special beds (known as **cholera cots**) allow patients with nearly constant diarrhea to rest without having to get up to use a toilet. Diarrhea can eventually exhaust the body of nutrients and hydration, leading to death.

As a bacterial infection, cholera is treatable with antibiotics. However, prior to the widespread acceptance among physicians of **germ theory** (i.e., the proposition that microorganisms unseen by the human eye can be the sole cause of disease), cholera was a rampant global infection that claimed millions of lives.

A classic story in epidemiology (there are many others) involves a scientist named John Snow and cholera prior to the acceptance of germ theory. Snow is considered the founder of epidemiology. Throughout this textbook, you will learn that epidemiology really is the backbone of public health! Consider that the term itself essentially translates as "what is upon the people." The essence of epidemiology is that sometimes we do not need to identify the microorganisms that cause disease. In the case of cholera, simple vital statistics (public records) saved the day, along with one extremely bold intervention. Using public records, John Snow was able to compare rates of new cases of cholera between homes (addresses) in London, England, that were being supplied with water by two different water companies. The differences in case rates were extreme, and based on the data, Snow speculated that the water from one company was far more likely to contain the cholera-causing germ than the water from the other company.

An 1854 cholera outbreak in the Soho district of London served as a second experiment and punctuated Snow's speculation in a convincing manner. He hypothesized that a particular well and its above-ground pump were heavily contaminated with the germ he believed was causing cholera. As death rates escalated, Snow removed the handle from this manually operated above-ground pump – and case rates and death rates began to subside. Snow mapped out recent cases that occurred in the geographic vicinity of this pump (known as the Broadwick Street pump or later the Broad Street pump). His maps showed that large clusters of cases were located in close proximity to the pump, thus solving the mystery of what was killing thousands of people during this period in history.

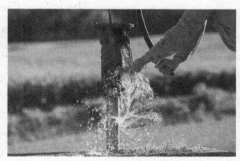

Photo 2.1   At one time, this was the only way most people could obtain water.
Source: sezer66/Adobe stock.

To truly function at a population level, public health addresses the root causes of disease and other forms of morbidity or premature death (e.g., unintentional injuries, childhood obesity, violence). As a function of searching for these root causes, public health is constantly unveiling common conditions that are highly implicated in morbidity and premature death. These conditions can be broadly thought of as **risk conditions** – meaning their presence poses hazards to the people who are exposed to them. Seven examples are briefly listed here:

- Inequitable socioeconomic conditions and lack of healthcare oriented around disease prevention (e.g., vaccinations, prenatal care, screenings for cancer)

- A lack of regulation regarding food and other products marketed to the public

- Easy access to products that place people at risk, such as guns, drugs, alcohol, and highly refined foods

- A lack of understanding in the public regarding the importance of daily health practices such as dietary and exercise habits

- The presence of social customs and practices that encourage and support ongoing behaviors that are harmful to the body, such as prolonged periods of sitting, excessive intake of food, and chronic daily stress

- A lack of regulation protecting the public from risk exposures such as antibiotics in meat, persistent organic pollutants in drinking water, and the effects of vaping/smoking

- An increasingly unhealthy physical environment created by climate change

Given these seven (and many other) **risk conditions**, a key responsibility of public health is to create and foster **health-protective conditions**: conditions that make it easy for people to choose safer options, as well as conditions that eliminate options in favor of default regulations that automatically confer protection to the public's health: for example, fluoride added to public water supplies, free contraceptive services offered to Medicaid-eligible females, and policies that regulate food additives. Other examples of health-protective conditions are:

- The mandatory use of collapsible steering columns in the construction of cars and trucks

- Fortifying table salt with iodine

- Regulating allowable amounts of toxic airborne emissions coming from factories and industrial plants

- The widespread implementation of laws that protect people from second-hand tobacco smoke

- The federal Clean Water Act, which protects our supplies of drinking water

- Bans and limits on the use of pesticides and herbicides applied to consumable foods

- Engineering outdoor public spaces for greater walkability for all people

As you reflect on these bullet points, it becomes clear that public health practice functions on multiple levels. Although old-school **health education** still has a role to play in public health, that role is minor in contrast to the tremendous potential of state and federal regulations and policy to ultimately create the conditions that lead to improved health of the people. At this juncture, it is important not to succumb to the common belief that we have little, if any, influence in altering state/federal regulations and policies. Keep in mind that all governmental bodies in the United States are formed – in the words of Abraham Lincoln – "by the people, for the people." To truly understand public health and the means to improve it, local action is inadequate; understanding and subsequent actions must be applied to all people.

Three Tenets of Public Health

The backbone of public health is the science of epidemiology.

The backbone of public health is the science of epidemiology. Ultimately, the methodology of epidemiology informs and shapes public health practice (although it is augmented by methodology from the social and behavioral sciences). Next, the implicit goal of public health is always prevention. This is in direct opposition to the implicit goal of medical care: healing. A final tenet of public health is that it must be applied at the population level, meaning it is designed for massive numbers of people.

Epidemiology: The Backbone of Public Health Practice

Let's begin by looking back at **Box 2.1**. John Snow's masterstroke (i.e., removing the pump handle to prevent cholera) was tested by a simple mapping of cases. In the parlance of epidemiology, this is known as **case findings**. Case findings are often a product of established **surveillance systems**. Surveillance is simply an organized method of tracking disease; typically, mandatory reporting to local and state health departments achieves this.

Because of surveillance, epidemiology can pinpoint unusual **outbreaks** of any given disease. Such outbreaks can be tracked to enable a public health response. Common examples include case findings of infectious hepatitis traced back to a **point source** such as a particular restaurant or fast food location. Identification of the source then enables public action in the form of swiftly closing the offending restaurant. This is a behind-the-scenes version of public health – one that is typically taken for granted in the United States.

Think about epidemiology as being tightly focused on counting. In addition to counting the occurrence of disease, it also counts the occurrence of **risk factors** that lead to disease. Risk factors are behaviors or various forms of pre-disease such as elevated blood serum cholesterol levels, hypertension, and elevated blood glucose levels. In fact, the science of epidemiology is credited with discovering all three of these risk factors as being forerunners to heart disease.

As you progress through this textbook, key terms from the science of epidemiology will often enter into the topics. **Table 2.1** is provided as a reference for future use.

It's All About Prevention!

Think of prevention as a three-tiered system, with the first tier being the most vital. This is labeled **primary prevention**. Primary prevention occurs when public health actions entirely avert a given disease or **health-compromising condition** (see **Box 2.2** for an explanation of what is meant by a health-compromising condition).

Consider, for instance, a simple and common health-compromising condition: dental caries (cavities). When public health dentists set up sealant programs for children residing in

Table 2.1   Useful terms and meanings from the science of epidemiology.

Term	Meaning	Example
Case rate	Number of cases/population at risk	The case rate in New Jersey nursing homes is 330 per 1,000 residents.
Association	Two factors are linked.	Smoking and lung cancer
Incidence	Number of new cases, expressed as a rate in a specified time period	The incidence of stroke among men under 50 was 12 per 1,000 in 2019.
Prevalence	Number of existing cases, expressed as a rate	The prevalence of COVID-19 was 390 cases per 1,000 in rural Iowa in 2020.
Relative risk	Incidence of a disease among those exposed to a given risk factor versus those not exposed	Cancer death is 3.2 times more likely in people using the herbicide called *Round-Up* compared to those not using it.
Randomization	The defining aspect of an epidemiologic intervention study	Volunteers were randomized to a treatment or placebo condition.
Placebo	An inert treatment, known to not prevent the disease	Volunteers randomized to the placebo group did not receive a real vaccine.

BOX 2.2 WHAT IS MEANT BY THE TERM "HEALTH-COMPROMISING CONDITION"?

As you learn about public health, you will inevitably also learn about diseases. However, there is more to consider than just disease! For instance, nobody would call teen pregnancy a disease, but (at a population level) it is an ever-present source of low-birth-weight babies, premature birth, and childhood poverty. Similarly, you would not think of obesity as a disease, but it is a risk factor for the onset of diabetes, heart disease, low-back pain, and some forms of cancer. An abbreviated listing of other health-compromising conditions is provided here:

- Memory loss and/or an inability to retain new information
- Addictions (even modest addictions) to drugs/alcohol
- Learning issues in children (often caused by toxic levels of heavy metals, such as lead and mercury)
- Childhood compromises in neurological development (iodine deficiency is a leading cause of this problem)
- Diminished respiratory capacity in survivors of COVID-19, heavy smokers, and people chronically exposed to air pollution

Also, as you progress through this textbook, be clear that the term **negative health outcomes** applies to any type of disease (chronic, infectious, or congenital) as well as all health-compromising conditions. Health outcomes, however, are distinct from the concept of risk conditions. To help you, think of risk conditions (one or several) as always preceding any given negative health outcome.

cultures and geographic areas characterized by high incidence rates of childhood dental caries, this is primary prevention. The sealants act as a barrier to sugar and other foods that are implicated in the formation of caries. So, in this case, one public health program aligns with *one form* of primary prevention.

Now, let's consider how one public health program could align with *multiple forms* of primary prevention. Entire cities (such as Philadelphia and New York City) have passed and implemented taxes on the sale of sugar-sweetened beverages. This singular public health action creates at least four significant outcomes: (a) meaningful and population-level reductions in body mass index (BMI); (b) meaningful and population-level reductions in blood glucose levels, translating to a lower incidence of adult-onset diabetes; (c) meaningful and population-level reductions in triglyceride levels, translating to a lower risk profile for cardiovascular disease; and (d) meaningful and population-level reductions in dental caries.

From a cost-benefit perspective, it is a wise practice to focus public health actions on a primary prevention target with the potential for yielding multiple positive outcomes. Thus, as shown in **Figure 2.1**, primary prevention exists at different levels. This figure provides a visual distinction of what public health does, in contrast to medical care (also known as healthcare). The figure uses the three prevention terms you will learn about in this chapter: primary, secondary, and tertiary prevention. This figure also makes a distinction between actions at an upper level (meaning entire populations) versus those at a lower level (meaning a one-person-at-a-time approach).

This contrast between the example with dental sealants and the example of taxing sugar-sweetened beverages sets up a vital distinction. As you certainly noted in reading both examples, only the second one uses the term "meaningful and population-level reductions." Even with an army of dentists applying sealants to children's teeth, making an impact across entire populations depends on how many parents consent to and support the sealant campaign.

Much like the national campaign to vaccinate at least 90% of all people against COVID-19, it is very likely that such ambitious targets will never be met. Indeed, it may be that parents with kids most at risk of dental caries are those least likely to sign up their children for sealants. Conversely, evidence strongly suggests that raising taxes on sugar-sweetened beverages has had an across-the-board (i.e., true population-level) effect on reducing consumption.

Public Health Is for Entire Populations

This tenet is vital for understanding what public health is all about. Just as public health is a public responsibility, it is also true that public health applies to everyone. Although the advantages of this are included as part of Figure 2.1, the tenet warrants further elaboration. As always, an example is useful.

Let's begin with a type of public health approach that was once widely advocated (and funded) by the Centers for Disease Control and Prevention (CDC). This approach is still in common use today; it is known as **community-based participatory research** (CBPR). The underlying concept is to involve members of the **target community** in all aspects of planning, implementing, and evaluating a specific public health program. These community members are, of course, volunteers. As volunteers, they are asked to sacrifice a great deal of their time and energy to be part of an advisory group that guides all phases of a given project. On its surface, CBPR appears to be a good idea. However, let's consider a few points below the surface:

- Any geographic community of density (population size larger than a small rural town) will not have a single monolithic community. The community, in fact, will be diverse, comprising subgroups of people who share much in common with each other on a within-group basis but few commonalities between groups. So, which subgroups are represented on the advisory council, and which are left out?

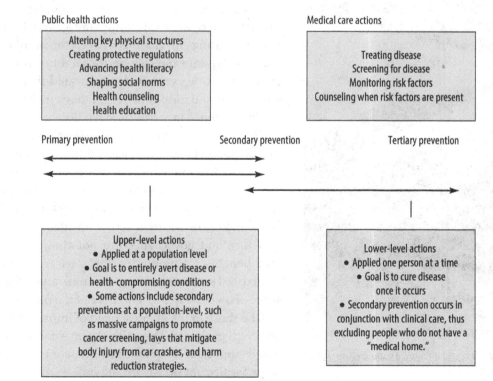

Figure 2.1   The difference between public health and medical care

- Advisory council volunteers are likely to be privileged people in that they have the time to donate to an unpaid, time-consuming activity that may last years. This may translate into a bias, given that people without this level of free time and energy are not represented.

- A key goal of CBPR is to inform and influence local policy: citywide ordinances, county-wide practices, and so forth. From a larger perspective, statewide – or even federal – regulations that can positively impact all people are not a realistic goal of CBPR. Thus, in its most successful form, CBPR would create added inequities in any given state, exacerbating health disparities.

Using the example of driving under the influence (DUI), consider the vast differences between a CBPR approach and a true population-level approach to the problem (one that inequitably kills teens). Given the disabilities and deaths that result from DUI, it is clear that public will and support to reduce these life-changing occurrences (see **Photo 2.2**) is strong. Thus, the focus is on finding the optimal course of action to achieve that goal. As opposed to pursuing and achieving local change one community at a time, a population-level approach would function at a state regulatory level to achieve goals such as tighter enforcement of prohibiting alcohol sales to minors, improved education for first-time offenders, stricter limits of locations of alcohol sales outlets, and laws prohibiting drive-thru alcohol sales.

Staying with the example of alcohol, consider the following study as an example of the potential for regulatory practices to improve population-level health. Chang, Wu, and Ying (2012) conducted a state-level analysis that enabled them to determine whether states with

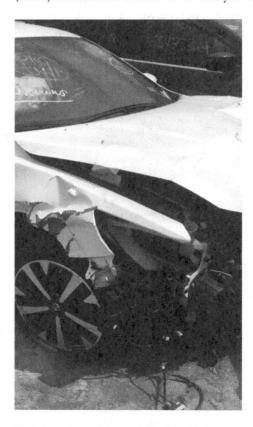

Photo 2.2 A typical DUI-related traffic accident leaves its mark on the world.

relatively more of nine assessed alcohol-related traffic laws had comparatively lower rates of traffic fatalities. Examples of these laws are taxes on beer sales, using 21 as the minimum legal drinking age, zero-tolerance policies, and open container laws. Their findings were intriguing and generally supported a strong correlation between the number of laws in each state and state traffic fatality rates. The evidence in this example demonstrated that state-level (i.e., population-level) regulations make a dramatic difference in terms of mortality.

Of course, it is perhaps unrealistic to expect that all public health practice will be predicated on passing legislation. However, it is entirely reasonable to expect that public health practices must transcend city and county borders such that privileged areas (towns, cities, etc.) with adequate infrastructure and governance are not the only areas that benefit. Communities that lack volunteers, shared and representative governance, and a shared sense of ownership in the welfare of the people may well be those in the greatest need of improved public health practices. Thus, the idea of a community-based approach to public health works well for some locales but poorly for others.

As opposed to pursuing and achieving local change one community at a time, a population-level approach would function at a state regulatory level

What Are the Tools of Public Health Practice?

Now that you know more about the tenets of public health practice, it is time to understand its basic structure. Simply stated, the structure is built in a sequential fashion. **Figure 2.2** displays this sequence from its starting point of education through its ending point of creating structural-level changes that can sustain public health improvements over time. This sequential model of the available tools to improve public health is one that you should learn carefully in this chapter, as it will be important to know the principles in each subsequent chapter.

At the heart of the sequence (middle box) is a web of regulatory and policy actions that are an important terminal point in their own right, as well as drivers of the structural-level changes needed to have large and lasting population-level effects on health. Underlying the entire sequence is an ongoing process of evaluation that informs adaptations to all three basic actions shown in the sequence. Now that you have a generalized understanding of the model, let's take a close look at each of its parts!

Education of Entire Populations and Key Policy Makers (Block 1)

A somewhat famous adage in public health practice is that *knowledge is a necessary but not sufficient basis for behavior change.* In less eloquent words, let's consider knowledge a forerunner to behavior change. To clarify, the term *knowledge* refers to health-related information that is of high relevance to one or more protective behaviors against disease or health-compromising conditions. In many cases, this role of knowledge may be quite strong: for example, the majority of the public reacted to COVID-19 prevention information by quickly adopting the behaviors of mask-wearing and social distancing. In many more cases, however, knowledge is nothing more than the first of many building blocks that may over time form a foundation of lasting behavior change.

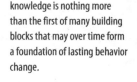

knowledge is nothing more than the first of many building blocks that may over time form a foundation of lasting behavior change.

Whether the role of knowledge, and the public health action of providing the education to acquire the relevant knowledge, is strong, mediocre, or weak is a function of two factors. The first involves differences among people in the target population. The ability to learn quickly, a desire to adopt self-initiated preventive actions, and the availability of needed resources to enact the preventive measures are all examples of these differences. Second, the complexity of the recommended health-protective behaviors has a tremendous influence on how much influence knowledge will ultimately exert on adopting lasting behavior change. Although this may seem complicated, in reality, the public action of knowledge provision is always important

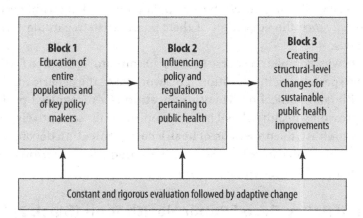

Figure 2.2   The basic tools of public health practice

to some degree, and thus it must be a part of a larger effort to protect and improve public health.

As noted in **Figure 2.2**, teaching and informing those who can ultimately *create and implement* regulatory actions and policy is another key tool of public health practice. As a subset of providing education, it is also vital to engage in planned efforts to provide advanced levels of highly relevant knowledge to all persons charged with *enforcing* regulatory and policy-related actions. This implies that public health education-based actions must often be specifically targeted and tailored to a defined need. As always, an example here may help you understand this concept more clearly.

Using America's opioid crisis for this example, it is important to note that most states have passed laws allowing pharmacies to sell needles and syringes to **people who inject drugs (PWID)**. The laws are important to public health because sales of new needles and syringes to PWID have been demonstrated to reduce their sharing of these items. Sharing is, of course, an issue because of the very likely event that any blood-borne infection within the first person to inject is transmitted to the next person using the same needle or syringe. These infections include both hepatitis B and C, with the latter being a common form of a chronic and debilitating infection in PWID.

Sadly, despite state laws allowing these sales to PWID, evidence from at least two states suggests that many pharmacists are reticent, or may even refuse, to make these sales (Meyerson, Davis, Agley, et al. 2018; Meyerson, Lawrence, Cope, et al., in press). As pharmacy employees, pharmacists are typically bound to follow established corporate (i.e., store-based or chain-store based) policies. Whether this occurs could be improved by providing targeted and tailored education to pharmacists relative to:

* Awareness of state laws relevant to the sales of needles and syringes to PWID

* Awareness and acceptance of corporate policy regarding these sales

* Enhanced understanding of addiction to injectable drugs, and thus the need for PWID to do so

* Basic skill acquisition pertaining to making these sales in the absence of stigma and/or judgment

As you can quickly discern from considering these four bullet points, the education in this example is geared toward the implementing policy. Similar efforts could be directed toward corporate executives relative to creating policies and also establishing methods of enforcing employed pharmacists following the established policy and working within established corporate guidelines to advance the education of their pharmacists regarding PWID and sales of needles and syringes.

Many students who complete a course such as this one are inspired to further their careers in public health by specializing in education. This work takes the generic form of either health education or health communication. **Health education** is a recognized profession, with the basic mission of providing health-related information and skills to relatively small segments of the population. In contrast, the profession of **health communication** devotes its efforts toward much larger-scale education campaigns, such as those frequently sponsored by the CDC (**see Box 2.3**) and similar public health organizations.

Regulatory and Policy-Based Public Health Tools (Block 2)

As perhaps the most essential tool in the repertoire of public health practices, it is vital to understand that creating and implementing regulations/policies is necessary to ensure population-level effects. Please note that this chapter will not attempt to draw distinctions

BOX 2.3 AN EXAMPLE OF A CDC-SPONSORED HEALTH COMMUNICATION PROGRAM

Without question, one of the most valuable health-protective behaviors is increasing daily consumption of fruits and vegetables, especially those that are unrefined: that is, foods remaining in their natural condition. To promote this behavior on a nationwide basis, the CDC created and implemented the *5-A-Day* media campaign and corresponding state-by-state information program (including technical assistance) designed to assist each of the 50 state departments of health in creating innovative programs for citizens most in need of improving their intake of fruits and vegetables. Thus, as you have already learned in this chapter (see Block 1 of **Figure 2.2**), this is an example of education being planned and delivered at two levels: (a) the education campaign was directed at the public in general, and (b) it was also directed at professionals tasked with helping local communities promote consuming five servings of fruits/vegetables per day while also providing funds to implement corresponding assistance programs at local levels. The photo shown here of CDC's *Action Guide for State Health Practitioners* is emblematic of how the national campaign reaches out to local professionals.

As part of this health communication campaign, the CDC makes various images available that can be used at local levels to promote consuming five servings of fruits/vegetables per day.

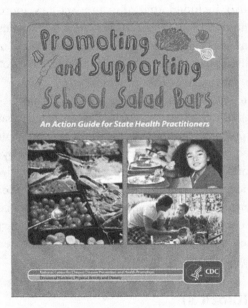
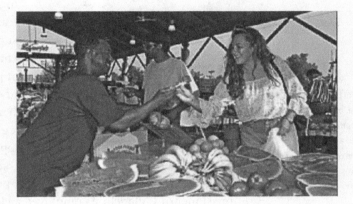

Source: U.S Department of Health & Human Services / Public_Domain.

between regulations, policies, and laws, as doing so would be cumbersome without any substantial advantage. For the purpose of learning basic public health practice, it is sufficient to consider (from this point forward) any formally sanctioned set of rules as being regulatory/policy-oriented. With this point firmly in mind, let's consider an example.

As you will learn in subsequent chapters of this textbook, one of the nation's leading culprits in causing population-level premature morbidity and mortality is the overconsumption of refined sugars (e.g., granulated sugars, high fructose corn syrup, honey). This overconsumption is largely a product of a food system constructed on quick energy and low-cost foods with long shelf-lives (i.e., they do not expire quickly). Sadly, and despite mounting evidence implicating sugar in the disease process, this trend in overconsumption is increasing at an alarming rate. It has been estimated that the average American in the early decades of the 2000s consumes just over 150 pounds of sugar annually, compared to two pounds annually in the 1800s. Of all the sources that provide Americans with this overconsumption habit, the one with the largest share of the blame has been labeled generically as **sugar-sweetened beverages** (SSBs).

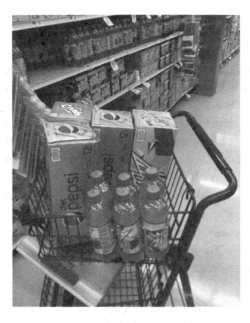

Photo 2.3   Soda sales comprise a large share of business of grocery stores.

Clearly, simply providing people with education about the harms of over-consuming sugar has not had a population-level impact on the problem. One regulatory/policy approach, however, is making a difference. This is an economics-based approach that simply levies a local tax on the purchase of SSBs. As mentioned earlier in this chapter, the city of Philadelphia was one of the first in the United States to implement and evaluate this tax.

Published in the *Journal of the American Medical Association*, the evaluation of the SSB tax for Philadelphia found that a 1.5 cents per ounce increase in sales tax created a population-level decrease in consumption of 1.3 billion ounces (Roberto, Lawman, & LeVassuer, 2019). Key findings also included that this modest tax increase translated into a 59% reduction in soda sales at supermarkets, a 40% reduction in sales at mass merchandise stores (e.g., Walmart), and a 13% reduction at pharmacies (e.g., Walgreens, CVS).

the evaluation of the SSB tax for Philadelphia found that a 1.5 cents per ounce increase in sales tax created a population-level decrease in consumption of 1.3 billion ounces

At this point in the chapter, you can now link the first block in **Figure 2.2** to this second block. This is because regulatory/policy changes in a democratic society are subject to some degree of public approval and a large degree of political support. Noteworthy, for example, is that the Philadelphia tax was adamantly opposed by some members of the public and by the group known as the American Beverage Association. As you can see in this case study, financial interests frequently compete with public health interests. Ultimately, the Health Commissioner of Philadelphia employed a clever tactic of pledging to use the added 1.5 cents per ounce tax revenue to fund early childhood education programs (i.e., preschool). Despite this tactic's great success, the city tax was passed only after a massive effort was devoted to educating both the public and their respective legislators.

Structural-Level Public Health Tools (Block 3)

The epitome of public health practice is creating sustainable structures that support long-lasting health-protective behaviors and discourage health-risk behaviors. In this sense, the term *structure* represents any planned intervention that takes the form of a permanent alteration to the physical, social, or economic environments that shape and promote health-protective behaviors. At this point in the chapter, you can now link the second block in **Figure 2.2** to this third block. This is because structural-level alterations are always predicated on underlying regulatory/policy changes.

the term structure *represents any planned intervention that takes the form of a permanent alteration to the physical, social, or economic environments*

Let's explore a good example that addresses both physical and social alterations: the *Atlanta Beltline*. To begin, it is noteworthy that our nation is sadly out of shape as a consequence of sedentary living. People largely rely on either fossil fuels or electric energy for their transportation to and from the workplace, to visit friends, to eat at restaurants, and even to use a gym. A clear public health priority is to create Block 3 interventions that structure urban life to make even modest human movement (such as walking to work) an easy option to adopt and maintain. It is not necessary for all people to be athletes, only for them to engage in what is known as **moderate to vigorous physical activity (MVPA).** The CDC recommends that most members of the public engage in at least 150 minutes of MVPA each week. Thus, improving population-level health involves integrating movement (even moderate exercise) into people's everyday lives.

In service of promoting MVPA, the city of Atlanta, GA (USA) dedicated a 22-mile stretch of old railways to become a common outdoor space for its residents. By paving this space, the city created what has become one of the most well-known outdoor recreation areas in the state of Georgia. On any given day, from dawn until after dark, it is common to see people walking, jogging, running, roller-skating, and biking the Beltline (see **Photo 2.4**). Many of the city's residents even use the Beltline as their route to commute to and from work using human movement rather than car or public transportation systems. Although athletes use the Beltline to enhance their aerobic capacity, it is far more populated by people of all ages and all levels of fitness as a method of keeping the body moving. It is also important that the Beltline was constructed with ample and close access to many of Atlanta's most-loved eating and drinking establishments. Thus, human movement is encouraged by the social life that has flourished on the sidelines of the Beltline. In many ways, this social aspect is perhaps a more significant factor motivating human movement on the Beltline than the idea of enhancing cardiorespiratory fitness. Regardless of the motivating reasons, Atlanta residents with access to the Beltline benefit from more frequent engagement in MVPA.

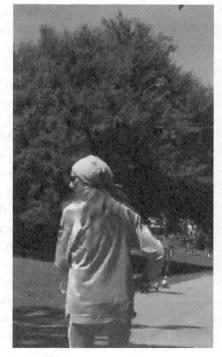

Photo 2.4   The Atlanta beltline attracts people of all ages who want to be outdoors and moving.

Let's consider for a moment what the structural-level aspect of the Beltline means to public health. First, the city maintains the paving of the Beltline on a permanent basis. This is the essence of a sustainable example pertaining to a public health intervention. Second, the Beltline has created a social norm – one that makes MVPA a normal part of everyday life as opposed to a chore or a fitness resolution. Third, the social capital created by the Beltline's construction has fostered a renewed interest and commitment among nearby residents to be outdoors and moving rather than being inside four walls and sitting. So, this population-level, long-term increase in MVPA was achieved without direct education of residents. In this example, public health education was directed at city legislators who supported the project. As you can imagine, Block 2 of **Figure 2.2** was also crucial in that the city had to approve numerous regulatory/policy changes that were needed to construct this massive urban project. The structural change to the city will improve the health of millions of people; this is in stark contrast to the medical approach to health, which is a one-person-at-a-time intervention.

Before moving to the next section of this chapter, it is worth noting that the Atlanta Beltline is only one of many examples of an urban-based intervention that promotes MVPA. United States cities are quickly learning that human movement is a method of reducing traffic congestion. For instance, New York City (despite its overcrowded nature) prioritized the construction of bike lanes along major commuting routes; this was the basis for the city's bike-to-work program (which also involved a huge investment in city bikes).

The Role of Public Health Research

Now that you have been introduced to the three basic tools of public health practice, it is time to learn about the role of public health research. Using the most recent example of MVPA, let's consider why this is being so strongly encouraged in public health practice.

Although dozens of recent research studies have investigated (and supported) the idea that even modest levels of physical activity promote cardiovascular fitness, the example used here is one of the earlier studies to arrive at this conclusion (Gutin, Zenong, Humphries, & Barbeau, 2005). As a public health research study, this example was highly focused on a prioritized population: adolescents. Also, as a public health research study, it included research volunteers of multiple races, as well as both sexes. As opposed to a medical study, the need for this study was based on a public health question: Is moderate physical activity adequate to promote cardiovascular fitness among adolescents?

Like all good public health research, the study used an outstanding set of measures, enhancing its validity. For instance, adolescents wore a device known as an *actigraph* (using a technology known as free-living accelerometry) just above the hip for seven days. The readings from this device were used to gauge their level of movement (low, moderate, vigorous). Cardiovascular fitness was assessed using a multistage treadmill test that continuously monitored heart rate and oxygen consumption as the workload (speed and incline) of the test intensified. Given the national attention to addressing childhood obesity, a second public health outcome was assessed: the percentage of body fat. This was assessed by using a technology known as dual-energy X-ray absorptiometry. So, as you can see so far, public health research is based on the same type of science as medical research. The exception with most public health research is that either a health risk or a health-protective behavior is also assessed (in our example, this is the level of activity as assessed by the actigraph).

The findings were highly supportive of a strong relationship between moderate physical activity and cardiovascular fitness. Although levels of cardiovascular fitness were significantly greater among those classified as engaging in vigorous activity, this conclusion had already stood the test of time and would not change public health practice. In contrast, the conclusion of a strong relationship between moderate physical activity and cardiovascular fitness carried several implications for public health practice: for example, promoting walking among adolescents as opposed to using fossil-fuel forms of transportation; and creating community recreation areas that allowed engagement in less athletic activities such as badminton, volleyball, and bowling.

Not all public health research supports the public health actions that we (i.e., the people) would support. In this example, the research team did *not* find a significant relationship between moderate physical activity and the percentage of body fat. But a significant relationship was found between vigorous physical activity and the percentage of body fat. Taking this finding to the level of public health practice, it becomes clear that the U.S. epidemic of childhood obesity will not be resolved through interventions such as increased hours of walking.

Throughout this textbook, you will be exposed to public health research studies as a method of helping you understand and appreciate that the tools of public health are only applied when ample science-based evidence demonstrates the value of a given intervention strategy. Public health practice is not dictated by morality, conventional wisdom, or even widely shared social values. For example, sitting is a widely shared social value.

Culture and custom dictate inviting visitors to a home or workplace to have a seat. The entire U.S. education system is based on students sitting in seats. Even outdoors, sitting is encouraged via park benches, amphitheaters, and lawn chairs. The problem with all this, as it turns out, is that sitting is simply not a healthy practice. We know this to be true as a result of public health research. For instance, an Australian study of more than 222,000 people showed a significantly higher level of cardiovascular risk factors for people sitting 11 or more hours per day compared to those sitting 8 hours or less per day (van der Ploeg, Chey, & Korda, 2012). So, let's take a moment to think about this! It is common for people to work an 8-hour day at a computer and then come home and sit 3 hours or more – 11 hours or more is an American norm. This is why a new phrase in public health is "sitting is the new smoking." Given this basic

public health research is based on the same type of science as medical research.

public health research, public health practice can begin to promote standing, movement, and so forth as health-protective practices.

In addition to informing public health practice, public health research is also valuable in determining whether practice strategies are working. This point takes you back to **Figure 2.2**, where you should now focus on the box that underlies the entire sequential model. That box is all about using a rigorous research process to evaluate and diagnose the success or failure of Block 1, Block 2, and Block 3. Public health research tells us what is working, what is not working, and what should be altered in terms of how public health practice is conducted. This is vital!

Why Is Public Health So Important?

The adage "an ounce of prevention is worth a pound of cure" sums up the evidence as to why our nation must increase its focus on public health practices. The alternative to public health is medical practice: that is, the treatment of disease after it occurs. Although this unwise course of action may be preferable to some people (consider, for example, people who refused the COVID-19 vaccine and were subsequently infected and hospitalized with the disease), from a national standpoint, it is foolish. This is because the costs of healthcare are already at an all-time high and increasing with each passing year.

In the past four decades (1980 through 2020), healthcare costs – as a portion of the gross domestic product (GDP) – have more than tripled! It has been estimated that spending on medical care makes up approximately 17% of GDP. To fully grasp what this means, consider the following:

- Inflation is not related to GDP.

- 70% of total GDP is *consumer spending.* The denominator used to calculate the 17% estimate was 100% of the GDP; thus an adjusted estimate brings the value closer to about one of every four dollars spent by consumers (25%).

- The budget for the entire Department of Defense (the U.S. military) is 3.2% of GDP. Thus spending on medical care is more than five times greater than spending on national defense.

- Medical care costs have increased at a pace that is greater than the growth of the economy (meaning the rising costs are *not* sustainable).

- By 2028, estimates suggest an increase in healthcare costs of 63%!

As you can readily guess, public health is a low-cost alternative to the medical paradigm. Yet medical care has become unfortunately ingrained in our culture. Every four years, during the U.S. presidential campaigns, it is all too common to hear Democrats and Republicans fiercely debate topics such as the right to select your own doctor or who should and should not be given Medicaid benefits. Sadly, these controversies rage without ever taking a detour in the direction of dramatically increasing spending on prevention (public health) as an investment in saving our population from laying out large portions of their income for medical care and/or medical insurance (a cost that also increases year to year).

medical care has become unfortunately ingrained in our culture.

At this juncture, you may expect this textbook to launch into a litany of all the things that must be done to fix the medical care system. But this book is not about fixing that problem. Moreover, it is suggested that inverting the entire approach – moving away from treatments and cures to a more progressive agenda of creating population-level conditions that constantly foster disease prevention – is the answer to a rapidly unaffordable and unsustainable medical system.

As this chapter comes to a close, it is again vital to remember that medical care is a "one patient at time" enterprise! Conversely, as you understand by now, public health is aimed at entire populations. **Table 2.2** briefly summarizes the critical differences between the two approaches.

One question you may now have is, "Why aren't prevention practices receiving far greater attention in the medical care professions?" Although the answers to that question could easily dominate another entire chapter, one important point is known as the **prevention paradox** (see **Box 2.4**).

Table 2.2   Critical differences between medical care and public health.

Medical care	Public health
Curing disease is the focus.	Preventing disease is the focus.
Recovery is the goal.	Advanced health is the goal.
People are responsible for their health.	Socioeconomics shape health.
Outcomes can be measured.	Outcomes are difficult to measure.
Investments needed are high.	Investments needed are low.

BOX 2.4 THE HUMAN SIDE

Human nature can be fickle. Often, for example, we have a hard time believing in things that are unseen. Thus, the old saying "seeing is believing" precludes the notion that seeing nothing is also meaningful. When a medical doctor places a stent in a coronary artery of an otherwise critically ill patient, that creates a "seeing is believing" cure – one that is quite tangible!

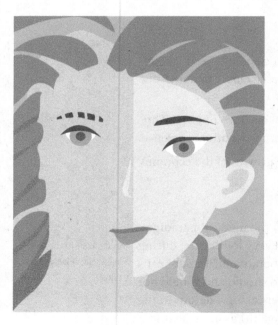

In contrast, when a city constructs massive bike-to-work trails and thousands of people improve their lung capacity and strengthen their heart muscles as a result of daily biking, there is no clear evidence that this public health program saves lives.

Let's consider a second – very different – example of this problem. Treating HIV/AIDS medically can prolong life for decades. Patients experience clear and convincing evidence of feeling well again. Yet the prevention of HIV infection in the first place (typically through the use of condoms) lacks a "seeing is believing" moment. The dutiful condom user can never really be sure that this health behavior paid off; perhaps they avoided HIV based on their choice of sex partners.

Each example illustrates what is known as the **prevention paradox**. People have a hard time giving credit to health behaviors as working because they cannot easily see a link between the health behavior and the absence of a disease or health-compromising condition. At a basic level, there is no tangible and/or immediate reward for engaging in many important health behaviors. Consider these three behaviors: reducing consumption of dietary sugars to avoid diabetes, reducing consumption of dietary sodium to avoid hypertension, and consuming ample dietary antioxidants to avert cancer. Each of these behaviors is a daily task that requires great attention and the purchase of foods that tend to be costly. But none of them provide any reward, leaving many people wondering, "Does it really matter? I'm fine."

On a larger scale, the prevention paradox works against making public health funding a priority. For instance, once public health efforts largely eliminate a given infectious disease, it is not unusual for governments to end the funding of those efforts (because the problem can no longer be seen). By preventing an otherwise visible occurrence of disease, public health efforts tend to fade into obscurity and thus do not typically attract continued funding.

Review and Key Terms

As you have learned in this chapter, public health is a public responsibility. As opposed to placing a sole focus on treatment, public health seeks to foster **health-protective conditions**. Further, public health seeks to minimize **risk conditions**. Although public health is not a profession, its underlying science of epidemiology is vital relative to **surveillance systems, case findings**, identification of **outbreaks**, and understanding **point-source outbreaks** of disease. Epidemiology is also the science behind **risk factor** identification – a necessary step in developing plans for the **primary prevention** of disease.

Ultimately, you learned in this chapter that public health is determined by creating conditions that allow for the health and welfare of "we the people" to prosper. A counterpoint involves recognizing and changing **health-compromising conditions**, such as those that are all too often found in workplaces, neighborhoods, and other settings and that foster risk behaviors. You also learned that the ambitious goals of public health typically require far more than mere community-level efforts. Thus, although **community-based participatory research (CBPR)** in public health may have a minor role to play, the bulk of lasting and substantial improvements to the health of people in the United States will occur through the implementation of regulatory/policy practices; these are also essential for serving communities that lack the ability to engage in community-level interventions. Rather than serving selected **target communities**, public health is broadly aimed at entire populations.

At the heart of this chapter, you learned about the three methods by which public health can best be improved. Using examples of specific populations, such as **people who inject drugs (PWID)** and the entire populations of cities or states via the taxation of **sugar-sweetened beverages (SSBs)**, you learned that public health practice moves through a sequence starting with education, proceeding to regulation, and ending with structural changes. As part of this model, you learned that **health education** and **health communication** are types of public health subsets supporting the larger role of education in public health practice.

Although many applied examples were included in this chapter, one that best illustrates the endpoint of public health practice (i.e., implementing sustainable structural-level changes) involves **moderate to vigorous physical activity (MVPA)**. In this regard, you now know that daily and prolonged movement of the body (including walking) is potentially just as valuable to preventing disease as intense periodic physical exercise. The example of the Atlanta Beltline was given as a structural-level public health intervention – one that creates conditions leading to the primary prevention of disease.

For Practice and Class Discussion

Practice Questions

1. Which example **best** illustrates primary prevention?
   a. Having a mammogram
   b. Being treated for early-stage cardiovascular disease
   c. Good oral hygiene
   d. Annually checking your blood cholesterol levels

2. The elimination of health disparities is **most** dependent on:
   a. Constantly improving clinical interventions
   b. Making health-related counseling and education widely available
   c. Creating highly effective interventions designed for individuals
   d. Changing inequitable socioeconomic conditions

3. Which example **best** illustrates how public health averts infectious disease?
    a. Regulating the tobacco industry
    b. Regulating carbon emissions
    c. Allowing needle/syringe exchange programs to function legally
    d. Taxing alcohol sales

4. Which example **least** illustrates a public health program?
    a. A program that helps diabetics control their disease
    b. A social media campaign designed to motivate less use of sodium in cooking
    c. Reducing the costs of organic produce
    d. Adding fluoride to drinking water

5. Which public health tool applies to the process of providing highly relevant and specific information to legislators?
    a. Education
    b. Regulatory/Policy changes
    c. Making structural-level changes
    d. All of the above

6. Which public health tool applies to the process of creating sustainable interventions?
    a. Education
    b. Regulatory/Policy changes
    c. Making structural-level changes
    d. All of the above

7. Why is a pump handle such an important part of this module?
    a. Removing the handle from just one pump was the key part of John Snow's intervention to prevent cholera.
    b. It was shown that these handles were a source of transmitting cholera.
    c. The old-fashioned water pump (used by hand) is a symbol of how easy it was to die of a water-based illness in the 1800s.
    d. This was the centerpiece of germ theory and the start of medicine.

8. Which one of the following is **least** illustrative of a risk condition?
    a. Social customs and practices that encourage and support ongoing behaviors that are harmful to the body
    b. Climate change
    c. Income inequality and socioeconomic disparities
    d. Having diabetes develop before age 40

9. As the science of public health, epidemiology serves multiple functions. Which one of the following examples is **least** related to the science of epidemiology?
    a. A restaurant chain is investigated for causing an outbreak of hepatitis A.
    b. A long-term study of factory workers identifies risk factors for chronic back pain.
    c. The role of political support is assessed regarding a program designed to control second-hand tobacco smoke.

10. As a share of the gross domestic product, U.S. medical care costs greatly exceed expenditures for the entire U.S. Department of Defense.
    a. True
    b. False

For Discussion (in class or small groups, or online)

11. Using the internet, locate a city that has constructed, or is currently constructing, a project similar to the Atlanta Beltline. Describe the project and then determine how many people you think may realistically avail themselves of increased MVPA as a consequence of having access to this structural-level intervention.

12. As you can imagine from reading this chapter, public health often conflicts with what people label as "individual freedoms." COVID-19 changed our lives, probably forever. An end to the pandemic may never come, but it is – so far—largely controllable through vaccinations. One of the many issues that have pitted individual freedom against public health involves people refusing or simply not taking the time to be vaccinated.

    Take a stand (in writing or orally to others) regarding whether vaccination against COVID-19 should be mandatory. In at least 100 words, describe your logic and reasoning for the opinion you offer. As much as possible, include keywords from this chapter in your argument.

13. As you learned in this chapter, public health is a public responsibility. Go online to locate and describe one clear example that illustrates this principle. For instance, many states have strict gun-control laws based on the overwhelming majority of voters who have responded to referendum questions on a ballot. Many of these laws originated from dedicated groups of citizens who are dedicated to changing the current reality of 300 deaths occurring each day in the U.S. due to guns. Once you have what you consider a great example of any action by the public to promote health, describe it to others in the class (and include the reasons you selected the example).

References

Chang, K., Wu, C. C., & Ying, Y. H. (2012). The effectiveness of alcohol control policies on alcohol-related traffic fatalities in the United States. *Accident Analysis and Prevention, 45*, 400–415.

Gutin, B., Zenong, Y., Humphries, M. C., & Barbeau, D. (2005). Relationships of moderate and vigorous physical activity to fitness and fatness in adolescents. *American Journal of Clinical Nutrition, 81*, 746–750.

Meyerson, B. E, Davis, A., Agley, J. D., Shannon, D. J., Lawrence, C. A., Ryder, P. T, Ritchie, K., & Gassman, R. (2018). Predicting pharmacy syringe sales to people who inject drugs: Policy practice and perceptions. *International Journal of Drug Policy, 56*, 46–53.

Meyerson, B. E., Lawrence, C. A., Cope, S. D., Levin, S., Thomas, C., Eldridge, L. A., Coles, H., Vadiei, N., & Kennedy, A. (2019). I could take the judgment if you could just provide the service: non-prescription syringe purchase experience at Arizona pharmacies, 2018. *BMC Harm Reduction* (in press).

Roberto, C. A., Lawson, H. G., & LeVassuer, M. T. (2019). Association of a beverage tax on sugar-sweetened and artificially-sweetened beverages with changes in prices and sales at chain retailers in a large urban setting. *Journal of the American Medical Association, 321*(18), 1799–1810.

van der Ploeg, H. D., Chey, T., & Korda, R. J. (2012). Sitting time and all-cause mortality risk in 222,497 Australian adults. *Archives of Internal Medicine, 172*(6), 494–500.

CHAPTER 3

THE EVOLUTION OF PUBLIC HEALTH PRACTICE

Think left and think right and think low and think high. Oh, the thinks you can think up if only you try.

—*Dr. Seuss*

Overview

As you learned in Chapter 2, public health is about creating conditions that foster health-protective behaviors and help to preclude people from engaging in risky behaviors that all too often lead to morbidity and premature mortality. Following the advice of Dr. Seuss, the evolution of public health practice has come from thinking differently! This chapter provides you with an intriguing chronology about past thinking and past strategies used to advance public health to its current state. This begins with a rather unsung hero who may rightfully be thought of as the founder of public health practice: Sir Edwin Chadwick. You will learn that, beginning in the 19th century, Chadwick's thinking was far ahead of his time.

As Chadwick's era became increasingly dominated by germ theory, public health took a turn toward being a subset of medical practice. Public health was seen as a way to distribute and administer vaccines. It also provided a type of reserve workforce that became a staple for responding to outbreaks of infectious diseases. This was a time when raging epidemics of gonorrhea and syphilis were common in the United States. In response, the U.S. public health system brought on **public health advisors** (PHAs), a workforce that eventually shifted to the Centers for Disease Control and Prevention (CDC) in Atlanta, GA.

As the 20th century progressed and infectious diseases were largely controlled through vaccines, public health turned its attention to preventing chronic diseases. Typically centered in county and state health departments, these public health efforts were based on the premise that people needed only to understand why and how they should adopt health-protective behaviors. At this stage in the evolution of public health, the suggested preventive behaviors focused on screening for early signs of pending disease or teaching people disease-specific information meant to alter behaviors and thus set the stage for primary prevention.

As the 20th century morphed into the 21st century, the thinking behind public health practice once again evolved. Public health began to bypass disease-specific health behaviors and, instead, embrace the concept of **actual causes of death**. The eloquence of this thinking was that many health behaviors were so important that

LEARNING OBJECTIVES

1. Explain the origin of public health as pioneered by Sir Edwin Chadwick.

2. Explain the history of public health from the perspective of vaccinations and outbreak responses by the government.

3. Describe the term *epidemiological transition*, and apply it to the rise and fall of local health departments as lead public health agencies.

4. Describe the phrase *actual causes of death*, and explain how this concept altered public health practice.

5. Explain the term *upstream thinking*, and apply it to public health practice.

6. Describe the scope of public health practice.

7. Understand that public health practice differs greatly between nations.

Understanding the Science and Practice of Public Health, First Edition. Richard Crosby.
© 2023 John Wiley & Sons, Inc. Published 2023 by John Wiley & Sons, Inc.

their adoption by the public could avert multiple forms of disease (for instance, a diet rich in antioxidants prevents several forms of cancer and greatly contributes to improvements in cardiovascular health, thus preventing heart disease). One task in this chapter is to gain a thorough understanding of these actual causes and begin to understand the corresponding public health challenges associated with these causes.

At the same time, public health practice shed its past thinking about the value placed on teaching people "why and how" and began to create conditions that fostered health-protective behaviors and helped preclude people from engaging in risky behaviors.

Roughly 200 years of evolving public health practices have culminated in what is best considered an open system – meaning the need for constant change and thus constant improvement is built into public health practices. As you can easily imagine, COVID-19 has, and will continue to have, a profound impact on the continued evolution of public health practice.

COVID-19 has, and will continue to have, a profound impact on the continued evolution of public health practice.

An Early Origin of Public Health Practice

History often repeats itself in a somewhat profound manner. That is certainly the case in tracing the origins of public health practice back to the 19th century and thinking about how that origin shaped today's public health practice. It began with an 1848 Public Health Law in the United Kingdom, authored by **Sir Edwin Chadwick**. Chadwick was considered a radical because he backed the idea that controlling disease meant "we the people" had to provide services that were lacking for the poor. These services were basic necessities that we now take for granted in cities. They included garbage removal, sanitary methods of removing sewage from homes and streets, and even the oh-so-radical idea of providing access to safe drinking water. He was widely criticized for suggesting that public dollars be spent to provide city sewage, clean water, regular trash removal, street cleaning, and even public bathrooms (as people otherwise urinated and defecated in the streets). As a reformer, Chadwick was the first to promote public health laws that channeled government spending into controlling disease.

At this juncture, it is worth pondering the following questions:

1. At the time, the **plague** was a raging pandemic. How did trash removal control the spread of its causative agent, *Yersinia pestis?*

2. How did public bathrooms and public sewage control the spread of *Yersinia pestis?*

3. How did something as simple as sweeping the streets each night (a practice that still occurs nightly in many U.S. cities, such as New Orleans) control the spread of *Yersinia pestis?*

4. What is a modern-day equivalent of Chadwick's approach to public health when it comes to controlling water-borne diseases (most of which cause severe or even deadly diarrhea)?

As you may have guessed, the answers to the first three questions center around rodent control. Rats are drawn to food sources, such as garbage, feces, and food remnants such as those found on dirty streets. Rats, in turn, carry fleas. The fleas, in turn, were a perfect host for the bacterium *Yersinia pestis*. But Chadwick's critics strongly believed that the poor were responsible for their own problems and that tax dollars should not be spent helping people who would not help themselves. Thus, in 19th century England, it first became apparent that debates would rage as to what extent public health is a public responsibility. Of course, as you know, these debates were ultimately settled relative to providing at least minimal sanitation services for all people, regardless of their income or ability to pay. Going back now to the fourth question, the answer is public sewage and wastewater treatment plants. A modern-day responsibility of public health departments across the United States is to regulate and monitor water treatment plants (aren't you glad?).

Following Chadwick's time, a host of other public actions became standard practice for public health. For instance, pasteurization became mandatory for commercially sold milk and milk products. Given the widespread popularity of drinking cow's milk (globally as well) combined with all the diseases that may be transmitted by drinking milk, you can readily understand why public health intervention was crucial. The basic options were to (a) tell people not to drink milk, (b) tax milk so people could not afford to buy it, or (c) treat milk in a way that made it safe. Of course, option c was the winner and led to the invention (by Louis Pasteur) of **pasteurization** (a method of thermal processing that heats the milk to the point of destroying **pathogens** – i.e., organisms that cause disease in humans).

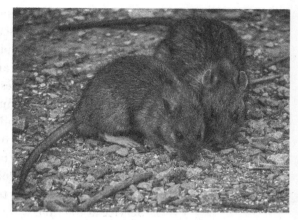

Photo 3.1   In the United States and throughout the world, rats are a leading carrier of disease.
Source: Pefkos/Adobe stock.

Vaccinations and Government-Based Outbreak Responses

At the very start of the 19th century, another bit of public history was in motion: vaccinations against smallpox (a viral disease that killed 3 of every 10 victims and typically left the remainder scarred by pockmarks for life). Although smallpox had been around for centuries, it was at this time that a vaccine first became available and widely distributed. The vaccine was a clear turning point in public health history. However, it took several decades to eradicate smallpox. Ever since, vaccination has been a staple of public health practice. This is another bit of evidence, often taken for granted, that public health is a public responsibility. Each summer, for instance, the CDC makes a data-driven determination about which three variants of the influenza virus are most likely to invade the nation in the coming flu season. This determination is ultimately translated into the mass production of the flu vaccine (which typically becomes available in September). This remains a vital public health practice because each year, there is a distinct possibility that a variant of influenza could infect and kill millions of people, as occurred during the 1918 influenza pandemic.

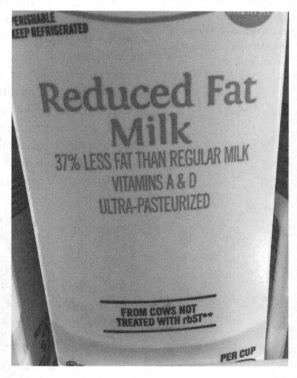

Photo 3.2   The pasteurization of milk is now a public health practice that most people take for granted.

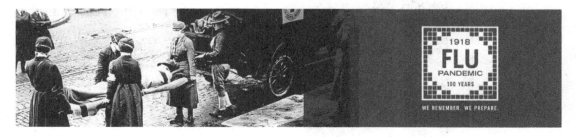

Photo 3.3   The 1918 influenza epidemic infected approximately one-third of the world's population, killing more than 50 million of its victims.
Source: U.S Department of Health & Human Services / Public_Domain.

Moving well into the 20th century, the United States found itself in an epidemic of two sexually transmitted diseases: syphilis and gonorrhea. Because these diseases are caused by bacteria (*T. pallidum* for syphilis and *N. gonorrhoeae* for gonorrhea), they were treatable with a relatively new invention: **antibiotics**. The problem was that both diseases could be largely asymptomatic in females and that males were often clueless about the symptoms (which were far more prominent in males). Consequently, people could be infected with one or both diseases and unknowingly spread the infection to their sex partners. The medical model was of little value in responding to the twin epidemics of syphilis and gonorrhea. Instead, a massive "find and treat" program was needed. This is precisely what occurred under the direction of the CDC.

In 1957, the U.S. Public Health Service transferred its division of Venereal Disease (VD, now known as sexually transmitted infections) to the CDC. A key feature of the Public Health Service at the time was the hiring and training of Public Health Advisors (PHAs). PHAs were committed to being always ready to go (Meyerson, Martich, & Naehr, 2008). This meant they might be sent to any hotspot in the world at a moment's notice to respond to a disease outbreak. PHAs were, in a sense, the disease cowboys of their time. When the CDC annexed the VD division from the Public Health Service, the PHAs became an invaluable public health asset against the epidemics of syphilis and gonorrhea. For example, PHAs regularly engaged in **contact tracing**. This typically occurred by starting with a single case (known as an **index case**) of either disease and efficiently treating the person with antibiotics, and then interviewing that affected person about their recent sex partners in an effort to obtain enough information to locate and possibly diagnose/treat these partners. Each partner of the index case who tested positive for either disease was then similarly treated and interviewed. This original model of contact tracing was applied nationally by CDC in the 1960s and remains part of the infrastructure in most local health departments. This same "find and treat" public health practice became a primary method of controlling the spread of COVID-19, especially in 2020 and 2021, prior to the majority of the public being fully vaccinated (see **Box 3.1**)

> When the CDC annexed the VD division from the Public Health Service, the PHAs became an invaluable public health asset against the epidemics of syphilis and gonorrhea.

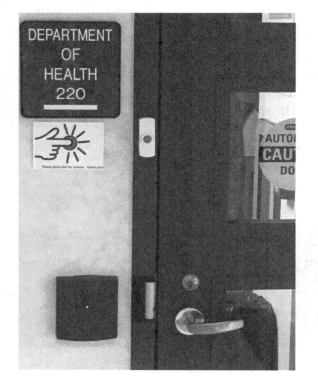

Photo 3.4   Local health departments are important assets for larger public health actions.

The Rise and Fall of Local Health Departments

As the 20th century came to a close, it became increasingly clear that many of the past challenges to public health were well-controlled and, therefore, no longer required urgent attention. As you have learned already in this chapter, these well-controlled diseases were all classified as **infectious diseases**, meaning their origin is a pathogen. When public health was focused on the prevention and control of infectious diseases, an underlying epidemic of chronic disease began to emerge. Chronic diseases are typically not related to pathogens (although exceptions exist). Instead, these diseases develop one day at a time in the body. Examples are heart disease, stroke, diabetes, cancers, and liver and kidney diseases. This shift from the majority of morbidity and mortality being

BOX 3.1 CONTACT TRACING WAS NOT NEW TO THE CDC WHEN COVID-19 ARRIVED

During the height of the U.S. COVID-19 epidemic in 2021, it was fortunate that the CDC could provide clear guidance to state and local health departments regarding contact tracing. Most of the U.S. public probably did not know that this public health practice was not newly developed for COVID-19. Instead, the art of contact tracing had been refined for more than 50 years through joint efforts of the CDC and state health departments. This art involves training already skilled interviewers to cautiously and diligently interact with suspected or confirmed cases (people) in a way that leads to honest responses. This is vital, because whether the disease is a sexually transmitted infection or COVID-19, not all people are eager or willing to cooperate with governmental officials when it comes to their personal habits and health.

The CDC guidance issued to state and local health departments early in 2021 provides only a superficial view of how complex the art of contact tracing can be for the public health workforce. And, of course, the COVID-19 precautions demanded that interactions be conducted remotely when possible. While this may seem straightforward, it becomes murky when considering that millions of Americans are not able to use Web-based conferencing, smartphones, or other technology-based methods of communication. Further, using telephones to contact suspected cases creates issues with confidentiality when leaving voice messages; therefore, repeated calls were needed until the suspected case answered the phone call placed by the public health worker. Fortunately, most state and local health departments had a cadre of skilled staff members with a vast amount of collective experience in applying contact tracing to another highly infectious airborne disease (tuberculosis) as well as a host of sexually transmitted infections such as syphilis, gonorrhea, and human immunodeficiency virus.

The following bullet points are taken directly from the CDC website that provides guidance to state and local health departments (https://www.cdc.gov/coronavirus/2019-ncov/php/contact-tracing/contact-tracing-plan/contact-tracing.html):

- State and local public health officials will decide how to implement these activities and how to advise specific people or groups of people to be tested.

- Contact tracing will be conducted for close contacts (any individual within 6 feet of an infected person for a total of 15 minutes or more) of laboratory-confirmed or probable COVID-19 patients.

- Remote communications for the purposes of case investigation and contact tracing should be prioritized; in-person communication may be considered only after remote options have been exhausted.

- Testing is recommended for all close contacts of confirmed or probable COVID-19 patients.

- Those contacts who test positive (symptomatic or asymptomatic) should be managed as a confirmed COVID-19 case.

Source: Adapted from Centers for Disease Control and Prevention (2021).

caused by pathogens to the vast majority being lifestyle diseases is known as the **epidemiological transition**.

The epidemiological transition proved to be a formidable challenge to the public health infrastructure – one dominated by local (i.e., county-level) health departments funded and regulated by state health departments.

The tasks of vaccinating, treating infections with antibiotics, and conducting contact tracing for sexually transmitted infections were the purview of health departments. However, with the transition, none of these functions applied to chronic diseases. The best tool for the prevention of chronic disease appeared to be health education. The idea was simple: if people could be taught *why* they should engage in a given health-protective behavior (daily exercise, for example), they would then only need some coaching as to *how* to engage in the behavior. Thus, health departments began to take on the role of community health educators, often following a behavior change model such as that depicted in **Figure 3.1**.

The **Health Belief Model** was at one time a staple of public health practice. It is worth providing a summary here to provide a glimpse of how this model informed practice. Reading

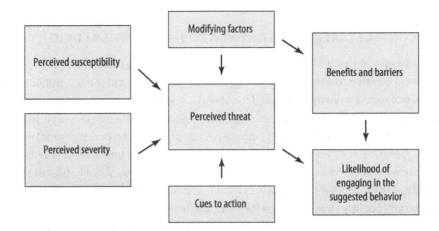

Figure 3.1   A depiction of the Health Belief Model

the model from left to right, you will immediately notice a distinction between *perceived susceptibility* (how likely a given person feels it is that they may develop the disease) and *perceived severity* (a judgment a person makes about how bad the disease may be). These perceptions combine to create the box labeled **perceived threat**. In turn, threat perceptions are altered by modifying factors such as age, gender, race, and income and by cues to action. These cues can be symptoms a person has already experienced, but they may also be social cues to adopt a given health-protective behavior. The Health Belief Model suggests that this construct of perceived threat directly influences the likelihood of engaging in protective behavior. The other direct influence is known as **expected net gain**. This is a balance of costs (defined broadly to include social costs as well non-monetary personal costs) and benefits (also defined broadly to include social rewards and self-satisfaction). Ultimately, the two main drivers of whether any given person engages in a recommended health-protective behavior are the terms shown in bold: perceived threat and expected net gain.

Ultimately, the model is a type of blueprint used to guide health education efforts. For instance, to promote the behavior of daily exercise, education may teach people about the risks of sedentary living and offer advice and tips on how to easily add exercise to a daily routine. The expected net gain may be further enhanced by teaching people about the benefits of exercise for their muscle tone and overall appearance.

As the 21st century dawned, it was becoming apparent that health education was not a panacea comparable to the tools used to control infectious diseases. Nonetheless, the guidance provided by tools such as the Health Belief Model did have some value in terms of promoting health-protective behaviors. Other models followed, most predicated on the two main drivers mentioned previously (perceived threat and expected net gain). As these other models were applied to public health practice, it soon became apparent that social rewards were often the primary driver of whether people engaged in health-protective behaviors. For instance, it was discovered that behaviors such as using bicycle helmets were, in essence, contagious, meaning that once a critical percentage of any given population adopted this habit, others would more readily follow. This concept of **social contagion** has since been applied to a massive number of efforts to promote health-protective behaviors (Crosby, DiClemente, & Salazar, 2013a).

Although health education did have a role to play in public health, an important realization began to permeate practice: that policy, regulation, and understanding how organizations function must be omnipresent in any planned approach to improving public health via behavior change. Known as the **Precede-Proceed Model**, this guide to practice was highly influential in planning community-based efforts to promote public health. (Crosby, DiClemente, &

Salazar, 2013b). Inspired by the dedication of PHAs, thousands of public health workers across the nation dedicated themselves to an ethic of taking on any and all challenges to preserve and protect health. Their mandates were, and are now, very much community-based. They deserve great praise and admiration for their tireless work, often in suboptimal conditions and typically for relatively low wages.

But the role of local health departments in the larger effort to promote and protect public health became smaller as the years progressed and the Internet spawned rapid and massive communications via social media. The most significant development in shifting emphasis away from the role of local health departments was an emerging body of evidence strongly supporting the point that making even small changes to physical, economic, social, or media-based environments could lead to large and population-wide improvements in the adoption of health-protective behaviors. This phenomenon was clearly described (and supported by evidence) in the book *Prescription for a Healthy Nation: A New Approach to Improving Our Lives by Fixing Our Everyday World* (Farley & Cohen, 2006).

> making even small changes to physical, economic, social, or media-based environments could lead to large and population-wide improvements

Embracing Actual Causes of Death

As public health practice expanded to fix our everyday world, an equally valuable trend began. This involved thinking differently about disease prevention by addressing the **root causes** (i.e., the root behaviors) of what could eventually develop into a chronic disease. As suggested by the opening quote for this chapter, public health relies on thinking differently about disease. Rather than thinking about the clinical aspects of any given disease or health-compromising condition, the task is to trace its origins back to a root cause. Indeed, accurate identification of the root causes of morbidity and premature mortality is vital to prevention. For example, kidney disease is increasingly common in the United States, and its clinical manifestations can be extremely difficult to control. But tracing the origin back to a source often finds that the root cause is **hypertension** (i.e., high blood pressure). In turn, a deeper root cause of hypertension is dietary sodium (typically consumed as sodium chloride, i.e., salt). So, this thinking reveals an opportunity that can be altered with the tools of public health! Now, consider that hypertension is also a risk factor for heart disease and stroke. The singular goal of a population-level reduction in sodium consumption warrants the attention and actions of public health practice. Tracing this root cause back up to its manifestations (kidney failure, heart disease, and stroke), it becomes accurate and insightful to conclude that sodium consumption is an important **actual cause of death** (see **Figure 3.2**).

Of course, sodium consumption is only one of many actual causes of death. To accentuate this point, let's take a quick look at sugar consumption. Considering that U.S. dietary guidelines recommend that females consume no more than 5 grams of sugar per day and males no more than 10, it is noteworthy that estimates suggest the average American consumes about 70 grams per day (see **Box 3.2**). This very clear over-consumption of refined sugars is perhaps one of the nation's leading actual causes of death. Evidence is rapidly emerging to suggest that this single health behavior leads to

- More rapid progression (growth) of cancer cells (ending in cancer)
- Atherosclerosis (ending in heart disease and stroke)
- Diabetes (also ending in heart disease and stroke)
- Depressed immune function (potentially ending in fatalities from influenza and pneumonia)

So, now that you understand the concept of actual causes of death, the question for you as a student becomes, what are the most important actual causes of death? Scholars have worked

Clinical manifestations

    Kidney disease
    Cardiovascular disease
    Stroke

Hypertension (high blood pressure)

Excess sodium consumption

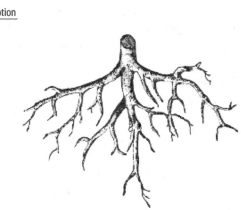

Figure 3.2   The example of sodium consumption as an important actual cause of death

BOX 3.2 THE HUMAN SIDE

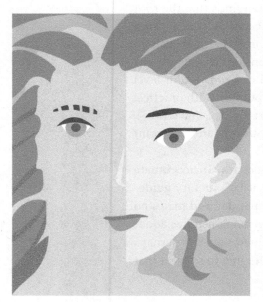

Think about when you were a child. Can you remember times when one or both of your parents rewarded you with food? Our culture has an embedded food-based reward system that features sugar. As a child, or even later in life, were you given foods such as ice cream, cakes, pies, or cookies as a reinforcement for a behavior? For instance, it is an American tradition to entice children to eat all of their regular meal (e.g., vegetables, proteins, salads) by withholding dessert on the condition of finishing the meal first. Desserts in our culture also tend to be a food-based reward for achievements such as weddings, graduations, and even turning one year older (i.e., birthdays). But the same highly refined sugars that make up most desserts are not a natural craving. Instead, this craving is learned. The human side to breaking sugar addiction is unlearning this reward system. Breaking the reward system is important because, as you know, adults (including college students) intuitively create their own reward systems, and many of these feature sugar. Typical systems may work something like this:

- "I made it through a very hard workday; I want a hot fudge sundae after dinner tonight."

- "After running my miles today, plus a few extras, I deserve to eat as many cookies as I want."

- "I have been depressed lately and find that ice cream and cake make me happy again!"

- "To give up drinking alcohol, I have been rewarding myself each day with a treat from the bakery – chocolate is an especially satisfying reward for me."

* "One motivation for me to get out of bed and go to work each day is having a nice doughnut from the coffee shop near my office."

If you can identify with one or more of these statements, you are probably following a pattern you learned as a child. The human side of over-consuming sugar is simply a habit that provides comfort and satisfaction. Both comfort and satisfaction are, of course, positive and productive emotions. These emotions set up what may become an impossible-to-break habit of self-rewards.

BOX 3.3 TEN EXAMPLES OF LEADING ACTUAL CAUSES OF DEATH OF SIGNIFICANCE TO PUBLIC HEALTH PRACTICE

In 2004, scholars from the CDC published a landmark paper in the *Journal of the American Medical Association* (Mokdad, Marks, & Stroup, 2004). Their work yielded a turn-of-the-century view of some of the most significant root causes of death in the United States. Although this venture was focused less on morbidity than death, it is noteworthy that the majority of these actual causes of death are also largely responsible for the morbidity that typically precedes death. Four root causes were found to account for an estimated 50% of all premature deaths. These were (in order of importance):

* Tobacco use
* Poor diet
* Physical inactivity
* Alcohol use

Each of these can be traced upward in **Figure 3.2** as being root causes of a host of chronic diseases, ranging from low-back pain and osteoarthritis to several forms of cancer and disease of the arteries. Other important actual causes of death are not related to one another in this same way; however, they collectively represent a vital opportunity for public health efforts to be channeled in a way that has an optimal impact on the health of Americans. These are:

* Microbial infections
* Toxins
* Motor vehicle crashes
* Firearms
* Risky sexual behaviors
* Substance abuse

In thinking about these six causes of death, you need to understand that ordering them from most to least important is *not* a useful endeavor, due to shifting trends in health risks in the United States. For instance, the opioid epidemic has made substance abuse a more important target for an actual cause of death than any before. Of course, with the onset of COVID-19, microbial infections were a leading actual cause of death in 2020 and 2021. It is also critical to note that many of these actual causes *do not* function through the onset of disease. For instance, homicide and suicide, as well as motor vehicle crashes, kill people instantly.

diligently to provide **empirically derived** (meaning the principles of scientific inquiry were followed) answers to this question. **Box 3.3** lists 10 examples of important actual causes of death and their urgency for the prevention of death and the resulting and related morbidity that may or may not precede death.

Before proceeding with this chapter, it is important for you to understand a bit of terminology. The science behind identifying actual causes of death is complex and can be unwieldy. Therefore, as an introductory textbook, this chapter will exercise a few liberties by simplifying two terms. You have already learned that risk factors are, in essence, one step back from disease acquisition. Further, you learned that these risk factors have root causes that are typically amenable to change. Thus, the term **actual causes** from this point forward in the chapter will be used to denote both risk factors and root causes. The second term that warrants simplification is **death**. Much of the evidence used to compose this chapter comes from an article published in the *Journal of the American Medical Association* (Murray et al., 208). That article is based on analyses that include both the outcome of death (i.e., mortality) and disabilities caused by disease before death occurs (i.e., morbidity). To keep your learning experience in this chapter manageable, the term **morbidity and mortality** will henceforth be used in place of the commonly used (but not correctly used) term **death**.

the term **actual causes** from this point forward in the chapter will be used to denote both risk factors and root causes.

As you continue to study this part of the chapter, keep in mind that public health cannot solve all the health issues that confront our nation. Instead, the intent of public health practice is to determine optimal priorities relative to protecting the quality and quantity of life. In this sense, the word **optimal** represents two key factors. First, the target of any organized set of prevention efforts (i.e., health-protective behaviors and the corresponding risk behaviors for a given disease or health-compromising condition) must be centered on a leading cause of morbidity and premature mortality. Second, the target must be highly amenable to improvement via the tools of public health that you learned about in **Chapter 2**. Both factors must have a high potential to provide significant payoffs for the public health efforts that will be expended. For instance, reducing the population-level consumption of tobacco and nicotine (the subject of **Chapter 4**) strongly addresses both factors. Reducing this risk behavior will lead to substantial declines in diseases ranging from cancers to heart disease and stroke. Further, all the public health tools can be applied to this goal. Thus, tobacco use is a leading actual cause of morbidity and mortality that has become a focal point of public health practice.

the intent of public health practice is to determine optimal priorities relative to protecting the quality and quantity of life.

Before proceeding to the next part of this chapter, consider again that massive amounts of research have informed public health practice in a way that makes the root cause the true target of intervention efforts. When a root cause (such as sodium consumption) leads to multiple clinical manifestations of disease or death, that cause becomes a more valuable target for making even small population-level changes relative to the actual causes of mortality and morbidity.

Shifting the Mean

As you learned in **Chapter 2**, public health focuses on entire populations instead of the medical approach of one-to-one intervention. In this highly ambitious approach to keeping people healthy, a key indicator of success or failure is the mean of a population. From high school, you know the mean as the arithmetic average of scores. Applied to public health, scores can be rewritten as indicators. As always, an example is useful. As you have already been introduced to the term *hypertension*, that example will work well here.

Also known as high blood pressure, hypertension is highly preventable. But let's begin with the basics. When somebody measures your blood pressure, you hear two numbers. The first is always of greater value than the second. This first indicator is known as *systolic blood pressure*. It is simply the pressure exerted by the heart when it forces blood into the circulatory system. The second indicator is known as *diastolic blood pressure*. This is the resting pressure recorded between heartbeats. Although values such as 120/80 (often considered normal) may be important for clinical reasons, from a public health perspective, the rule is simplified: the lower the better, as long as the person remains healthy! The public health goal is to lower blood pressures across entire populations. What matters is the mean of all systolic and diastolic blood pressures in a given population. To understand this approach, it is important to know that not everyone's indicators are measured. Instead, epidemiological studies recruit a representative sample of the population and use the indicators from the sample to make inferences about the mean of the population.

The concept of the mean can be tricky when it comes to shifting it in an entire population. This is because even seemingly small changes signify substantial improvements. For instance, a mean reduction in systolic blood pressure of even a few points across the population of an entire state (such as 129 to 126) can significantly reduce the public's risk of coronary artery diseases, stroke, and so forth. This "thinking big" approach to public health helps everyone instead of simply identifying persons at extreme risk of health issues based on very high systolic blood pressures. So, those at the extremes in terms of how the mean is influenced are a worthy target of population-level intervention, especially because efforts such as sodium reduction will provide much greater improvements in blood pressure for them compared with people who have much lower systolic pressures. But at the same time, people with lower readings who also engage in efforts to reduce their blood pressure benefit as well. Think of population-level intervention as an "everybody wins" approach. In a thoughtful academic book review of *Prescription for a Healthy Nation: A New Approach to Improving Our Lives by Fixing Our Everyday World*, one scholar of public health summarized the core meaning of population-level intervention:

> Preventive education has largely targeted individuals at high risk such as people with high-fat diets who are thus at a higher risk for having a heart attack, while neglecting the much larger population of individuals with moderate- or low-fat diets who have a lower risk for heart attack. By absolute numbers, more lower-risk people will suffer heart attacks than high-risk individuals; therefore, consuming less fat will reduce everyone's risk. (Rull, 2005)

At this point, truly inquisitive students should be thinking, "Why not be more judicious and economical by focusing intervention efforts on those at the extreme end of a curve that plots blood pressures for people in a given population?" This was once the standard public health approach – one that functioned somewhat in harmony with medicine by targeting only people with clinically meaningful warning signs of impending disease. Let's change the example to the risk behavior of smoking. A somewhat tainted legacy of public health is that massive sums of public funds were once expended on tobacco cessation programs for persons considered heavy smokers. Sadly, the vast majority of these programs failed. However, for the sake of argument, let's focus on the idea that some of these programs worked for some people. Letting this play out in your mind, think about what would define success. Would you declare success if one-third of heavy smokers became tobacco-free for one year? This is a very tempting proposition – it sounds like a worthy goal! But the problem is that tobacco companies are committed to increasing sales, and they are highly cognizant that heavy smokers die; thus, they must be sure that replacement customers soon become heavy smokers. As you can imagine, every time a public health success occurs with heavy smokers, they are plenty of new heavy smokers to take their place at the extreme level on the risk curve. Focusing only on those at most risk necessitates a never-ending cycle of intervention, most of which comes too late in life to avert morbidity and mortality.

Upstream Thinking

Now that you understand shifting the mean, let's consider why it is so vital to focus on improving health indicators for everyone rather than just those at extreme risk. The concept of **upstream thinking** comes from a relatively well-known metaphor in public health practice. Imagine a gently flowing river that becomes increasingly turbulent as it approaches a huge waterfall. At first, the gentle flow is deceiving because it is enjoyable for swimming and paddling small boats. In this part of the river, people ignore signs and warnings that the waters will soon become turbulent. Choosing to stay in the water to enjoy themselves, the swimmers and paddlers don't notice the change in the speed of the water's current. But the current gets progressively faster, and the water soon becomes difficult to manage. Now some swimmers want to return to shore, and many reach shore safely. Others desperately need assistance – but assistance may not be found. Ultimately, the gentle stream becomes a roaring river, the waterfall appears, and nothing can be done to save these people from going over the craggy rocks covered in white raging water. Townspeople below the waterfall set up first-aid stations and hire and train specialized rescue squads to save from drowning those who survive the fall. Rescue squad members become highly respected members of the town and are revered for their heroism. Meanwhile, as time goes by and the problem of people going over the falls does not improve, a few citizens erect fences in places that were popular for entering the gently flowing upstream waters. As more fences are built, fewer people wind up going over the falls and dying or needing to be rescue. The people building fences are not revered or even thanked, but their work turns out to be the real solution.

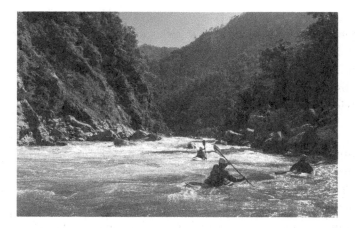

Photo 3.5   Saving people from raging waters will never be as easy as preventing them from entering the seemingly calmer waters upstream. Source: robertharding/Adobe stock.

To accentuate this metaphor, think about a college student who smokes on occasion (usually at parties) but is not yet addicted. This is the gently flowing water upstream, and it is time for this person to quit entirely (i.e., come to shore). As the same college student goes through the next 10 years of life, the waters are noticeably less gentle, and quitting can still be a life-saving effort. As another 10 years or more go by, the person is a steady customer of the tobacco companies and considered a heavy smoker (i.e., the waters are turbulent). Intervention is still possible, but these efforts are more intensive and costly. One day, this once-recreational smoker has an episode of cardiac arrest and survives, but at great expense to the medical establishment (i.e., the rescue squad). So, returning to the concept of population-level intervention, the idea of upstream thinking and building fences is very much the essence of public health practice. The fences comprise regulations against smoking that discourage forming the habit in the first place (i.e., getting into the gentle waters) and laws that preclude younger people from easy access to cigarettes. Fences further downstream (but not near the falls) comprise workplace and health department programs that offer free cessation services to smokers who want to quit the habit. And downstream, the training of physicians, the construction of hospitals, and the maintenance of rescue squads commands massive public funding and great recognition.

the idea of upstream thinking and building fences is very much the essence of public health practice.

The Scope of Public Health Practice

Thus far in this textbook, you have learned that public health practice is designed to avert morbidity and mortality. Additionally, you have learned about health-compromising conditions that are an equally important target of public health efforts. Moreover, you now understand the concepts of actual causes of death and upstream thinking. With all this firmly in mind, it should be apparent to you that the scope of public health practice is largely defined by the greatest needs for improvement that also offer high chances of being amenable to primary prevention via the definition of public health practice you learned about in **Chapter 2** (i.e., creating conditions that control and even reverse the tide and trajectory of any one nation's current epidemics).

At this point in your learning experience, it becomes valuable to elucidate the exceptions to these general guidelines of what constitutes public health practice. Two extremely important exceptions are substance abuse and unintended pregnancy, neither of which fits the disease mold.

Why Substance Abuse Prevention?

As you will learn in **Chapter 7**, America's opioid crisis quickly became a larger crisis of stimulant use and caused people to lose their homes, significant aspects of their mental capacities, their freedom, and often their lives. Broadly speaking, the negative outcomes characterizing the lives of those who chronically abuse substances are more about a loss of quality of life than about medically diagnosed morbidity or death (although death from an overdose of opioids is all too common). Given this, many would argue that treating substance abuse is a medical endeavor and prevention should simply be a matter of increased law enforcement, followed by incarceration. But these approaches have seldom worked.

the negative outcomes characterizing the lives of those who chronically abuse substances are more about a loss of quality of life than about medically diagnosed morbidity

Once again, remember that public health is not a profession per se; it is a set of public actions. Because substance abuse is frequently a **co-occurring problem** (meaning it coincides with behaviors such as gun violence), and because it leads to conditions that spawn health-risk behaviors (such as poverty, homelessness, and social marginalization), public health is improved by reducing the number of people entering into chronic addiction. The public health approach to substance abuse is very much characterized by upstream thinking and upstream actions.

Why Unintended Pregnancy?

As you will learn in **Chapter 13**, the earth's resources are finite, and overpopulation of humans on this planet threatens to exacerbate the depletion of these resources. Moreover, you will learn that for millions of women (and girls), unintended pregnancy limits and sets boundaries on the control they have over their immediate environments. This translates to conditions such as not being able to afford healthy foods, engage in daily exercise that is also recreational and enjoyable, or have autonomy in marriage or long-term relationships. Similar to substance abuse – but in very different specific terms – unintended pregnancy spawns conditions that may work against having ample support and control to engage in health-protective behaviors.

A related concern is teen pregnancy. Teens tend to be more likely than their adult counterparts to report unintentional conception. Further, they tend to be less prepared to engage in a full range of prenatal care and precautions (such as quitting smoking), becoming more likely than adults to give birth prematurely and give birth to a low-birth-weight (LBW) baby. Babies born prematurely and LBW babies require intensive care in neonatal units of hospitals, often at extremely high costs. This form of morbidity is certainly a concern to public health, especially given its significant potential for primary prevention.

This very brief introduction to the reasons why pregnancy prevention is a core aspect of public health practice deserves continued emphasis on the concept of upstream thinking. The ease of obtaining low-cost, highly reliable contraception is an excellent example of upstream actions that have tremendous impacts on reducing downstream issues. Further, as these downstream issues are averted, medical resources are preserved for other issues that are not nearly as amenable to primary prevention (e.g., several common forms of cancer, degenerative arthritis, traumatic brain injury). Upon reflection, you should now understand that one great advantage of public health is that it greatly reduces the burden on the medical service sector of society.

> The ease of obtaining low-cost, highly reliable contraception is an excellent example of upstream actions that have tremendous impacts on reducing downstream issues.

Public Health Practice Is Unique in Each Nation

As this chapter comes to a close, you should have a clear vision of the central nature of policy, regulation, and general structural changes to our everyday world that predominate today's approach to improving the health of the public. Given this understanding, you can also understand the interrelated nature of public health practice and local and state governments as well as the federal government (as was particularly true in the early years of the COVID-19 pandemic). This does not imply that public health must always work in harmony with governmental bodies. Instead, public health is best considered opportunistic, meaning its actions occur at all possible levels. These levels range from simple health education to community-based campaigns regarding a specific health issue to changes in public policy and related laws. None of these actions can occur without a thorough understanding of culture, how people will react to health promotion efforts, or how state and local governments can be efficiently persuaded to protect the public's health. Thus, it is not possible for this textbook to be all-inclusive when it comes to public health taken from a global perspective. The disparities and challenges that constantly define and redefine public health practice in the United States are unique, just as they are for each nation. In that regard, public health — once again — is a "we the people" endeavor.

Although each nation has its own unique needs and approaches to its national public health issues of greatest priority, a strong need exists to think globally when it comes to two key aspects of public health: climate change (see **Chapters 12** and **13**) and infectious diseases (especially COVID-19). The former is true because drawing down carbon must be a shared responsibility of all humans. The latter is true because microorganisms can quickly spread from one nation to another, as you discovered in **Chapter 1**. Therefore, while the majority of the remaining chapters in this textbook focus on the United States, global health concerns will also be presented when applicable.

Review and Key Terms

This chapter has provided a mix of history and thinking differently about public health practice. You learned that **Sir Edwin Chadwick** was a 19th century revolutionary of sorts, given his radical ideas about improving public health through structural-level changes. Chances are, you had never wondered or understood why milk is **pasteurized**; now you know that this was emblematic of a public health intervention designed for the primary prevention of disease. The chapter also taught you an important term: **pathogen**. For the remainder of this textbook, keep in mind that any microorganism capable of causing disease in humans is called a **pathogen**. For instance, a major concern when a new species of bacteria is discovered is whether it is pathogenic!

As the brief chronology continued, you learned about the use of **public health advisors** by the CDC and how they greatly influenced the art of **contact tracing**, a process that begins with an **index case**. The chapter also introduced you to the concept of the **epidemiological transition**, meaning a massive change from a predominance of death by infectious disease to a predominance by chronic disease.

As the burden of disease shifted to chronic illness, public health began to emphasize health education, using the concepts of **perceived threat** and **expected net gain** from the **Health Belief Model**. This highly cognitive approach to altering risk behavior and promoting health-protective behavior was later augmented by the idea of making health-protective behaviors **socially contagious**. However, public health practice evolved into a much more ambitious set of actions, focusing on **root causes** of **morbidity and mortality**. Known more formally as **actual causes of death**, the value of identifying these **empirically derived** behaviors lies in guiding and prioritizing the scope of public health practice. Sodium consumption, for instance, is an actual cause of death when considering the link between excess sodium and **hypertension** (hypertension is sometimes known as "the silent killer").

Finally, you learned about the public health concerns of substance abuse and unintended pregnancy. Specifically, you learned that substance abuse is often a problem that co-occurs with a host of health-risk behaviors and that unintended pregnancy greatly contributes to the overpopulation crisis of the planet. The close of this chapter taught you that a balance exists between each nation having a unique approach to its public health priorities and the need to have nations work together relative to the control of climate change and infectious diseases.

For Practice and Class Discussion

Practice Questions

1. The plague would have been much worse had it not been for the public health efforts of Chadwick. Which one of the following was *not* included in these efforts?
   a. Cleaning public streets
   b. Installing fire hydrants
   c. Removing garbage on a regular basis
   d. Removing human waste from public spaces

2. Which one of these early public health actions was responsible for the control of smallpox?
   a. Vaccination of entire populations
   b. Pasteurization of milk
   c. Improved public sanitation services
   d. Improved health education

3. All of the following terms except one apply to VD control in the middle of the 20th century. Which term does *not* relate to this set of public health actions?
   a. Antibiotics
   b. Public health advisors
   c. Vaccination
   d. Contact tracing

4. As pathogenic diseases subsided and chronic disease became the leading causes of morbidity and mortality, health education became a job of local and state health departments.
   a. True
   b. False

5. The Health Belief Model relies on two main concepts. These are:
   a. Perceived susceptibility and perceived severity
   b. Expected net gain and perceived threat
   c. Perceived threat and modifying factors
   d. Social contagion and cues to action

6. Kidney failure is increasingly common in the United States. Of the options listed, which would be the most significant in terms of a root cause?
   a. Hypertension
   b. Inadequate health care
   c. Poverty
   d. Sodium consumption

7. Public health practice cannot do everything. Instead, it must prioritize its efforts. This occurs by:
   a. Selecting actual causes of morbidity and mortality that can be changed through population-level intervention
   b. Following the advice and wisdom of congressional mandates
   c. Targeting only the leading forms of death
   d. Selecting health behaviors that can be altered by policy changes

8. Shifting the mean implies all of the following *except*:
   a. Creating a population-level impact
   b. Upstream thinking
   c. Focusing on those most at risk
   d. Targeting actual causes of morbidity and mortality

9. Which action is the *least* upstream in terms of public health practice?
   a. Taxing tobacco
   b. Providing free childbirth services to teens
   c. Regulating the food industry's use of sugar and sodium
   d. Using massive social media campaigns to promote daily walking for all people

10. All of what forms public health practice is global in terms of the actions needed to create conditions that avert morbidity and mortality.
    a. True
    b. False

For Discussion (in class or in small groups, or online)

11. In Greek mythology, two gods are highly relevant to this chapter. One is a female figure: Hygieia. The other is a make figure: Asclepius. Your task is to go online and read about both of these gods and then describe how they are relevant, using keywords from this chapter.

12. As you read this chapter, you likely felt it was a bit harsh toward the medical profession in terms of the rescue squad. But the chapter did not include the financial costs of this downstream care. Using the Internet, select one downstream procedure from the following list. Then, determine the most recent average cost of that procedure. In one paragraph, describe the procedure and its costs, and include your source for the information you obtained. Share this (via web-posting or other electronic methods) with other students taking this course.

- Coronary bypass surgery

- Angioplasty

- Colectomy

- Mastectomy

- Yearly cost of dialysis

13. The political resistance to Chadwick was characterized by the ethic of "everybody receives what they work for," implying that the poor were to blame for the unhealthy conditions that defined their existence. Is this – even to a small degree – a sentiment you agree with? Or do you disagree with this idea? Create a short list of bullet-point statements that illustrate your thoughts. Using your list, be prepared to debate with others taking this course.

References

Crosby, R. A., DiClemente, R. J., & Salazar, L. F. (2013a). Diffusion of innovation theory. In R. J. DiClemente, R. A. Crosby, & L. F. Salazar (Eds), *Understanding and changing health behavior: A theory-based multidisciplinary approach*. Jones & Bartlett Learning.

Crosby, R. A., DiClemente, R. J., & Salazar, L. F. (2013b). The PRECEDE-PROCEED planning model. In R. J. DiClemente, R. A. Crosby, & L. F. Salazar (Eds), *Understanding and changing health behavior: A theory-based multidisciplinary approach*. Jones & Bartlett Learning.

Farley, T., & Cohen, D. (2006). *Prescription for a healthy nation: A new approach to improving our lives by fixing our everyday world*. Beacon Press.

Meyerson, B., Martich, F. M., & Naehr, G. P. (2008). *Ready to go: The history and contributions of the U.S. Public Health Advisors*. American Social Health Association.

Mokdad, A. H., Marks, J. S., & Stroup, D. F. (2004). Actual causes of death in the United States, 2000. *Journal of the American Medical Association, 291*(10), 1238–1245.

Murray, C., and the U.S. Burden of Disease Collaborators. (2018). The state of U.S. health, 1990–2016. Burden of diseases, injuries, and risk factors among U.S. states. *Journal of the American Medical Association, 1319*(14), 1444–1472.

Rull, R. (2005). Book review: Prescription for a Healthy Nation: A New Approach to Improving Our Lives by Fixing Our Everyday World. *Environmental Health Perspectives, 113*(9), A632.

CHAPTER 4

HOW DOES PUBLIC HEALTH WORK? THE EXAMPLE OF TOBACCO CONTROL

Today's teenager is tomorrow's regular customer, and the overwhelming majority first begin to smoke while still in their teens . . . The smoking patterns of teenagers are particularly important to Phillip Morris.

—*Philip Morris, Special Report, "Young Smokers: Prevalence, Trends, Implications, and Related Demographic Trends," March 31, 1981, https://the84.org/get-the-facts/tobacco-executive-quotes/*

Overview

Phillip Morris is one of four tobacco companies that were taken to court by the attorney generals of 46 U.S. states in what ultimately became known as the *Master Settlement Agreement*. The success of this court action in 1998 brought somewhat of an end to the previously unrestricted times when tobacco companies could freely spend huge sums of money enticing teenagers to smoke, thereby creating a never-ending supply of lifetime customers for their product. This battle between an industry and state governments exemplifies the upper-level view of public health when it comes to **cause and control**. The quote from Phillip Morris documents also indicates why the vast majority of the public health response to the tobacco epidemic is based on efforts to prevent teenagers from ever taking the bait and starting to smoke (or use tobacco in other forms such as dip, snuff, chew, etc.). Indeed, a major emphasis of a medical sub-discipline known as Adolescent Health is placed on preventing addiction to nicotine.

The purpose of this chapter is to describe tobacco control as an example of how public health practice and policy can (and should) function to create widespread improvements in the health of the public. This chapter will introduce you to the concepts that have been applied to make dramatic reductions in the consumption of tobacco among Americans. To punctuate how important these reductions are, the chapter provides several tutorials on the physiological effects of tobacco – primarily nicotine – on the human body. More importantly, the chapter will demonstrate the power of behavioral science to shed light on how public health practice can best be applied to help understand and control tobacco use. The chapter will also describe how within 20 years after the Master Settlement Agreement, the tobacco industry found a new way to revive its old profit margins: vaping. The chapter concludes by laying out a framework – one learned from the lessons of

LEARNING OBJECTIVES

- Understand the effects of tobacco (particularly nicotine) on the human body and how these effects culminate in chronic disease.

- Explain how the four tenets of the *California Tobacco Control Program* and how it became highly successful.

- Summarize the principles of the Master Settlement Agreement, especially as applied to the control of environmental tobacco smoke.

- Apply social cognitive theory as both a cause and a control measure relative to smoking initiation among U.S. teenagers.

- Articulate the differences between smoking tobacco and vaping, and describe the known effects of vaping on disease development.

- Understand a general framework (based on the California Tobacco Control Program) that can be applied to the control of daily behaviors that place people at risk of premature morbidity and mortality.

Understanding the Science and Practice of Public Health, First Edition. Richard Crosby.
© 2023 John Wiley & Sons, Inc. Published 2023 by John Wiley & Sons, Inc.

tobacco control – that can be applied to other seemingly intractable public health issues arising from a competition between corporate America and people's daily health behaviors.

The Effects of Tobacco Use on the Human Body

Inevitably, people believe that the major health risk from smoking is developing lung cancer. Most people may fail to appreciate that the cardiovascular system suffers immediate and long-term damage with each cigarette smoked. So, let's begin there!

First, it is vital for you to understand that tobacco contains thousands of harmful compounds. Collectively, these compounds – other than the actual drug found in tobacco (i.e., nicotine) – are referred to as **tars**. It is not the tars that contribute to damage and a decline in cardiovascular health. Instead, nicotine is the culprit. For instance, nicotine is a **vasoconstrictor**. This term is easy to understand. *Vaso* is a root for blood vessels, and you are most likely aware that *constriction* refers to the narrowing of a space. When applied to the cardiovascular system, vasoconstriction means arteries (which carry oxygenated blood) and veins (which carry blood with the waste product of carbon dioxide to the lungs for exhaling) constrict. This constriction forces the blood to move faster, given that it must reach its same target cells using a much narrower roadway. The result – much like placing your thumb over the end of a garden hose to make a spray of water – is an increase in pressure. This increase in blood pressure may reach levels classified as hypertension. Even in the absence of hypertension, fleeting increases in blood pressure are harmful to the cardiovascular system.

Now, let's consider what nicotine does to the walls of your arteries. Again, these are effects that occur immediately rather than developing over long periods. Blood platelets normally move easily through the arteries, slipping through even smaller arteries rapidly. This rapid movement is vital to health. Nicotine has a negative effect on platelets. That effect is best described as making the platelets likely to adhere to artery walls. As they accumulate – particularly on artery walls scarred by elevated blood pressure – plaque forms. Much like the plaque that a dentist may remove from the enamel of your teeth, this arterial plaque is resistant to change; it will not simply disappear. As arterial plaque accumulates, portions of any given artery become progressively narrower (again leading to elevated blood pressure). The threat is that if the area open for blood flow becomes so small that a blood clot lodges there (i.e., get stuck), any cells reliant on this blood flow will be cut off from oxygen and begin to die. When the affected artery feeds the most important muscle in the body (the heart), this is known as a **coronary occlusion**. When this occlusion reaches a crisis level, it results in the death of muscle tissue in the heart – a **myocardial infarction**.

Next, it is important to understand that nicotine stimulates the **sympathetic branch** of the nervous system. The nervous system is divided into the sympathetic and parasympathetic branches, and the sympathetic branch creates physical conditions responsive to stress. For instance, dilated pupils of the eyes, increased adrenaline, increased blood sugar levels, and increased heart rate are all natural responses to stimulating this branch of the nervous system (stimulating the parasympathetic branch has the opposite effects). Thus, one of the greatest illusions held by smokers is that it helps them relax. While this may be true at a psychological level, it is certainly not the case physiologically. When nicotine is inhaled, thus stimulating the sympathetic nervous system, the elevated functions – especially heart rate and blood sugar levels – take a toll on the body. An elevated heart rate, for example, leads to elevated blood pressure. Elevated blood sugar levels create risks related to obesity, which further compounds issues with cardiovascular health. The problem is that typically, as nicotine levels drop and the body's physiology returns to normal levels, the smoker has a craving for more nicotine and thus repeats the process. For some smokers, this repetition occurs during most waking hours.

tobacco contains thousands of harmful compounds

This increase in blood pressure may reach levels classified as hypertension

As arterial plaque accumulates, portions of any given artery become progressively narrower

Table 4.1   Cancers having tobacco tar as a cause or a contributing factor.

Tars as a cause	Tars as a contributing factor
Lung	Cervix
Stomach	Pancreas
Breast	Bladder
Head and neck	Lymph nodes
Kidneys	Liver

The result becomes a chronic state of high alert in the body, which creates conditions leading to both myocardial infarctions and occlusions in the main arteries supplying blood to the brain (thus causing **strokes**).

Given your new appreciation of how nicotine creates immediate and long-term negative health effects on the cardiovascular system, let's go back to tars and consider cancer. *Cancer* is a generic term used to describe the uncontrolled growth and spreading of abnormal cells. As a rule, almost every known type of cancer has the tars of tobacco as one of its causes. **Table 4.1** provides you with a partial listing of cancers caused, in part, by tobacco tars.

As shown in **Table 4.1**, it is difficult to think of a type of cancer that is not linked in some way with tobacco use. This is because tars constitute compounds that can lead to cellular mutations that subsequently become dominant in cellular reproduction. They are known generically as either **carcinogens** (left column in **Table 4.1**) or **co-carcinogens** (right column in **Table 4.1**). This is why even second-hand smoke (i.e., passive smoking) can lead to cancers, particularly of the lungs. Here, however, the effects of smoking are long-term in contrast to the immediate effects described relative to cardiovascular disease. This is problematic from a public health perspective because far too many young people begin smoking as teenagers and have a complete absence of even precancerous signs or symptoms for one to two decades. This absence of apparent negative effects reinforces personal beliefs along the lines of "It won't hurt me." Armed with what they consider evidence that they are immune to the effects of smoking, people continue the habit – fed by a powerful physical addiction – unabated. It is noteworthy that while tars cause cancers, nicotine drives the addiction. As described by the U.S. Surgeon General in 1988, nicotine rivals both cocaine and heroin in its addictive powers (Estill, 1988).

> As a rule, almost every known type of cancer has the tars of tobacco as one of its causes

> while tars cause cancers, nicotine drives the addiction

Understanding the California Tobacco Control Program

Figure 4.1 shows the main components of the California Tobacco Control Program. It further displays, in each corner, the applicable levels of intervention: that is, whether the intervention implications occur at the intrapersonal level, the interpersonal level, the community level, the institutional level, or the policy level. Based on the outstanding record of success for this program, and its adoption for use in other U.S. states, the model shown in this figure warrants significant attention. Let's begin with the upper-left corner and proceed clockwise.

Limiting Access

A primary task of any control program designed to eliminate a health-risk behavior is to limit **access** to any product associated with the risk behavior. This is where governments (local, state, and federal) must play a strong and decisive role. For instance, having laws against minors purchasing tobacco is one thing, but enforcing these laws is the key to limiting access by minors. So, think of this as a three-pronged approach, with the first being relatively simple in words but difficult in practice: passing effective legislation that limits access.

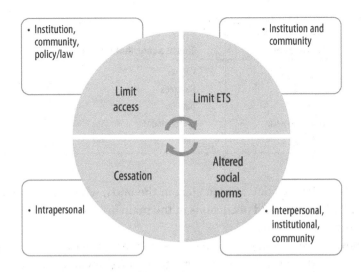

Figure 4.1   Components of the California Tobacco Control Program

Next is the ongoing task of education. The task is to inform both merchants and law enforcement officials about state and local legislation governing tobacco sales to minors. The final task is to design and fund ongoing actions to enforce these laws. As always, an example is helpful.

Consider a small-town gas station that is licensed to sell cigarettes. The owner is Mr. Smith, a businessman who is always eager to make a profit when anyone comes into the store. In his state, the laws pertaining to minors and tobacco sales are very clear. His state follows the federal *Tobacco Free Youth Act*. This act restricts the sales of tobacco and vaping products to anyone under the age of 21 and, in parallel, makes it illegal for anyone under the age of 21 to purchase these products. Mr. Smith engages in the education of the public about this law and posts signs in prominent locations so that teenagers are well aware of the law. But many of the check-out clerks working for Mr. Smith don't take the time to ask suspected teens for ID cards, or they simply don't agree with the law and opt not to enforce it. So, the process meant to cut off the endless supply of new lifetime customers to the tobacco industry is subverted by the whims or rushed nature of people working in low-paying jobs. The public health solution to this problem is elusive because it would have to involve partnerships with local law enforcement agencies or local health departments that would have the legal ability to suspend store licensures. Because of the need to involve local enforcement, a broad-sweeping public health response is problematic.

Although preventing easy access by minors may be a local issue, from a larger

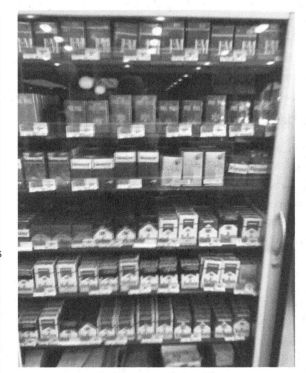

The public health solution to this problem is elusive because it would have to involve partnerships with local law enforcement agencies

Photo 4.1   Stores that sell cigarettes and other tobacco products are subject to multiple regulations, but enforcement is a problem.

perspective – influencing a much broader population – a vital policy-level intervention to limit access involves raising taxes on all tobacco products. In the California program, this added state revenue was used to fund nearly every aspect of the efforts shown in **Figure 4.1**; thus, the program was self-funded. The basic concept underlying the premise of raising taxes to limit access (one widely applied in behavioral economics) is known as **price elasticity**: as price goes up, consumer demand goes down. As a rule of thumb, a 10% increase in tobacco tax will produce a 3 to 5% decrease in sales. Thus, in progressive tobacco cities such as New York City, tax codes have been shifted to charge as much as $1.50 in added tax for each pack of cigarettes sold. This form of public health taxation has worked well in that city and many others.

Access can also be limited based on the concept of **product placement**. When a product (in this case, tobacco) is easy to find and convenient to purchase, people will naturally be more likely to buy it. Using the reverse of this concept, limiting the types of places where tobacco products can be purchased is another key part of interventions – this involves all three levels shown in the upper-left corner of **Figure 4.1**.

Controlling Environmental Tobacco Smoke

Moving in a clockwise direction around **Figure 4.1**, let's consider the success of controlling **environmental tobacco smoke** (ETS). A great advantage of the approach is that it has two very positive effects: (a) it protects non-smokers against the harmful effects of **passive smoking** (see **Box 4.1**), and (b) it creates barriers to smoking; thus, smokers become more prone to quit or at least attempt to quit by entering tobacco cessation programs. Largely under local control, creating regulations in workplaces (i.e., the institutional level) and communities has been the public health practice used in this regard. Of course, a more comprehensive approach, such as passing ETS laws in an entire state (e.g., California), has effects that are more far-reaching and may also prompt people to enter into cessation. Features of such a comprehensive approach include:

- Providing outdoor (not indoor) designated areas for smoking that are at least 50 feet from a building entrance

- Providing free tobacco cessation services to employees who smoke

- Posting rules and regulations in prominent places regarding ETS

- Prohibiting (without exception) all smoking in bars, restaurants, hotels, and all forms of public transportation (buses, taxis, trains, and airplanes)

- Regulating tobacco use in outdoor public spaces/places (e.g., streets, parks, bus stops, and parking lots)

These measures work! For instance, despite initial objections from restaurant and bar owners about ETS laws negatively impacting business, these concerns have not materialized into actual loss of business because the laws are universally applied. Statewide surveys have typically found a significant decline in restaurant/bar exposure to ETS immediately following the implementation of statewide ETS regulations.

However, the most important intervention point for implementing ETS policies involves the

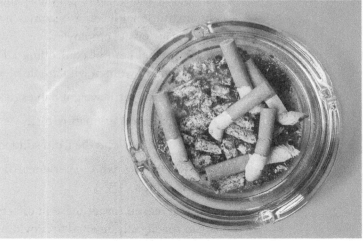

Photo 4.2 The smoke emanating from ashtrays contains a higher level of carcinogens than the smoke being exhaled by a smoker.
Source: BillionPhotos.com/Adobe stock.

BOX 4.1 WHAT IS PASSIVE SMOKING?

Although seemingly straightforward, the concepts and health consequences associated with passive smoking are complex. Let's consider a bonfire burning in your backyard on a cool fall evening. At first the fire is weak, burning but not blazing. At this early stage, the relatively cooler temperatures of the fire fail to fully incinerate all of the wood particles, so the unburned matter becomes a thick cloud of smoke constantly rising from the fire. As the fire matures and becomes hotter, it reaches temperatures exceeding 700 degrees Fahrenheit. These higher temperatures are much more efficient at burning the wood, which means far fewer unburned particles are spewed out as smoke.

Bringing this back to tobacco, consider a basic principle of fire: it needs oxygen. When a person inhales a cigarette, they bring oxygen into its tip, stoking the fire. If you watch a smoker taking puffs at night in darkness, the act of inhaling makes the cigarette tip glow bright red with heat. Once the inhaling ends, the red color fades, meaning a much lower temperature at the tip, translating into more unburned tobacco particles that rise (recall that all heat rises) as smoke.

With this metaphor in mind, let's divide passive smoking into two categories. The most dangerous is **sidestream smoke**. The smoke is released from the tip when the smoker is not inhaling (i.e., when the tip is burning cooler). Less dangerous, but still a culprit in diseases in non-smokers, is **mainstream smoke**. This is the smoke exhaled from the smoker's lungs when they inhale fresh oxygen to stoke the fire at the tip of their cigarette. As you know from the metaphor, this smoke has fewer unburned particles (known as **particulate matter**). Both sidestream and mainstream smoke have been heavily implicated in disease development for non-smokers in relatively close proximity to people who smoke. These diseases are most likely to affect the cardiovascular system (including heart attacks and stroke); however, emerging evidence suggests that a range of other diseases and conditions are probably caused by passive smoke, including most cancers that smokers disproportionally experience, lung infections, upper respiratory infections, asthma, and a host of issues relative to fetal development and infant health in the first few years of life.

Now that you have a better understanding of passive smoking, let's complicate things by noting that it is also known as **secondhand smoke**. There is also **thirdhand** smoke: residual smoke, mostly from sidestream smoke that permeates porous surfaces such as clothing, draperies, upholstered furniture, rugs, carpets, and objects like stuffed animals that children play with and hold close to their faces. Given its distinct tobacco scent, thirdhand smoke is mostly a nuisance to non-smoking adults. This is one reason many hotel rooms are now off-limits for smoking (with large fines for violators). However, the real threat from thirdhand smoke involves children and asthma. Accumulating evidence implicates chronic exposure to thirdhand smoke – as might occur in some home-based daycare centers – as a substantial risk factor for the development of childhood asthma, as well making existing cases of childhood asthma even worse.

one public place where people spend the vast majority of their time: the workplace. Thus, at the institutional level, it becomes important for large employers to install and enforce ETS policies for onsite employees.

A special case of controlling ETS applies to pregnancy. Overwhelming evidence shows that pregnant women who inhale second-hand smoke are much more likely to:

- Have low-birth-weight babies (less than 5 pounds at birth)

- Experience a premature birth

- Have babies who die from sudden infant death syndrome (**SIDS**)

- Have babies who experience (into childhood) issues such as **asthma**, pneumonia, and bronchitis

The reason for all these ill effects on fetal development involves the **placenta**. This is an organ specifically devoted to providing nutrients and oxygen to the fetus (as well as taking away waste products), right up until birth. It was once thought that the placenta could screen out all toxins from the mother's blood supply. The dominant medical thinking even in the mid-1900s was that nicotine and tars from tobacco would not cross the placenta, and thus the fetus would be protected against any possible effects of maternal smoking. Of course, none of this thinking was true. Video imaging shows that the effects of nicotine reaching the fetus may even exceed the damaging effects experienced by the mother who is directly inhaling the smoke and nicotine. This is because the fetus is tiny, so the relative concentration of nicotine in the fetal cardiovascular system is very high. The take-home lesson here is that most drugs – including nicotine – have a distinctly negative impact on the developing fetus. The negative effects of compounds in tars may be equally damaging. Carbon monoxide, for instance, is toxic to the fetus and is present in tobacco smoke.

Recalling what you have learned in previous chapters of this book, it is notable that public health practice often stems from community-based efforts. Controlling ETS is a great example because local regulations, policies, and laws carry the day when it comes to prohibiting smoking in public spaces. Restaurants/bars are a prime example because the municipality where the restaurant resides issues and controls the licensure of the establishment and thus can suspend or remove a license as a method of enforcing local health codes. Across the United States, ETS regulations and laws have largely come about based on the work of county, city, and state governments. Because local control is vulnerable to public pressures, ultimately, public health policy and laws will not achieve 100% smoke-free indoor and outdoor environments. Instead, reaching the 100% goal will be a function of altering social norms to the point that non-smokers can freely correct smokers when they infringe on the right to breathe clean air. Again, this is one reason public health is a public responsibility.

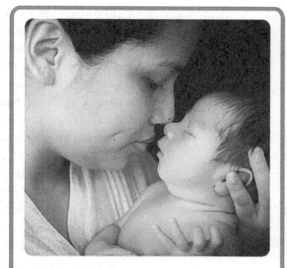

BABIES WHOSE MOTHERS SMOKED
DURING PREGNANCY OR WHO ARE EXPOSED
TO SECONDHAND SMOKE AFTER BIRTH
ARE MORE LIKELY TO DIE OF
SUDDEN INFANT DEATH SYNDROME (SIDS)
THAN ARE BABIES WHO ARE NOT EXPOSED.

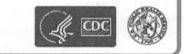

Photo 4.3   The CDC has created large-scale campaigns to keep pregnant women from smoking.
Source: U.S Department of Health & Human Services / Public_Domain.

Altering Social Norms

Again moving clockwise around **Figure 4.1**, this third component of the program is likely the most important to its success, and it is certainly the most daunting challenge. Social norms are best thought of as local cultures. Age groups, neighborhoods, and entire communities (both virtual and in person) have subtle rules and unwritten regulations pertaining to what people should believe, how they should act, and even what health behaviors they embrace or eschew. To put this in terms of tobacco use, think of it as the public health version of advertising/marketing. The tobacco industry spends about $25 million *each day* attempting to alter social norms to make tobacco use appear sexy, rugged, satisfying, and so on. The tobacco industry specifically targets youth 12 to 17 years of age. As an example of how blatantly the tobacco industry tries to manufacture social norms supporting tobacco use, consider one of its prize cartoon characters from the 1990s: Joe Camel. You can quickly google *Joe Camel* to see that the tobacco industry cleverly designed a camel's face in the approximate shape of a very large penis and scrotum, thus sending a not-so-subtle hidden message to young males that linked the product (Camel cigarettes) with masculinity. The vast majority of young teenage boys felt pressured to establish and enhance their masculinity, and thus Joe Camel was highly effective – so effective that the logo was banned as part of the Master Settlement Agreement, described later in this chapter.

The challenge to public health practice – and more specifically to the California Tobacco Control Program during its developmental period – is to counter the power of advertising from the tobacco industry on a much smaller budget. Again, keep in mind that the goal is altering social norms. In this regard, a signature achievement of the California Tobacco Control Program is the Truth Campaign. This was a dramatic and exciting departure from previous anti-smoking campaigns that largely focused on facts and details of how tobacco harms the body. The reasoning behind these health-based campaigns was that if people – specifically, teenagers – knew it was bad for them, they would never begin to smoke or would quit smoking. Of course, this type of approach did not work, probably because very few teens experienced any noticeable health issues from their early-in-life tobacco use. One school-based tobacco information program failed so miserably (Peterson, Kealy, Mann, et al., 2000) that the tobacco companies subsequently endorsed it! (See **Photo 4.4**.) This endorsement from the tobacco industry was a clever public relations move because it expressed a "we care" sentiment to the public, relative to America's teenagers.

Distinct from health-based or information-based programs, the Truth Campaign is designed based on the premise that people (especially teens) do not tolerate the deliberate attempts of big business to deceive the public. Further, the campaign is premised on the point that the tobacco industry profiles potential customers by race, ethnicity, and gender, exploiting and thus magnifying unwarranted stereotypes. Teens view these stereotypes as yet another form of injustice on the part of what they are likely to view as dirty big business. The campaign also reveals how the tobacco industry has attempted to fabricate evidence counter to the mountains of epidemiological evidence demonstrating the harmful effects of nicotine and tars on the human body. Beyond this fabrication, the industry has also been caught lying to Congress, covering up harmful production practices, and threatening the lives of former employees who turn against the tobacco companies. So, the Truth Campaign is about creating *social outrage* among young people toward the tobacco industry – and it worked in California! This success was subsequently replicated in other states, such as Florida.

> the campaign is premised on the point that the tobacco industry profiles potential customers by race, ethnicity, and gender, exploiting and thus magnifying unwarranted stereotypes

Altering social norms through programs such as the Truth Campaign is indeed a matter of changing culture. Making something un-cool or just plain ugly is a good way to change part of a culture. In terms of being un-cool, think about the social norms in U.S. cities where the number of people who smoke tobacco is extremely low; in these cities, there is an ethic that people who smoke are not as successful, confident, or well-adjusted socially. This same ethic is unlikely to exist in villages, towns, or cities where smoking is common. In either location, though, smoking is likely to serve an important social function: in places where smoking is not popular or accepted, lighting up with a friend or two serves as a bonding experience against the larger norms of the social setting. In places where smoking is accepted and widely normative, this same social cohesion from the shared experience of smoking can be highly reinforcing.

If you wonder why this chapter has highlighted smoking as a reinforcing social experience, let's take a brief look at how a popular theory applies to smoking. **Social Cognitive Theory**

Hutchinson Smoking Prevention Project: Long-Term Randomized Trial in School-Based Tobacco Use Prevention—Results on Smoking (FREE)

Arthur V. Peterson, Jr. ✉, Kathleen A. Kealey, Sue L. Mann, Patrick M. Marek, Irwin G. Sarason

JNCI: Journal of the National Cancer Institute, Volume 92, Issue 24, 20 December 2000, Pages 1979–1991, https://doi.org/10.1093/jnci/92.24.1979

Photo 4.4   This article described the evaluation of a school-based smoking cessation program that failed and was thus endorsed by the tobacco industry.

(SCT) is a psychology-based theory that has been widely applied to public health practice. A key tenet of this theory is that the social environment largely shapes human behavior. This occurs through what is known as **positive reinforcement**. For instance, when a young boy watches an older man – someone he may be modeling himself after in terms of masculinity – smoke, he is likely to feel a shared sense of identity in someday becoming a man who smokes. As the boy ages and begins to smoke, his friends may reinforce this as an act of defiance, independence, or brazen masculinity. This is a type of social reward for the boy, who may continue to smoke to build his perceived rugged identity. All this, of course, is programmed into our society by carefully created messaging in movies, television, sporting events, and advertising. SCT further suggests that any other type of reward for smoking (e.g., the feeling of alertness and heightened mental states from nicotine) will promote repetition of the behavior.

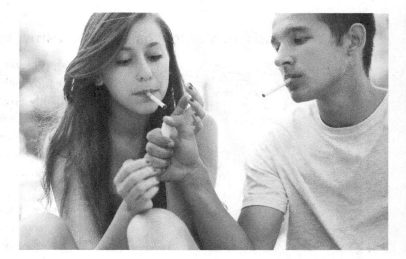

Photo 4.5   Smoking with friends is a reinforcing social experience.
Source: pikselstock/Adobe stock.

Taking SCT as a framework, the CDC and other government-based agencies have wisely used the concept of social reinforcement to promote the behavior of *not* smoking. This is achieved by altering social norms to suggest that healthy and successful teens (for example) have optimal fitness and lung capacity, and creating images of teens enjoying life and staying smoke-free. Unlike the well-funded tobacco industry, government agencies cannot, for example, fund mini-series that glamorize non-smoking teens as smart and cool; however, a large-scale use of media to reinforce abstinence from smoking (and vaping) among America's teens may become part of the future public health strategy against tobacco use. The inherent problem is that positive reinforcement of smoking is immediate (i.e., social recognition and peer bonding), whereas the concept of positive reinforcement does not aptly apply to the behavior of *not* smoking (see **Box 4.2**).

Tobacco Cessation Programs

Moving now to the final quadrant of **Figure 4.1**, the California program also spent millions of dollars at the intrapersonal level (recall that this means "the person"). This part of the program was about helping people break their addiction to nicotine (again, a drug as addictive as heroin or cocaine). Much as with heroin addiction, breaking a person's dependence on nicotine typically requires professional assistance, especially pharmacotherapeutic approaches (*pharm* = drug, *therapeutic* = therapy). The most valuable of these is the **nicotine patch**. Based on the same concept used to help heroin addicts withdraw from that drug, the nicotine patch delivers a low dose of nicotine on a constant basis to circumvent the brain's craving and signals to take in new nicotine supplies via tobacco. Although far from adequate in its own right, the patch makes a highly effective adjunct therapy to counseling-based efforts aimed at smoking cessation.

Counseling-based therapy is also somewhat successful, independent of the nicotine patch, as an individual-level intervention for ending tobacco dependence. This type of therapy typically relies on behavioral theories such as the **transtheoretical model of change** (TMC). The TMC was specifically designed and refined for use by therapists conducting one-to-one smoking cessation efforts with clients. To give you a sense of how these types of theories work, look at **Figure 4.2**. Starting at noon and moving clockwise

BOX 4.2 THE HUMAN SIDE: THE PROBLEM WITH POSITIVE REINFORCEMENT

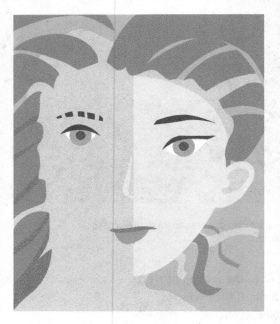

A key principle of positive reinforcement is that it must occur in close time proximity to the behavior that is being rewarded. For instance, diligently brushing and flossing your teeth before hooking up or going on a date gives a sense of self-confidence related to kissing and perhaps other mouth-to-body experiences. Thus, the reward for this hygiene is relatively immediate. Similarly, the daily health behavior of monitoring and limiting caloric intake may help you stay trim, thereby promoting a good sense of body image; this feeling of satisfaction with your body is a reward for not over-consuming calories. Doing something actively (e.g., exercising, weightlifting, or refraining from binge drinking at a party) is typically tied to a short-term outcome that is desirable to you!

So, what happens when the reward does not occur in close time proximity to the behavior? This is true of most vital health behaviors such as avoiding excess sugar and sodium consumption, increasing aerobic fitness to become fortified against heart disease, and avoiding exposure to carcinogens to avoid cancers. In each case, the reward for the behavior is *not* immediate. The reward may never be realized simply because so many health behaviors only reduce the risk of disease onset. It is generally impossible to know for sure whether, for example, the long-term rewards of avoiding an animal-based diet to avert cardiovascular disease ever materialize. The human side is that people seek and even need some form of immediate reward or gratification for engaging in health behaviors, but this is not always possible given the way most chronic diseases occur over a span of years.

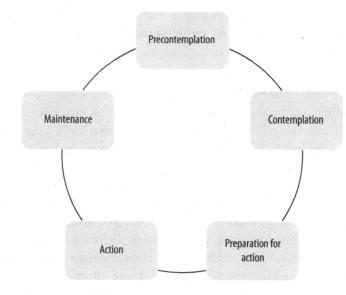

Figure 4.2   The stages of change involved in the transtheoretical model

in this figure, you can see how the theory helps a person progress from not seriously thinking about tobacco cessation (a stage known as **precontemplation**) through a series of distinct steps that ultimately culminate in the long-term maintenance of total cessation from tobacco use. The second stage (**contemplation**) is particularly important to public health practice because this is an ideal intervention point relative to providing medically accurate information that can greatly favor movement to the next stage (**preparation for action**). The success of the fourth stage (**action**) largely depends on how thoroughly a person prepares for this action: for example, obtaining professional assistance, joining a support group, or finding and purchasing a form of nicotine replacement. Typically, the entire process of moving through these stages is fraught with setbacks, second and third attempts, complete failures, and even occasional but fleeting success experiences. To be considered successful, the theory posits that a person must abstain from all forms of tobacco use for at least six months (known as **maintenance**). Funding these counseling programs so they become easy to access and low-cost, or no-cost, to smokers is a key part of the California Tobacco Control Program as well as similar statewide programs that followed in its wake.

One advantage of devoting attention and funds to cessation efforts goes back to altering social norms. Although you may wonder, based on **Chapters 2 and 3**, how cessation for those who are tobacco-dependent fits into a public health paradigm of prevention, there is a clear answer: one involving social norms. In a nutshell, the fewer adults who smoke, the less likely it is that young people will begin the habit and develop an addiction.

In a nutshell, the fewer adults who smoke, the less likely it is that young people will begin the habit

Key Principles of the Master Settlement Agreement

Although it was not met with much fanfare, public health history was made in 1998 when the largest civil litigation ever in the United States concluded with what quickly became known as the **Master Settlement Agreement** (MSA). The states bringing this legal action against the largest manufacturers of tobacco products sought financial compensation for the billions of dollars in medical care costs paid for by state-based Medicaid and Medicare funds. The essence of this agreement was that states would not hold the tobacco companies liable for these medical costs if the companies, in exchange, agreed to make annual fixed payments to each state, with this money being devoted to prevention programs aimed at reducing tobacco use. This annual payout to the 46 states was gradually increased to $9 billion dollars in 2018, at which point the amount stopped increasing, but annual payments will continue in perpetuity (forever). These payments have been used wisely by some states (such as California) and rather foolishly by many others (including use not related to the goal of reducing population-level tobacco reduction). Unfortunately, many of the 46 states have spent less than 3% of these funds on tobacco-related prevention programs.

The MSA also restricted how tobacco companies were allowed to advertise their products. For instance, cartoon characters in advertising were banned as part of the MSA. Ads specifically directed toward teens were also banned, as well as ads directly or indirectly targeting pre-teens. The use of billboards and other prominent forms of outdoor advertising was banned except for outdoor advertising near stores selling cigarettes and other tobacco products. Further, branded merchandise and sponsored events (such as sporting events and car racing events) were banned as part of the MSA. Also noteworthy is that the MSA included agreements by the tobacco companies to refrain from distributing false or mitigating information about the harms of nicotine and smoking (a previously widespread practice). This final point warrants attention because it is important that you understand the term **junk science**.

Accusing the science of public health of being junk science is a common practice of the tobacco industry. This stems from the all-too-common practice of the industry becoming involved in what they have called "sound science." **Box 4.3** provides an example one directly related to tobacco.

BOX 4.3. THE "SOUND SCIENCE" PROGRAM OF PHILLIP MORRIS

This story begins with two public health researchers who obtained internal documents from tobacco giant Phillip Morris. The ploy used by Phillip Morris was simple. The company worked tirelessly to redefine what it means to practice "sound science." Its work on this was designed to set standards of proof for cause and effect (such as whether exposure to environmental tobacco smoke causes lung cancer in non-smokers) to unobtainable levels. The company's redefinition of what it means to prove cause and effect had the parallel effect of allowing it to relabel all other studies (conducted using standard methods of scientific practice) as junk science. In turn, the junk science refrain became a new rallying point for discrediting hundreds of excellent epidemiological investigations showing a strong association between exposure to ETS and ill-health effects among non-smokers.

According to the two researchers, Phillip Morris began its efforts to discredit science in 1993, one year after the U.S. Environmental Protection Agency (EPA) declared second-hand smoke a group A carcinogen. (Ong & Glantz, 2001). The company began by orchestrating the creation of what became known as The Advancement for Sound Science Coalition (TASSC). This coalition consisted of people with profit motives reaching beyond tobacco, including representatives protecting the interests of other companies being regulated by the EPA. Ultimately, the TASSC produced what appeared to be a set of standards that greatly advanced the rigors of conducting and publishing epidemiological research. However, as any well-trained and experienced epidemiologist knows, these proposed standards were not practical or even, in most cases, possible to achieve. The true goal of the TASSC was then clear: making all routine science seem weak and not capable of proof. In the absence of proof, the TASSC could freely claim the FDA-imposed regulations were unfair and should be removed.

One example from the proposed set of standards is noteworthy: "Odds ratios of 2 or less should be treated with caution, particularly when the confidence intervals are wide. There is likelihood that the odds ratio is artefactual and the result of problems with case or control selection, confounders, or bias" (Ong & Glantz, 2001, p. 1751). To understand this, think of an odds ratio as the odds of winning a bet. Let's say you have a chance to win $100 by guessing a person's political party affiliation. Rather than taking a 50/50 chance (i.e., guessing Democrat or Republican at random), you ask for one clue. Let's say that the clue is whether the person is male or female. Knowing only this clue, you make your guess. The question is, how powerful is the clue? To illustrate, let's say that a study found an odds ratio of 1.7 relative to predicting a party affiliation of Republicans among males. This means your odds of being correct in guessing Republican increase by 70% if you know the person is male. So, do you feel that the 1.7 odds ratio would be useful to you in this hypothetical contest?

Returning to public health, a 70% increase in being correct or incorrect relative to whether a given disease will develop based on a risk factor (i.e., the clue) is generally considered valuable science. The exception would be if the study had a very small sample size (which would create the wide confidence intervals cited by the TASSC). As for the selection of human subjects, confounding, and bias, all three issues are omnipresent in any studies of humans; this is an acceptable sacrifice that protects the ethics of human subject research (they must, for example, freely volunteer, and confounding is a result of normal individual variations in behavior and physiology).

The U.S. Vaping Epidemic: The Tobacco Industry Strikes Back

Not unlike the ever-popular *Star Wars* trilogy, it is fair to say that the tobacco industry is alive and well and (much like the Empire) has re-emerged in full force. At the time of the MSA, nobody from the side of public health practice could have envisioned a time when nicotine would be distilled from tobacco and placed into gas-filled cartridges that produce a vapor-like smoke mimicking that from using cigarettes. Tobacco is used only as the source for obtaining the nicotine, thereby entirely bypassing the MSA because it was predicated on tobacco use.

Sadly, the empire did strike back, making vaping a type of epidemic in the United States. The most vital concern is that young people who vape (formally known as using an electronic nicotine delivery system) will be more likely to begin using cigarettes to boost their increasing nicotine dependence. Again, recall that nicotine rivals the addictive power of cocaine and

Tobacco is used only as the source for obtaining the nicotine, thereby entirely bypassing the MSA

heroin. Recent studies document a complete lack of evidence that vaping is useful for smoking cessation. Yet (and this is a subtle point) studies also do not provide direct evidence that disproves the idea that vaping is a legitimate method of becoming less dependent on nicotine. This creates a classic gap for companies (such as the tobacco industry): they can legitimately claim that their product has *not* been *disproven* to help people quit.

Generally speaking, vaping has been a workaround on the part of the tobacco industry. It sidesteps the MSA because tobacco is no longer the product – only nicotine. Again, however, this is where the Truth Campaign comes into play (note: it is funded by the MSA). The campaign brings to the public's attention that e-cigarettes are as harmful as tobacco cigarettes with respect to the effects of nicotine on the cardiovascular system and adolescent brain development. The campaign has a strong focus on vaping and teens. Particularly dominant in this campaign is the JUUL e-cigarette. The manufacturer of JUUL provided data showing that a single JUUL cartridge has as much nicotine as an entire pack of cigarettes (Willet, Bennett, & Hair, 2018). JUUL exemplifies the return of the tobacco industry by showing us that the basic drug – nicotine – remains the primary approach to creating an entirely new generation of people who are dependent on it. Dependency, of course, breeds spending money to stay on the drug, which creates an ever-lasting profit margin of billions for the industry. Again, as per the opening quote of this chapter, teens are the target because their lifetime addiction is highly valuable to the goal of making money. This focus on teens and pre-teens is obvious in the marketing of e-cigarettes with flavors such as fruit, candy, desserts, and mint.

From a public health perspective, it is entirely fair to declare vaping an epidemic among America's teens. Approaching the problem from this viewpoint of urgency is vital because estimates suggest that rates of vaping among American teens are growing astronomically. For instance, the DC reports that in 2020, approximately 3.6 million U.S. middle school and high school students had vaped at least once in the past 30 days (Park-Lee, Ren, Sawdey, et al., 2021). Among these 3.6 million, the CDC estimates that just over 2 million used e-cigarettes at least 20 of every 30 days, with 27.6% of high school students and 8.3% of middle school students being daily users. The CDC has also noted that e-cigarette use increased by 900% between 2011 and 2015, with continued increases in the rate of use by teens and pre-teens also reported for 2017 and 2018. In 2018, one of five U.S. high school students was a current user. Through an extensive surveillance system, the CDC constantly monitors the U.S. tobacco problem among American teens, creating a type of blueprint for public health action (see **Figure 4.3**).

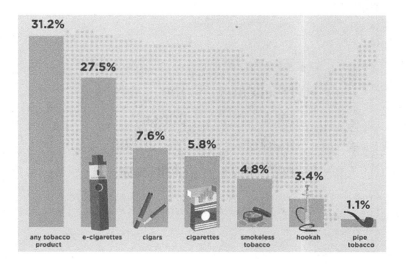

Figure 4.3   Tobacco product use among high school students.
Source: CDC / Public Domain.

These very recent eye-opening estimates led U.S. Surgeon General Jerome Adams to state, "The recent surge in e-cigarette use among youth, which have been fueled by new types of e-cigarettes that have recently entered the market, is a cause for great concern. We must take action now to protect the health of our nation's young people" (Park-Lee, Ren, Sawdey, et al., 2021, p.1).

What Are the Public Health Lessons Stemming from Tobacco Control?

By this point in the chapter, you have probably realized that big business is all too often in control of the daily choices (including health behaviors) that people make. The tenets of the California Tobacco Control Program work both ways, meaning principles such as altering social norms in favor of tobacco products and enabling easy access to tobacco products have been successfully applied by the tobacco industry. This is apparent with respect to the great success of the tobacco industry with e-cigarettes.

Compared to the tobacco industry, public health is funded for pennies on the dollar. Of course, other large-scale industries can follow in the footsteps of the tobacco industry. The food industry – driven by agribusiness – is a primary example. Also consider the massive challenges of slowing climate change (see **Chapters 12 and 13**), as presented by the automobile and oil industries. Although not an industry per se, it is also important to consider the billions of dollars that flow from the sale of illicit drugs to the American public. For public health to take on all these industry-driven causes of risk to Americans is simply not realistic. Instead, public health will need to change the paradigm by redefining the rules of the game. Driven by supply-and-demand principles, the United States exists in what is known as a **market economy**. However, the principles of a market economy include government regulation and controls on what can be done within fair boundaries of decency and respect for the health and welfare of society. Think of this as a steady tension between two extremes: a completely unbridled marketplace (absence of regulations and controls) and a primary focus on the health and welfare of society (with a general disregard for the ability of industries such as tobacco to generate billions of dollars in annual revenue). **Figure 4.4** helps envision this tension.

Returning to an earlier premise of this book, it is important to remember that "we the people" form the American government. Further, and as provided in the preamble of the U.S.

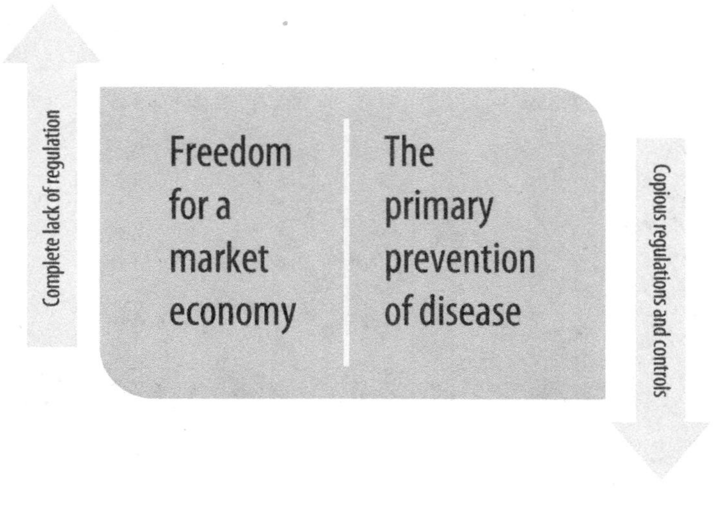

Figure 4.4 Market economy vs. a focus on health and welfare

Constitution, the government has an obligation to protect the public's general welfare. Once your generation comes of age and begins to dominate the political landscape of this nation, remember how the MSA, for example, once brought tobacco companies to a breaking point. Also remember that taxing cigarettes led to lower population-level consumption of this product and saved millions of lives. And remember that the Truth Campaign worked so well because it exposed unethical practices of big business – a type of boundary line that most Americans will not tolerate others crossing, regardless of their wealth and power.

Beyond ethics, one highly applicable and important term to learn is **negative externalities**. Often described as the real cost, a negative externality is simply a cost to society incurred by the manufacturing or use of a product stemming from industry. Consider, for instance, the costs to Medicaid and Medicare of nicotine addiction among the people in their 20s (such as most of the students reading this chapter) as they progress through life with various cardiovascular disorders caused by the accumulating damage of the drug. This cost of the tobacco industry doing business is placed on the shoulders of American taxpayers rather than companies such as Phillip Morris. And this is where public health practice increasingly involves economists! Economists use modeling techniques to skillfully determine the monetary values of nearly any negative externality related to disease onset and progression. Examples include:

> a negative externality is simply a cost to society incurred by the manufacturing or use of a product stemming from industry

- The manufacturing and massive distribution of high fructose corn syrup relative to America's diabetes epidemic

- The cost to the U.S. healthcare system of America's habit of consuming fast foods (e.g., Burger King, McDonald's, Wendy's) that are exceptionally high in fat and cholesterol

- The economic burden (including lost lives, permanent disabilities, lost wages, and lost jobs) of driving while intoxicated in states that allow the drive-through purchase of liquor and cold beer

- The probable costs of cancers (including treatment and loss of life) in geographic areas close to manufacturing plants that emit known carcinogens into the environment

The purpose of calculating dollar values related to negative externalities is to ultimately hold the offending industries financially responsible. As you have already learned in this chapter, this is the origin of the MSA. Remember that the MSA was brought about via a lawsuit (by 46 states) against the large tobacco companies, and the complaint was focused on the costs of tobacco relative to state Medicaid and Medicare bills pertaining to smokers.

Ultimately, the most important public health lesson gained from tobacco control is that regulation and legislation is the approach that will create population-level improvements in health. The concept of school-based education programs teaching youth about the risk of tobacco use did not fare well. Similarly, community-based anti-smoking programs were, at best, only partially effective and in only very limited geographic areas. The departure from risk education to a comprehensive approach such as the California Tobacco Control Program sets an example for future directions of public health practices relative to a broad array of health behaviors (e.g., controlling sugar and sodium intake, limiting overall alcohol consumption at a population level, and even controlling the U.S. opioid epidemic). Although this type of **comprehensive approach** does involve some education (e.g., the Truth Campaign is designed to teach teens about the deceitful and corrupt practices of the tobacco industry), its backbone is regulation achieved through means such as taxation and withholding licensures, and legislation (local, state, or federal laws passed and enforced in service of population-level declines in the use of products/substances that are strongly tied to disease). Thus, the comprehensive approach shown in **Figure 4.1**, for instance, can be modified from a tobacco-based application to nearly any other application that involves a ubiquitous health-compromising behavior.

As a close to this chapter, think back to what you have learned in this book about the difference between upstream and downstream approaches. Recall that the upstream approach is far more focused on entire populations! This is a vital point because it punctuates the idea that controlling huge health problems (e.g., tobacco addiction, alcoholism, the opioid epidemic) must not occur at the individual level. The all-too-common tendency is to assume that unregulated industries are not the problem and that the real problem is the weak character of people who choose to smoke, drink heavily, or use opioids. This is a convenient paradigm for the industries, but it is simply incorrect. Advertising works! Knowing this, industries such as tobacco constantly invest millions of dollars in ensuring that their customer base stays at a high level. The CDC has estimated that about 7 million people die from smoking each year (this is a global estimate). Thus, you can be sure that the tobacco industry's investment in addicting pre-teens and teens is being made on a large-scale (population-level) basis to replace these deceased customers. To have a fighting chance to compete with this type of industry-based, population-level promotion, public health practice must be on the same playing field, meaning it must also function at a population level. It is inadequate to compete against tobacco with brochures in doctor's offices and other individual-level approaches to cessation when cessation is far less the issue of concern compared to the massive numbers of new customers recruited by the industry every day. Thinking about the problem in this population-level paradigm applies to all the most pressing public health issues of our era.

> To have a fighting chance to compete with this type of industry-based, population-level promotion, public health practice must be on the same playing field

Review and Key Terms

With this first topical chapter in this book firmly in your grasp, you have learned how public health can succeed (and fail). You began by learning about some of the basics relative to tobacco and health. You should now know the difference between **tars** and **nicotine** and how each affects the body differently. You should understand how nicotine triggers the **sympathetic** nervous system to cause **vasoconstriction**. Ultimately, **coronary occlusions** – leading to **myocardial infractions** – will result from nicotine use, as will **strokes**. Conversely, tars act as carcinogens and co-carcinogens, thereby accounting for a large portion of the annual cases of cancer.

Turning attention to the control of tobacco, you learned about four key tenets of the California Tobacco Control Program. In so doing, you gained insights into why control efforts must prioritize teenagers, especially relative to limiting access. Think about the key concepts you learned in that part of the chapter, such as the use of **price elasticity** and the application of **Social Cognitive Theory**, focusing on the role of **positive reinforcement**. You also learned about strategies such as **product placement** and the process of altering **social norms**. Social norms are an especially important leverage point relative to ETS regulation. Hopefully, this chapter inspired you to go online and learn more about the Truth Campaign; it remains a vital part of the current U.S. tobacco control strategy.

Although less vital regarding tobacco control for teens, another public health strategy has been applying the **Transtheoretical Model of Change**, with its five stages as applied to tobacco cessation: **precontemplation, contemplation, preparation for action, action**, and **maintenance**. You also learned about the tremendous importance of **nicotine replacement** in this process of quitting. You may have been surprised to learn that evidence does not yet fully condemn the use of vaping as a type of nicotine replacement. Science is an objective process and often a slow one. Relatedly, bear in mind that science is not perfect; however, it is well-established and has served public health for more than a century. This is in contrast to the great efforts by the tobacco industry to discredit science as being junk science.

At the end of this chapter, you gained insights into how controlling tobacco created lessons learned that can be applied to an endless number of equally challenging public health problems. These include taking on the food industry, the alcohol and bar industry, and powerful cartels that dominate America's flow of opioids and other illicit substances that cause premature morbidity and mortality on a widespread basis. Key concepts in this regard are **negative externalities** and the use of a **comprehensive approach** to these otherwise intractable problems facing Americans.

For Practice and Class Discussion

Practice Questions

1. Which one of the following is *not* true about nicotine?
   a. It is at least as addictive as cocaine.
   b. It is extracted from tobacco for use in e-cigarettes.
   c. Nicotine is carcinogenic, especially in the trachea and lungs.
   d. It stimulates vasoconstriction and increases the adhesiveness of blood platelets to artery walls.

2. A true public health approach to preventing death from tobacco would involve each of the following actions *except*:
   a. The widespread distribution of brochures in clinics and doctor's offices
   b. Funding community-based organizations to pass ETS policies/laws
   c. Changing entire cultures relative to smoking and other forms of tobacco use
   d. Taxing all tobacco products

3. In a few words, the concept of price elasticity refers to:
   a. A degree of tolerance in price that, when exceeded, translates into a decrease in demand
   b. The price point at which a company no longer makes a profit on the product
   c. A method of keeping consumers happy by placing limits on tax increases for any given product

4. The state of New Hampshire would like to mimic the California Tobacco Control Program. This state, however, has limited funds and wants to begin with an effort that will yield the greatest impact for the amount of funds allocated. Which one (*best*) approach should the state use?
   a. Provide funding to support the costs of the nicotine patch for people on Medicare who want to end their dependence on tobacco.
   b. Adopt the Truth Campaign as part of the statewide health curriculum for high school students and even middle school students.
   c. Train high school teachers to teach students basic facts about the harmful effects of tobacco and vaping.
   d. Develop and fund a statewide network of social media experts who can then build websites that teach teens the harmful effects of tobacco use and vaping.

5. Given the high costs associated with paying for employees' healthcare expenses, a large company has recently created an employee education-based program designed to help people end tobacco dependence. Which one company policy would be *best* suited to also help this effort by its influence on social norms?
   a. Provide smoke-free break rooms
   b. Refuse to pay for health insurance for employees who smoke

    c.   Provide the nicotine patch at no cost, upon request

    d.   Prohibit tobacco use and vaping on all company property

6.   The California Tobacco Control Program relies *least* on which level of intervention?

    a.   Intrapersonal

    b.   Interpersonal

    c.   Institutional

    d.   Community

    e.   Policy/law

7.   When a pregnant woman inhales secondhand smoke, several effects occur on the fetus. These effects can all lead to issues with fetal development. Which of the following is the *least* likely of these issues?

    a.   Premature birth

    b.   Low birth weight

    c.   Compromised fetal immunity

    d.   Subsequent childhood risk of asthma

8.   The Master Settlement Agreement currently provides states with millions of dollars, yet only a small portion is used to fund tobacco use prevention programs.

    a.   True

    b.   False

9.   A key philosophy of the Truth Campaign is:

    a.   Teens need to know the facts about how smoking harms their bodies.

    b.   All people deserve access to medically accurate information about tobacco.

    c.   The hidden injustices of the tobacco industry must be exposed.

    d.   Taxing tobacco products will greatly reduce teen smoking.

10.   The public health approach of making health-compromising products – such as nicotine – too expensive for people to easily afford is based on the economic principle of:

    a.   Supply and demand

    b.   Price elasticity

    c.   Market justice

    d.   A comprehensive approach

For Class Discussion

11.   This chapter frequently referenced the food industry as the next tobacco. Of course, the food industry is much larger, so let's consider just the industry of selling chicken meat. Go online to find out what federal regulations are currently applied to the chicken industry. Then, in less than two pages, compose a summary of what you learned. Include any issues you see as lacking (and thus favoring the industry over public health). Send this to at least three other students taking this class, and then have the group engage in an agree vs. disagree discussion about what each person found and concluded was missing.

12.   One of the most urgent public health challenges regarding tobacco involves maternal smoking. Imagine that you have been hired to create and produce a YouTube video that will be shown to pregnant women who smoke. In outline form, describe at least four objectives and key scenes you will include in this video. Compare your outline to that of at least one other student taking this class. What did you leave out? What did the other person leave out?

13. The tobacco industry rose again with the invention of e-cigarettes. This increase in wealth was based almost entirely on customers who were pre-teens and teens. The industry used candy flavors to make the smoke more appealing to kids. It also engaged in altering social norms such that vaping became sexy and a sign of being young and smart. In bullet-point format, describe how the industry's overall promotion of e-cigarettes violated (or nearly violated) the MSA. Compare your list to as those of many other students taking this class as possible. Discuss the difference between these lists, and try to conclude what the most egregious violations have been.

References

Estill, J. (1988). *Surgeon General says smoking is addictive.* AP News. https://apnews.com/article/758ad3 d40dd12dea234f19ecd7b6de2c

Ong, E. K., & Glantz, S. A. (2001). Constructing "sound science" and "good epidemiology": Tobacco, lawyers, and public relations firms. *The American Journal of Public Health, 91*(11), 1749–1754.

Park-Lee, E., Ren, C., Sawdey, M. D., Gentzke, A. S., Cornelius, M., Jamal, A., &Cullen, K. A. (2021). *Notes from the field: E-cigarette use among middle and high school students.* National Youth Tobacco Survey, United States, 2021.

Peterson, A. V., Kealy, K. A., Mann, S. L., Marek, P. M., & Sarason, I. G. (2000). Hutchinson smoking prevention project: Long-term randomized trial in school-based tobacco use prevention – results on smoking. *Journal of the National Cancer Institute, 92,* 1979–1991.

Willet, J. G., Bennett, M., & Hair, E. C. (2018). Recognition, use and perceptions of JUUL among youth and young adults. *Tobacco Control Published Online First, 18.* https://doi.org/10.1136/ tobaccocontrol-2018-054273

AMERICA'S OBESITY AND CARDIOVASCULAR DISEASE EPIDEMICS: POSSIBLE PUBLIC HEALTH SOLUTIONS

It's bizarre that the produce manager is more important to my children's health than the pediatrician.

—*Meryl Streep*

Overview

As you learned in **Chapters 2–4** of this textbook, public health takes a very different approach than the medical sciences to protecting the quality and quantity of human life. This is particularly true when it comes to America's number-one cause of morbidity and premature mortality: **cardiovascular disease** (**CVD**). The U.S. epidemic of CVD has arisen in tandem with the U.S. obesity epidemic. The two epidemics are linked in many ways; however, the actual causes of each are also somewhat distinct.

Past public health scholars have referred to both epidemics as "wicked problems," meaning resolving either may be an unsolvable challenge. In this century, however, emerging approaches to solving these epidemics are becoming increasingly realistic and practical. For the first time in history, our nation has a fighting chance at reducing the severity of both epidemics. This is because of thinking differently (as you learned in **Chapter 3**) and an increased reliance on applying public health practice via regulatory and policy-based actions (as you learned in **Chapters 2 and 3**). The bold steps needed, for example, to reduce the prevalence of childhood obesity are nicely embodied in the quote from actress Meryl Streep. Indeed, the foods parents provide for their infants, toddlers, and young children lay a foundation of sorts. Part of the foundation is physical. Plant-based whole foods avert obesity, protect against the formation of CVD, and nourish the brain and immune system. That foundation is also related to how children form and maintain the food preferences that will carry into adulthood.

As you read this chapter, you will most likely be surprised at what you learn about the role of **movement** (i.e., keeping the body in motion) as a second pillar of health-protective behavior – one that is just as important as the pillar of food choices. Of course, the public health actions pertaining to both pillars (i.e., healthy eating and movement) are quite different. But these approaches share the concept

LEARNING OBJECTIVES

1. Explain the magnitude of the U.S. epidemics pertaining to CVD and obesity.

2. Explain metabolic syndrome, and describe its four factors.

3. Describe the phrase "obesity is contagious." and explain how this concept altered public health practice.

4. Describe public health efforts to regulate the food industry.

5. Learn about the farm-to-table movement and its value to public health.

6. Explain what is meant by the phrase "sitting is the new smoking."

7. Understand the public health approach to promoting daily movement and exercise.

8. Appreciate the value of upstream interventions occurring early in life as opposed to being applied after clinical signs of CVD occur or obesity is diagnosed as a health problem.

of intervention occurring primarily at the regulatory and policy levels, emphasizing the actions needed to change social and physical structures to create the conditions that enable healthy eating and daily human movement.

The interventions you will learn about in this chapter are not easy to implement. Further, they are not easy to finance. Ironically, the depth of commitment and the extent of financial resources needed to realize the potential of public health to reduce these wicked problems is a point of contention among policy-makers and politicians who hold the power to make these changes. The irony lies in the costs of the alternative – particularly the existing downstream approach to CVD, which consumes an abundant share of the annual gross domestic product of the United States. Thus, this chapter lays out a challenge for you as a young citizen of this nation, regardless of whether you support an upstream or downstream emphasis to the prevention of CVD and obesity. Remember that the phrase "we the people" includes you! Do you have the courage and foresight to recognize that daily choices (such as the one alluded to in the opening quote of this chapter) are more crucial than doctors and hospitals when it comes to CVD and obesity?

The Magnitude of the CVD and Obesity Epidemics

Without question, CVD is the leading cause of death in the United States. Each year, about 650,000 people die from CVD. To put that number into perspective, consider that in the early summer of 2021, approximately 1.5 years after the start of the COVID-19 pandemic, the United States passed 600,000 deaths caused by this virus. At a relatively predictable 650,000 deaths per year, every year, you can begin to appreciate the magnitude of mortality from CVD. Unlike COVID, though, the death toll from CVD garners little, if any, attention in the media and seems to have become an accepted form of morbidity and premature mortality in the United States. You may ask, "Isn't CVD what people die from when they die of old age?" To answer this question, it is important to gain a deeper understanding of CVD.

CVD is a broad term encompassing any of the arteries that make up the circulatory system. This means CVD may affect the heart directly or the most valued part of the human body: the brain. About one of every six deaths from CVD is attributable to a stroke. When the arteries providing blood to the brain become occluded (i.e., clogged), brain tissue quickly dies. This is known as a **stroke**. Similarly, when the arteries that provide the blood supply to the heart muscle (i.e., the coronary arteries) become occluded, heart muscle begins to die. This occlusion results from plaque buildup on the walls of the arteries (see **Figure 5.1**). This plaque may begin to form early in life – even in childhood—as a result of dietary factors you will learn about in this chapter. As you learned in the previous chapter (**Chapter 4**), plaque is also a result of nicotine use. Sadly, once plaque forms, it is irreversible.

Returning to the question of dying from old age, it is not unusual for people to live well into their 90s or even reach age 100. But the average age of death from CVD is approximately 65 for males and around 72 for females. Although the average for females is later in life, they are not as likely as males to survive their first heart attack (Harvard Health Publishing, 2016). The challenge to public health lies in increasing the average age of first attacks by several years for both males and females. Contrary to what many people expect and what may be suggested by a medical care approach, the biological evidence indicates that this form of prevention must begin relatively early in life instead of middle age or older (Liu et al., 2012). This means most people attending a college or university (such as yourself) are currently shaping the outcome relative to what age they will be when they might have a first heart attack. Noteworthy is that, in autopsy-based studies, people less than 35 years of age have been found to have relatively advanced plaque buildup in their arteries. This is why it is not uncommon for people to have a

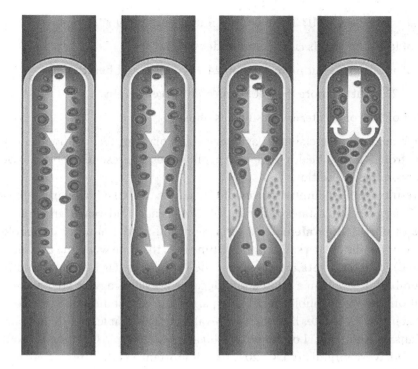

Figure 5.1   Plaque accumulation on the walls of a coronary artery
Source: Centers for Disease Control and Prevention. Heart disease facts / Public domain.

heart attack or stroke prior to 45. So, as you may guess, the idea of increasing the mean age of the first attack must begin with people in their second and third decades of life (i.e., teens and young adults), and thus any immediate public health progress toward reaching this goal will take several more decades to realize. In essence, understanding that the efforts of public health to prevent heart attacks (and strokes) cannot be evaluated easily is critical in terms of maintaining these efforts over several decades.

At this juncture, let's turn our attention to the point that CVD leads to a massive amount of morbidity in the United States. Thus, although CVD is costly (more than $200 billion per year) and tragic, its annual death toll is not the entire story. The rest of the tale involves the loss of function that people experience when they survive a heart attack or stroke. Convalescence from either can take years, adding billions in cost to a largely preventable cause of morbidity.

Let's now consider the magnitude of America's obesity epidemic. As you proceed through this part of the chapter, be aware that obesity is a **health-compromising condition** (recall that you first learned this term in **Chapter 2**) that can lead to several forms of morbidity and mortality. These include the all-too-common issues chronic low-back pain, kidney disease, some forms of cancer, diabetes, and –as you might guess—CVD.

Obesity is defined based on what is known as **body mass index** (BMI). BMI can be calculated using a person's height and weight measurements. The equation is based on metric measures (kilograms for weight and meters of height). The equation is simple division, with the numerator being a person's weight. The denominator is a bit complex because the person's height must be squared. In summary form, the equation looks like this:

Weight (in kilograms) / Height (in meters)^2

For instance, a person weighing 135 pounds would have a numerator of 61.23 kilograms. If this same person was five feet tall, the denominator would be 1.527 meters, which squares to 2.33. Dividing 61.23 by 2.33 gives a quotient (BMI) of 26.27.

understanding that the efforts of public health to prevent heart attacks (and strokes) cannot be evaluated easily is critical in terms of maintaining these efforts over several decades

So, what is a healthy BMI? The CDC has four classifications:

- A BMI of less than 18.5 is considered **underweight**.

- A BMI of at least 18.5 but no more than 24.9 is considered **healthy.**

- A BMI of 25.0 but no more than 30.0 represents **overweight.**

- Any BMI of 30.0 or greater is classified as **obesity.**

*from a public health perspective, only **obesity** presents a problem because it is a health-compromising condition*

Although some people classified as **overweight** may not feel confident in their physical appearance, from a public health perspective, only **obesity** presents a problem because it is a health-compromising condition.

Using results from a biannual survey of U.S. adults, the CDC regularly publishes maps of the United States depicting states with relatively low-range, mid-range, and high-range **prevalence rates** of obesity. **Prevalence** is a term representing the number of people having any given disease or condition at a single point in time (i.e., the time when the prevalence estimates were assessed). The term **rate** indicates that the prevalence has been adjusted by estimating the total number of people in a population. Because prevalence rates are adjusted for the size of a population, they allow public health comparisons across states, for example. Consider, for instance, that in 2019, 12 states had obesity prevalence rates of at least 35%: Alabama, Arkansas, Indiana, Kansas, Kentucky, Louisiana, Michigan, Mississippi, Oklahoma, South Carolina, Tennessee, and West Virginia (CDC, 2021). Of importance is that the prevalence rates for all 50 states have been steadily rising for more than 30 years! For example, even as recently as 2011, no state had 35% or more of its population classified as obese. America's obesity epidemic is becoming progressively worse, thus serving as a harbinger of the disease epidemics caused by this health-compromising condition. Fortunately, public health research has cast a great deal of light on the culprits of the obesity epidemic. The best summary of these dietary causes is simply that animal-based products are culprit #1 and refined sugars are culprit #2. The role of wheat-based products is an emerging culprit #3 (more about sugar and wheat in **Chapter 6**).

Metabolic Syndrome and Its Four Factors

A **syndrome** is best thought of as a collection of physical issues in the body. In the case of **metabolic syndrome**, four distinct factors contribute to the development of CVD:

- Central obesity

- Hypertension

- Unfavorable lipids (fats) in the bloodstream

- Elevated levels of blood sugar

This part of the chapter introduces each of these four factors, with less emphasis on elevated blood sugar levels because that topic is a mainstay of **Chapter 6**. This brief tutorial aims to prepare you to better understand the wisdom and benefits of the public health actions that will be described in the remainder of this chapter.

Central Obesity

Most obesity is known as **central obesity**. This means the excess fat in the body is stored around the waist. Generally speaking, obesity – especially central obesity – overworks the heart. The heart, of course, is a muscle. Take a moment to lay one hand over your heart and feel its beat. This beat began long before you were born and will continue until you die (it is part of how death is defined). Therefore, as a muscle, the only rest the heart receives is between beats. For example, a heart that beats 60 times per minute will have more rest and live longer than one consistently beating at 90 times per minute or more. Because obesity implies more body tissue and thus more cells that must be nourished by blood, the total blood volume is inflated in obese people. This requires the heart to work abnormally hard (beating more times per minute) to keep up with the body's needs.

Further, obesity negatively influences the natural filtration system in the kidneys. Your kidneys regulate blood pressure by removing sodium from the bloodstream. Therefore obesity – especially central obesity – as a health-compromising condition leads to the second issue in metabolic syndrome: hypertension.

Hypertension

Recall that **Chapter 3** provided you with a basic introduction to hypertension. As you learned in that chapter, the goal of public health is less concerned about a given threshold that defines people with hypertension and is instead focused on lowering blood pressure across entire populations. The physiology can be boiled down to this short list:

* Reduced use of salt **on and in** foods

* Increased levels (minutes per day) of vigorous exercise (e.g., doubling the heart rate for at least 60 minutes at a time)

* Reduced instances of stress response throughout any typical day

* Reduced BMI

At this point, the role of salt in terms of public health practice warrants extensive consideration. Again, remember that the **sodium** in sodium chloride is the issue. The vast majority of the sodium that most people eat comes from hidden sources. This is because the food industry values your business and wants you to love the taste of their products (and humans have an affinity for the taste of salt). To help you better understand these hidden sources, take a long and thoughtful look at **Table 5.1**.

As you study **Table 5.1**, keep in mind that foods such as tomatoes are not naturally high in sodium. In fact, fresh fruits and vegetables have negligible amounts of sodium. For instance, one 8-ounce serving of fresh green beans contains only 1 mg of sodium. In contrast, a 4-ounce serving (i.e., half a cup) of canned green beans contains a whopping 300 mg of sodium (see **Photo 5.1**). Also, as you study **Table 5.1**, be aware that the recommended daily sodium intake limit is 1500 mg. As you might easily surmise, most people greatly exceed this recommended limit: it has been estimated that the average American consumes twice this amount (i.e., 3,000 mg) of sodium daily (Illades, 2021).

Unfavorable Lipids

Lipids are various types of fats circulating in the bloodstream. Many lipids are highly beneficial to the body. In fact, fats from most plant-based sources provide a great deal of long-term value to the body's organs and systems. These benefits include preventing some cancers, regulating blood sugar levels, and providing essential

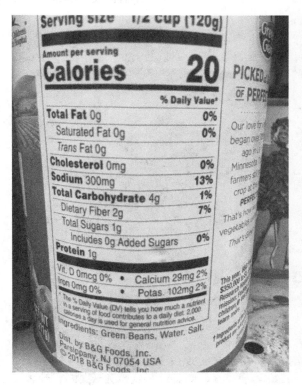

Photo 5.1   A typical 8-ounce can of green beans is two servings of half a cup each.

Table 5.1   Sodium content of typical foods

Food	Serving size	Sodium (in mg)
Hot dog	One	700
Deli ham	One slice	300
Tomato juice	One 8-ounce can	700
Ketchup	One tablespoon	150
Soy sauce	One tablespoon	1,000
Spaghetti sauce	One cup	1,000
Flour tortilla	One 10-inch piece	500
Canned tuna	Three ounces	300

Source: Adapted from Illades, C. (2021).

nutrients for the endocrine system. However, other lipids are damaging to the body. The most well-known of these offenders is **cholesterol**; however, **triglycerides** are equally important to consider. Understanding lipids is an essential part of understanding public health practice, so pay close attention to this section of the chapter. Because lipids most often (but not always) come from the same general class of foods (i.e., animal products), both cholesterol-laden foods and those high in triglycerides are typically found in the same meal. It becomes a somewhat artificial and academic exercise to distinguish which animal-based foods are the highest in either cholesterol or triglycerides. Also, before proceeding, it is noteworthy that foods do not contain cholesterol; rather, the lipids in foods such as eggs, beef, and pork produce cholesterol in the body.

Now that you know a bit about lipids, this chapter can introduce you to a relatively famous study in CVD and nutrition: ***The China Study***. Published in 2005, *The China Study* was the initial academic work suggesting that a plant-based (and whole food) diet can somewhat reverse CVD (Campbell & Campbell, 2005). The study was prospective (over 20 years) and included people from 65 countries. Its data and conclusions have been widely reviewed by academics and have held up under this scrutiny. The premise of the study's overall conclusion is that **plant-based diets** that are also designed to preserve foods in their **whole food** form are the upstream approach to CVD and obesity. Those two terms were subsequently merged to become a **plant-based whole food** (PBWF) diet.

To begin your understanding of a PBWF diet, it is important to clarify the latter part of the term. A **whole food** is simply one that lacks any processing. Fresh green beans, for example, are a whole food, whereas canned green beans (see **Photo 5.1**) are not a whole food. An even better example is beets. In its original form, a beet is loaded with micronutrients, favorable phytochemicals, antioxidants, fiber, vitamins, minerals, and so on. But let's consider how most beets are consumed in the United States and globally. The most common variety of beet grown is known as the sugar beet.

The American Sugar Association estimates that U.S. farmers produce approximately 4.5 million tons of sugar annually by extracting sugar from the root of the beet plant. Thus, sugar is a plant-based food; however, it is certainly not a PBWF. This distinction is vital to understand on a general basis because simply eating a plant-based diet is not a valid public health approach to preventing CVD

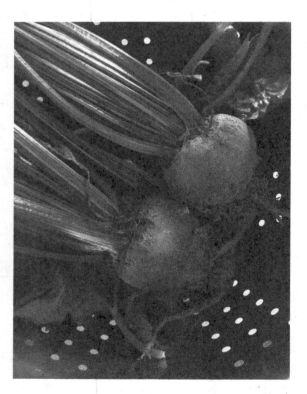

Photo 5.2   This entire food is highly nutritious – both the root and the leaves.

and obesity. To emphasize this point, consider that (staying with the same example) eating a whole beet is good for you, but eating only its refined sugar is one of the primary causes of CVD and obesity. This same rule applies to a host of plant-based foods, such as these:

simply eating a plant-based diet is not a valid public health approach to preventing CVD and obesity.

- Rice
- Wheat
- Olives
- Potatoes
- Carrots
- Corn
- Oats
- Apples

At this point in your introduction to metabolic syndrome, you may feel a bit overwhelmed by the heavy emphasis on lipids. More information is shown in **Box 5.1** as an add-on to this part of the chapter.

BOX 5.1. A TUTORIAL ON ATHEROSCLEROSIS

As you already know, **atherosclerosis** refers to a narrowing diameter of the arteries. This condition is especially dangerous when it comes to the arteries feeding blood to the heart (i.e., the coronary arteries) or the brain (i.e., the cardioid arteries). Fortunately, the human body has defense mechanisms against the formation of the plaque that causes this problem.

One of these defenses is **vascular endothelial cells**. These are cells within arteries that neutralize factors leading to atherosclerosis; thus, these cells help avert CVD. An even more important defense is based on the biochemistry of **free radicals** and **antioxidants**. Free radicals are a form of stress in the arteries (technically known as **oxidative stress**). Antioxidants have the unique ability to bind to free radicals, thereby rendering them harmless to the arteries. This is one reason, among many, why you may have read and heard so much about foods that are rich sources of antioxidants. In a visual form, you can think of antioxidants as being a type of barrier to oxidative stress.

Free radicals circulate in the arteries.   Antioxidants may be present.

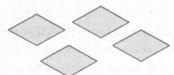

If so, the antioxidants bind with the free radicals.

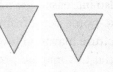

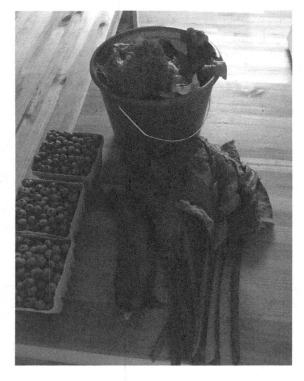

Photo 5.3   T typical daily bounty from a home garden in New England

Elevated Blood Sugar Levels

A chronic state of elevated blood sugar levels is perhaps the most insidious of the four issues that make up metabolic syndrome. Of the four, this one has been the subject of intense public health research. In terms of CVD, this research implicates refined sugars as a primary cause of elevated triglyceride levels as well as central obesity. In short, the copious consumption of refined sugars by Americans is a leading cause of CVD. Further recent evidence strongly implicates refined sugars as a more prominent cause of obesity than fats. This is important and intriguing because estimates suggest that the average American consumes 57 pounds of refined sugar each year! Sugary foods are used as part of celebrations in American culture (e.g., birthday cakes, Valentine's chocolates, Christmas cookies, summer ice cream, Halloween treats). However, the vast majority of this 57 pounds comes from everyday foods such as condiments for burgers, cornbread, pies, milkshakes, sauces, and – most importantly – soft drinks and energy drinks. All of this will become clearer to you in **Chapter 6**; as noted previously, this chapter does not discuss sugar in detail. Nonetheless, a key point relative to sugar is a simple one: foods in their natural state do not have sugars that can harm the body (see **Photo 5.3**)!

Obesity Is Contagious

the copious consumption of refined sugars by Americans is a leading cause of CVD

In a now-famous public health study, Christakis and Fowler (2007) used data from the largest prospective study of CVD in the United States (known as the **Framingham study**) to learn about the effect of social connections on obesity. Based on a sample of more than 12,000 people who were assessed repeatedly between 1971 and 2003, these researchers determined that obesity (defined as a BMI of at least 30) was found in what they called **clusters** of people. Defined by social ties, these clusters were highly predictive of whether people met or exceeded the BMI criteria for obesity during any given assessment interval. For instance, having a close friend who was obese during any given assessment interval increased the odds of the person interviewed being obese by about 57%. Similar findings applied to siblings and married persons in that having a brother, sister, or spouse report a BMI classified as obese during an assessment period also increased the odds of the person interviewed being obese.

So, the take-home point from this study of social ties and obesity is that people who share a given food culture may tend toward the norms of that culture. Thus, some clusters of people bonded by social ties may be protected from obesity based on shared values and behaviors relative to exercise and diet. Conversely, other clusters may share values and behaviors that tend toward high-calorie diets of non-PBWFs and a largely sedentary lifestyle.

Regulating the Food Industry

Estimates indicate that up to 90% of the American food supply is produced by less than 15% of all farms. Here, it is important not to think about a farm in terms of past farms or the farms you may have seen in movies such *Field of Dreams*, with Kevin Costner. Instead, think of farms as large-scale companies. These companies have become known as **agribusiness**. In 2009, the movie *Food Inc.* became popular and remains valuable today. This documentary described and showed the inner workings of the farms that provide food to most Americans. The movie is a reasonable landmark in recent history to pinpoint a time when agribusiness first received intense scrutiny from the public as well as non-governmental watchdog agencies. Using graphic video footage and live interviews, the documentary makes it clear that the health of the American public is at risk based on relatively common agribusiness practices. For instance, viewers learned vital and hidden facts such as cows being fed a corn-based diet (which is not natural) and how that translates into a risk of *E. coli* infection for humans. Americans learned that chickens are raised almost artificially, with their bodies pumped full of hormones and antibiotics. They learned that giant corporations spawned widespread poverty among farmers and farm workers through patents on seeds. Further, viewers learned that the states must rely on the U.S. Congress to pass laws to protect an otherwise vulnerable public from a cadre of health risks imposed due to greed and a lack of ethics in the food industry.

A prime example of agribusiness is the company **Monsanto**. This company is a leader in creating **genetically modified organisms** (GMOs). The motivation behind GMOs is greater crop yields and thus greater profit margins. For example, one of the most commonly consumed GMOs in the United States is corn. Through genetic modifications, this crop is robust to drought, destruction by insects, and so on. Consequently, corn is a low-cost food that is used widely by agribusiness to make products ranging from breakfast cereals and breads to pancake mix, salad dressings, tortilla chips, soft drinks, and even peanut butter. In each of these highly processed foods, a key ingredient is high-fructose corn syrup (see **Box 5.2**).

Let's focus on a term you just read about in Box 5.2: the verb **subsidize**. When the U.S. government subsidizes crops such as corn, wheat, rice, and soybeans, farmers are paid to grow these crops. These payments, of course, are in addition to the income farmers receive from

> When the U.S. government subsidizes crops such as corn, wheat, rice, and soybeans, farmers are paid to grow these crops

BOX 5.2. HIGH FRUCTOSE CORN SYRUP

Unless your diet consists mostly of whole foods, you probably consume more corn-based products that you can imagine. Beef, for example, is a corn-based product. This may surprise you and even cause you to re-read the sentence to be sure you understood. Beef is corn-based because agribusiness has found that cattle grow more efficiently if they are fed a diet of corn rather than their natural diet of grass (of course, this practice raises other issues, such as the use of antibiotics in cattle feed because they are not animals that can stay free of disease on a corn-based diet). Moreover, fast food hamburgers are often "bulked up" with corn to make the product more cost-efficient to produce.

A landmark book titled *The Omnivore's Dilemma: A Natural History of Four Meals* (Pollan, 2007) provides compelling detail about the ubiquitous use of corn as a "filler" ingredient and primary ingredient in the majority of the products sold in most U.S. grocery stores. Most remarkable is that agribusiness has thus far succeeded in saturating the U.S. food market with a corn-based sweetener known as **high fructose corn syrup**. Collectively, eating meat from corn-fed animals, eating a predominance of corn as a grain (especially in cereals, snack foods, and corn tortillas), and consuming large amounts of high-fructose corn syrup are implicated as causative agents in developing CVD, obesity, diabetes, and tooth decay and even as potentially causative agents in some forms of cancer (Pollan, 2007).

Now for the kicker: the U.S. Department of Agriculture provides several billion dollars each year to subsidize corn production in the United States. This keeps prices low and thus greatly increases access, especially for people who have a limited budget (or no budget) for food. So, the corn products we eat are by design of policy passed in Washington DC, not by design of public health experts. Certainly, the advantage is that these low prices keep many people from experiencing food insecurity. The cost, however, is that millions of Americans are experiencing negative health effects due to these government subsidies. Ultimately, the U.S. government is funding the massive growth of a crop that produces considerable morbidity and mortality.

Source: A landmark book known as The Omnivore's Dilemma: A Natural History of Four Meals (Pollen, 2007).

Table 5.2   What should people look for on food labels?

What to look for	Why it is important
Total calories per serving*	This is important for weight control.
Fiber content	Fiber is good; it keeps the calorie count low and helps prevent CVD.
Fat content	
Unsaturated fats	This type of fat is the least likely to cause CVD.
Saturated fats/Trans fats	These are primary causes of CVD.
Sodium content	Excessive sodium leads to hypertension.
Total carbohydrate	Look for sugar content under this heading, as sugars are implicated in both CVD and obesity.

*Because all entries in this table are based on a per-serving amount, this phrase is only shown once.

selling the crops. Thus, it is logical to ask, "Why not promote public health by ending subsidies for crops such as corn?" If this is a question you are asking yourself as you read this chapter, you are in good company; but unfortunately, the answer is based on political action committees from agribusiness having a huge influence over maintaining the subsidies given to farmers. Consequently, the seemingly simple upstream approach to preventing CVD and obesity in the United States has yet to gain any real traction.

Although not as powerful as eliminating subsidies, a more realistic public health approach to regulating the food industry involves labeling laws, prohibiting the use of antibiotics in some animals, and prohibiting the use of growth hormones in pigs, chickens, and turkeys. **Table 5.2** provides a bit of detail about labeling laws that pertain to CVD and obesity. As you read this table, keep in mind that the information shown on food labels is based on a serving size selected and specified by the manufacturing company. This can be deceiving when serving sizes are artificially low, such as 1 ounce or half a cup.

Of course, the concept of regulating the food industry by passing and enforcing food labeling laws relies on consumer education and the will of people to take the time to study their foods. Food labeling also implies that consumers must be able to read and understand the information. Sadly, evidence suggests that the majority of people purchasing food products with labels do not read the information provided. Those who do take time to read labels often are looking for something very specific (e.g., total calories) and may not fully understand what they are reading or what it means relative to CVD and obesity risk. Regulating the food industry to prevent CVD and obesity must be extended far beyond this relatively benign practice.

the concept of regulating the food industry by passing and enforcing food labeling laws relies on consumer education

As for using antibiotics, this practice remains legal in the United States, provided that the antibiotics are used to avert disease rather than promote growth. At issue in this practice is the global problem of antibiotic resistance. Although this issue is not germane to CVD or obesity, it warrants mention at this point in the textbook. This resistance occurs because bacteria residing in cows, poultry, or pigs eventually mutate to survive, and these variants then become dominant until a different type of antibiotic is used. When the animals harboring these resistant bacteria are slaughtered, intestinal waste becomes a hazardous by-product, with bacteria often inadvertently entering the packed meat during production. Further, the manure of these animals (especially dairy cows and beef cattle) compounds the spread of antibiotic-resistant bacteria when it contaminates crops of fruits and vegetables.

Finally, it is noteworthy that any pork products or poultry sold in the United States must – by regulation of the Food and Drug Administration – be from livestock that was not given hormones of any kind. Unfortunately, this same regulation does not apply to dairy cows or beef cattle. Dairy cows are routinely given a growth hormone to stimulate milk production; this practice is common throughout the United States. Beef cattle are given hormones (often via an implant in their ears) throughout most of their lives. These hormones are used to essentially speed up production, meaning the cattle can be slaughtered for their meat sooner. The health effects of indirectly consuming these hormones by eating this meat are, as yet, unknown, but the indirect consumption by humans of these hormones **may** be a contributing factor to CVD and/or obesity.

A final set of regulations that this chapter considers involves fast-food chains. Regulating the fast-food industry is especially important given that estimates suggest the average American spends one-third of their food budget at fast-food chains. In the 1990s, federal laws were passed requiring fast-food companies (such as Burger King, Wendy's, and McDonald's) to post the calorie, fat, sugar, and sodium content of each product appearing on the menu. This (at least for some Americans) offered a chance to more fully understand the real cost of eating fast food. **Real cost** in this sense means trade-offs exist between the low prices paid for these foods and their very high levels of unhealthy ingredients designed **only** to enhance flavor and consumer satisfaction. As an example, let's deconstruct the Burger King Whopper. The Whopper with cheese contains 740 calories, most of which (57%) are in the form of fats. So, from the standpoint of obesity, this common entree is a culprit in America's problem with weight gain. Thinking now about CVD, the Whopper unduly impacts metabolic syndrome through its high cholesterol content (111 mg.), high sodium content (1,339 mg), and high levels of saturated fat (15.8 g). This sandwich also contains 11 g of sugar, more than twice the daily suggested limit for females and past the 10 g suggested limit for males. Combined with the high calorie count, it becomes easy for you to see that all four issues involved in metabolic syndrome are largely exacerbated by fast foods such as the Whopper. As a caveat, and to punctuate the public health problem of fast foods, also consider that most people have more than just a sandwich when eating fast food. Changing examples to the McDonald's Triple Thick Shake, this beverage has about 50% more calories (1,160) than the Whopper. For millions of Americans, the burger and shake alone provide more than enough calories for their daily needs; any additional calories are stored as fat. Quite separate from exceeding a balance of calories and energy expenditure is the point that the burger-and-shake routine is very much a causative agent of CVD. But Americans spend billions of dollars on fast food each year, with more than four of every five families eating fast food at least once each week. One reason may be the **comfort factor** (see **Box 5.3**).

Regulating the fast food industry is certainly a mammoth challenge for the future of public health practice. For now, the only real progress in this area has come from local municipalities. Cities and towns have the legal authority to control whether any given business (including fast-food chains) can operate in any given location. For decades, fast-food outlets have been strategic in placing their restaurants in easy-to-reach (swing in and swing out by car) locations to tempt people to buy their foods on the way to work (quickie breakfast sandwiches) and on the way home from work (pick up dinner in a box). At a local level, zoning ordinances can go a long way to end this practice.

Emerging Programs That Promote Improved Population-Level Nutrition

One of the most intriguing aspects of public health is that its landscape is constantly evolving to meet the ever-changing needs of people. The **farm-to-table** movement in America is an excellent example of this public health evolution. The concept of the farm-to-table movement is entirely consistent with what you have learned so far in this chapter. **Figure 5.2** provides a visual illustration of the tenets involved in farm-to-table programs.

BOX 5.3. THE HUMAN SIDE

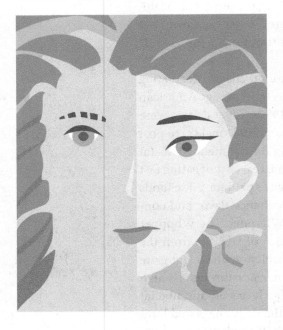

Children often learn that some foods are given to them for the express reason of being happy. Known as **comfort foods**, meals that have lasting taste and keep the brain in a state of satiation (meaning the hunger center of the brain sends out signals to indicate a full stomach) are an American favorite. Extra-crispy fried chicken and creamy mashed potatoes, for example, are a common comfort food for kids, and this habit may easily be carried into adulthood and even the senior years of life. Similarly, desserts such as ice cream, pies, and cakes are prized comfort foods in U.S. cultures. Perhaps the all-time-favorite comfort food – pizza – dominates the fast-food market.

The science behind comfort food is relatively simple. Mounting evidence suggests that comfort foods stimulate the pleasure centers of the brain and may mimic (although to a lesser degree) the same neuropathways triggered by drug addiction. In the sense of being a type of drug, comfort foods allow people to freely self-medicate issues such as depression, loneliness, and fatigue. These forms of self-medication may even become habitual. The sense of extreme pleasure and happiness induced by so many comfort foods may also become a type of self-reward. In this regard, people incentivize their own hard work or successful efforts with a jolt of a drug-like substance (i.e., comfort food) to the pleasure centers of the brain.

Thus, the human side of CVD and obesity is that people are not perfect; they medicate their psychological pains with fats, sugars, and high-sodium foods. Further, they stimulate the reward center of the brain in a way that is not only socially acceptable but also socially rewarded (e.g., comfort foods like potato chips and burgers at outdoor parties). Whether the foods associated with comfort, and therefore pleasure, are those that people learned to love during childhood is a question that has yet to be answered. The more important question for adults, however, is "How can the brain be redirected to respond to healthy foods as though they were comfort foods?"

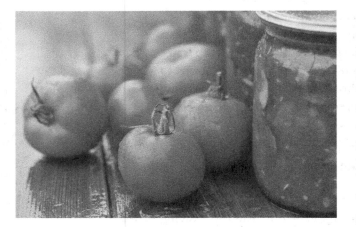

Photo 5.4   Home canning tomatoes is a common method of preserving summer's bounty for winter months.
Source: ortodoxfoto/Adobe stock.

Starting in the top-right corner of this figure, the concept that foods should be fresh is deceptively simple. To make this tenet a reality, farm-to-table programs must be planned to optimize the use of local farms and minimize the travel distance between these farms and the population served by the program. This planning ensures that PBWFs can be preserved in their natural state given a close proximity to the people who will consume them. As a rule, foods that best nourish the body have a short shelf life: they must be consumed within 7 to 10 days after harvest. Of course, this point raises the ultimate issue with farm-to-table programs: they can only provide fresh foods during the growing season (which in some parts of the United States is only a few months). An old-school solution to this involves home canning – a labor-intensive process that requires a great deal of energy (i.e., heat to boil water) and thus is costly (see **Photo 5.4**).

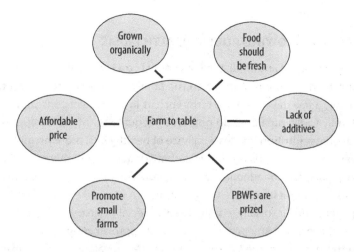

Figure 5.2   Tenets of the farm-to-table movement in America

An alternative to canning is freezing. Like canning, this is a process and thus removes the food a bit from its natural state. Nonetheless, most PBWFs maintain their nutritional integrity during the freezing process. A more affordable alternative to canning and freezing involves farm-to-table foods that naturally stay preserved. These include black-eyed peas, beans (kidney, lima, pinto, navy, etc.), butternut squash, spaghetti squash, and pumpkins.

Regardless of how locally grown foods are stored for consumption, the mere act of keeping the foods in the same geographic area where they were raised is also vital to public health in terms of stemming the tide of climate change. Many people consider food as having its own carbon footprint, meaning it becomes progressively more of a carbon liability as it travels farther from its source. This is why, for example, PBWFs that are fresh but out of season (e.g., strawberries, lettuce, spinach, and sweet corn in the winter months) are not compatible with the culture that has been created relative to the farm-to-table movement.

Moving clockwise around **Figure 5.2**, the tenets of minimal to no additives and prizing a PBWF diet are paramount in farm-to-table programs. Generally speaking, food additives can present health problems to enough of any population to make the additives an overall liability. The farm-to-table movement recognizes this and thus does not engage in the for-profit action of extending the shelf life of foods with preservatives of any kind. This concept of respecting food and not altering its natural state is part of the farm-to-table culture. From a larger perspective, the concept of prizing a largely PBWF diet is catalyzed by the farm-to-table movement. This is not to suggest that farm-to-table eschews meat, dairy, cheese, eggs, and other animal-based products. Instead, the farm-to-table movement is simply a logical home for people who value the health benefits of a PBWF diet.

Again moving clockwise around **Figure 5.2**, the farm-to-table philosophy embodies the American ideal of local farmers independent from agribusiness. Milk is a great example. An independent dairy farmer is likely to lose money every day. For instance, the cost of producing 100 pounds of milk is about $22.50, while the sale price for 100 pounds of milk typically falls between $15.00 and $19.00. Thus, producing milk actually costs the farmer money. The following quote is taken from the Farm Aid website (Farm Aid, 2018):

Since 1970, the number of American dairy farms has dropped by more than 93 percent, from more than 640,000 to around 40,000 today [2018]. In an industry dominated by corporate interests, family farms are constantly at risk of going under. A consistent, severe slump in milk prices in recent years has pushed many dairy farm businesses beyond the point of survival.

> most PBWFs maintain their nutritional integrity during the freezing process

BOX 5.4. FOOD INSECURITY IN AMERICA: A GROWING PUBLIC HEALTH CRISIS

Broadly defined as "less than reliable" access to food (of any kind), the concept of **food insecurity** is about conditions such as those often occurring for families near the end of the month, when the family income is received on the first of the month. Hunger may be transient – lasting only a few days – or long-term, such as in the case of consistently spending less on food to the point where people in a family (or living alone) do not have adequate nutrition to support healthy daily activities and neurological functioning. Adequate nutrition implies a balance of healthy fats, proteins, and complex carbohydrates. The term further implies that diets largely comprising simple carbohydrates (e.g., highly refined breads, pastas, and foods based largely on corn or refined sugars) are not adequate and therefore constitute food insecurity.

Given its intimate link with poverty – as you might imagine – this public health issue (like so many others) disproportionately impacts persons who are economically and/or socially marginalized, especially persons of color. Food insecurity is an ongoing problem for approximately one of every five Americans. This value of approximately 20% was derived after the start of the COVID-19 pandemic; prior to the pandemic, the U.S. estimate for the prevalence of food insecurity ranged between 13% and 17%. That 20% of the population is consistently placed in harm's way because a lack of nutritious food creates a corresponding lack of immunity, issues with chronic disease, and even safety issues relative to efforts to obtain food. Food insecurity further exacerbates threats to public health as a consequence of its devastating effects on senior citizens, who are often faced with overwhelming medical bills, and on children, given that basic learning skills needed for school are compromised when nutrient intakes are lacking.

The relationship of food insecurity with CVD and obesity is a strong one! This involves both agribusiness and fast-food chains. Agribusiness products such as high fructose corn syrup (see **Box 5.2**) and boxed macaroni and cheese create sustenance to keep people alive, but without the benefit of antioxidants or other heart-protective properties. Because they are highly refined, these same foods tend to cause obesity. Inexpensive fast foods such as burgers and fries give people temporary relief from hunger at the expense of creating an unhealthy lipid profile, as well as increasing other indicators of metabolic syndrome such as blood pressure (via the high sodium content) and central obesity (via the high levels of mass-produced meat).

Ultimately, because locally produced foods – and even beverages such as wine and beer – are not part of the agribusiness empire, they can be both produced and sold to consumers at a price far below similar products made available through the hands of large corporations. Thus, the farm-to-table movement puts the business of feeding America back in the hands of local farmers who are not indebted to corporate monopolies. The greater level of affordability to consumers is also a tremendous advantage in addressing the wicked public health problems of CVD and obesity. The advantage involves making healthy diets a realistic possibility for people with very limited food budgets. This is a vital aspect of public health practice because of the massive food insecurity in the United States (see **Box 5.4**).

Finally, the farm-to-table movement embraces the ethic of growing food organically. To be certified as organically grown, plant-based foods cannot be raised using synthetic fertilizers or synthetic pesticides. Further, the seeds must not be genetically modified. And certified organic food cannot be irradiated at any time (the food industry frequently uses radiation to kill bacteria in foods). Certified animal-based foods must come from livestock that were not fed any type of animal by-product and were raised in the complete absence of synthetic hormones and antibiotics. Further, the livestock must have had access to the outdoors, and grass-eating animals (e.g., cows, sheep, goats) must have had access to pasture.

A twist on being certified as organic applies to the farm-to-table movement in that low-income farmers may practice all the ethics involved in raising organic plants and animals but lack the formal certification conferred by the government. This, of course, does not compromise the food in any way.

Sitting Is the New Smoking

As you know by now, public health research is critical to understanding how upstream actions can best be used to avert morbidity and mortality. Some of the most important recent public health research implicates chronic sitting as a health risk behavior for both CVD and obesity. Specifically, this emerging evidence implicates sitting as a cause of lowering the metabolic rate in the body: the body adopts an **inactivity physiology**, which means it adjusts (in a bad way) to doing nothing by slowing down its metabolic needs. This inactivity physiology leads to CVD, obesity, and diabetes. The altered physiology is reversible, but only with a renewed routine of daily movement. Otherwise, for people who sit eight hours or more each day, this inactivity physiology becomes the new normal for their body.

Without overwhelming you with detail, the basis for implying that sitting is a risk behavior on par with smoking involves the concept of **metabolic equivalents** (METS). METS are personalized ratios based on the amount of energy needed for a person to do nothing but sit. One MET is the unit of energy it takes to just sit for a defined period of time. Two METS double that energy expenditure by engaging in activities such as walking. As a person's movement becomes more vigorous, the METS increase accordingly.

Given this basic information about METS, let's dive a bit deeper into the subjects of movement and exercise. **Sedentary** behaviors are those that involve sitting and very low levels of energy expenditure (1.0 to 1.5 METS). METs of 1.5 to 2.9 are considered relatively sedentary yet somewhat active, such as moving around a house while cleaning, doing laundry, grocery shopping, walking at a gentle pace, and engaging in everyday actions such as cooking, using stairs, and so forth. Therefore, this 1.5 to 2.9 range is distinguished from just plain sitting and is considered moderate physical activity. Exercise behaviors begin at 3.0 METS and go as high as 8.0! Vigorous exercise such as cycling, running, and swimming raises METS to 5.0 or more for most people. The public health value of knowing this is that people can benefit from even modest movement (1.5 to 2.9 METS), but even mild exercise (e.g., 3.0 to 5.0 METS) is much better. With this knowledge firmly in mind, you can appreciate why a vital upstream approach to CVD and obesity is focused on promoting daily movement and even moderate exercise.

But as much as the public health goal of promoting movement makes sense, it is clear that U.S. culture encourages sitting. People are typically sitting when they commute to work. For many people working in white-collar jobs, their workplace is loaded with chairs; and sitting is normative, even expected, during meetings. Upon returning home from work to the domestic environment, sitting is a built-in part of what millions of Americas do during their leisure time. Watching television, movies, or streaming video are all actions paired with sitting. Similarly, using a computer and even talking or texting on phones is often a sitting-based activity.

A logical question you should have by now is, why is there a new emphasis on avoiding sitting behaviors? The answer involves our modern environment. Think about all the things that are designed into our daily lives!

- Most white-collar jobs demand long hours of computer use (from a METS perspective, this is no different from TV viewing).

- Reading is no better than TV viewing, as most people read while sitting.

- Even new forms of transportation (e.g., micro-transportation) encourage very little energy expenditure. Walking is often discouraged for reasons involving time, safety, or weather.

- Leisure-time activities increasingly involve screen time. For example, Netflix, FaceTime, Zoom, video games, internet use, and cell phone use all encourage sitting rather than movement.

- Some states and municipalities do not invest in outdoor (or indoor) recreational facilities, leaving it up to the individual to find a way to be active rather than making activity an easy daily option.

Promoting Daily Movement and Exercise

A built environment is designed and engineered to attract and entice people to use it for its intended purpose

As a means of achieving population-level reductions in the mean BMI and obtaining population-level increases (i.e., delays) in the mean age of first heart attacks or strokes, the public health success story is all about **built environments**. Think back to **Chapter 2**, and remember (or reread) what you learned about the Atlanta Beltline. This is a stellar example of a built environment. A built environment is designed and engineered to attract and entice people to use it for its intended purpose. The concept of enhancing **walkability** was the initial goal of built environments. Walkability implies that the walking path/area is safe, has ample lighting, is aesthetically pleasing (e.g., green space, trees, shrubs, absence of trash or other eyesores), and serves a purpose in terms of its location (provides on-foot transportation to places that otherwise would be accessed by car, bus, train, etc.). As walkability became progressively more popular, the concept of built environments was extended to running, cycling, and other METS-intensive forms of movement.

urban planning and development can be informed by public health practice

With the concept of built environments firmly in your grasp, you can now consider this statement: urban planning and development can be informed by public health practice. Again, you learned in **Chapter 2** that public health is not a profession per se; instead, it is a shared responsibility of all people. On the other hand, urban planning is a profession that can and would greatly benefit from people like you (given your familiarity with public health) bringing an upstream perspective to the planning process. To accentuate this point, let's consider a tale of two cities.

City A has a population of 350,000 in the space of about 100 square miles. This city has invested in over 1,000 miles of paved asphalt running/biking trails, 30 playgrounds, 4 city parks large enough for dog-walking and soccer fields, and over 50 other public recreation areas such as tennis courts, baseball fields, river walks, and mountain climbing trails.

City B has a population of 300,000 in about 122 square miles. This city has invested in a single paved asphalt running/biking trail just under 10 miles long. It has a collection of 22 playgrounds, but most of them are outdated and located in dangerous places. All other forms of recreation (indoor and outdoor) are privately owned and operated, such as tennis clubs, indoor gyms, and rowing clubs.

Ultimately, *City A* will be a far more attractive place for people to live and buy real estate (even at prices much higher than those in *City B*). As the people in *City A* become progressively more accustomed to using their built environment, it is likely that population-level indicators such as blood pressure, blood sugar levels, BMI, and so on will improve. *City A* may eventually attract retirees as well as young people to become residents, thereby raising the tax base and creating added funding to maintain and expand the built environment. In short, *City A* is far more likely to thrive than *City B*, and the people of *City A* are likely to live longer and healthier lives than *City B* residents.

This brief introduction to built environments raises another question for you to ponder: "Should municipal governments pay for built environments, or is it better to let the free market dictate outdoor (and indoor) recreation opportunities?" This is, of course, the ultimate controversy pertaining to built environments. Astute voters and informed citizens need to understand the public health advantages of such funding. At a federal level, the advantages have been spelled out clearly by the United States Prevention Services Task Force; this body is a respected part of the U.S. Public Health Service, and it strongly advocates that governments invest in built environments to reduce health care costs and, by extension, increase the quality and quantity of life for residents.

A Cautionary Note: Preventing CVD and Obesity Involves People Making Lifetime Commitments

So far, this textbook has not used the term **wellness**. This is because the term is relatively amorphous and thus of little value. However, CVD and obesity are an exception, meaning the concept of **wellness** is applicable and appropriate. Rather than being defined as the absence of disease, wellness is conceptualized as the polar opposite of disease. For instance, just as a person may have mild clinical symptoms of CVD, someone of the same age may have relatively low levels of triglycerides, cholesterol, blood pressure, and fasting blood sugar. From a medical care perspective, this same-age, relatively healthy person would simply be called **normal** (meaning at or below any clinical indications of CVD). But the medical perspective misses the point of the bell-shaped curve.

In science, the bell-shaped curve has been used to characterize almost every trait or physical aspect of humans. It has been applied to intelligence, weight, height, gender conformity, and physiological characteristics such as heart rate, blood pressure, and so on. The eloquence of the bell-shaped curve lies in its mirror-image effect. In essence, for every person at the far-right end of the curve, there is a person at the mirror opposite position on the far-left end of the curve. So, let's apply this to CVD and the concept of wellness.

Figure 5.3 provides a useful visual relative to the concept of wellness as it relates to CVD. Suppose a risk index for CVD is administered to 1,000 people. The index assesses the various risks that make up metabolic syndrome. The scores obtained for the population of 1,000 people range from a near-complete absence of risk (i.e., scores of 2) to extremely high risk (i.e., scores of 18). As shown, the portion of the curve at the greatest clinical risk of stroke and heart attack (i.e., the extreme right-hand portion of the curve's total area) has a mirror opposite on the left-hand side. The people at this mirror opposite end are likely to be marathon runners, triathletes, distance swimmers, and so on. They are not merely normal when it comes to CVD risk; they are greatly fortified by having very low levels of overall risk. They personify the

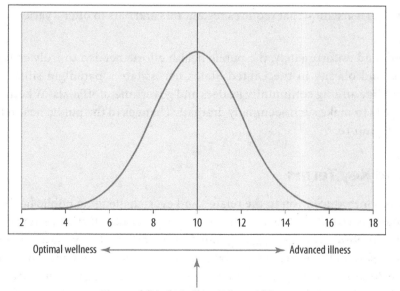

Optimal wellness ← → Advanced illness

↑
Absence of clinically significant indicators of disease

Figure 5.3   A visual depiction of wellness

concept of wellness because they are distinct from what would be considered normal (with **normal** being the curve's height, where the vast majority of the 1,000 people are located in the figure (i.e., scores of 10).

As applied to CVD and obesity, the concept of wellness can be extended to habits and actions rather than being relegated to only physical indicators. Thus, a person who has consumed a PBWF diet for several decades would be at the far-left end of the curve for both CVD risk and obesity risk. The take-home point is that public health practice does not lump people into the categories of normal versus diseased. Instead, when it comes to CVD and obesity, public health practice encourages lifelong habits that confer significant protection against ever crossing into a clinically defined zone such as being diagnosed as obese, having elevated cholesterol, or having hypertension.

Now that you are familiar with the concept of wellness, let's take a final look at the primary prevention of CVD and obesity. Without question, the ethic of preventing CVD and obesity is that daily health-protective behaviors must begin early in life and continue indefinitely. The idea of crossing far into the right-hand extreme in terms of CVD risk on a curve such as **Figure 5.3** and then moving back to the far left is wishful thinking. This is not to say that some highly motivated, well-resourced people cannot turn this wishful thinking into reality. But remember that public health is about entire populations rather than individuals per se. So, on a population-wide scale, efforts to reverse CVD and obesity after people cross into the illness side of the spectrum will not be nearly as effective as equally applied efforts to keep as many people on the far left of the spectrum as possible. These efforts would involve public health actions such as these:

the ethic of preventing CVD and obesity is that daily health-protective behaviors must begin early in life and continue indefinitely

- Subsidizing plant-based agricultural practices

- Making locally grown, whole foods a benefit of public assistance programs

- Helping municipal governments design and build structures that promote movement and walkability

- Taxing highly processed foods, especially those with direct links to CVD and obesity

- Creating local legislation that requires restaurants and bars to offer a variety of low-sodium foods/drinks

Ultimately, and unfortunately, the public health efforts needed to truly change the prevalence of CVD and obesity in the United States necessitate a paradigm shift requiring bold action and courage among community leaders and government officials. Whether this level of willingness exists to make such seemingly dramatic changes to the public health landscape is a question for the future.

Review and Key Terms

This chapter has introduced you to the related and ever-challenging public health problems of **cardiovascular disease** and obesity (particularly **central obesity**). A primary term in all of this is **metabolic syndrome**. Comprising four factors, this syndrome lays out a public health agenda that can save millions of lives and billions of medical care dollars. This agenda features **plant-based whole foods** (PBWFs) naturally low in sodium, sugars, and unfavorable **lipids** such as **cholesterol** and **triglycerides**. *The China Study* firmly established the outstanding value of a PBWF diet in the primary prevention of both CVD and obesity.

A second and equally viable public approach to reducing the four factors of metabolic syndrome involves daily **movement**. Although more vigorous exercise – consuming at least

3.0 **metabolic equivalents** – is important, promoting ongoing daily movement consuming 1.5 to 2.9 METS is a worthy public health agenda. A currently successful (and expanding) public health approach to promoting both movement and exercise is based on the concept of **built environments**. Even making public spaces more user-friendly for walking (i.e., **walkability**) has significant potential to help reduce population levels of **BMI**, thereby addressing America's epidemic of being **overweight** and obese. Separate from its part in metabolic syndrome, the epidemic of obesity is perhaps the most prevalent **health-compromising condition** in the United States.

Other valuable public health approaches to the primary prevention of CVD and obesity involve regulating **agribusiness** and **subsidizing** PBWFs rather than animal-based foods, as is currently common in our nation. An especially paramount aspect of regulating agribusiness pertains to **genetically modified organisms**. The extent of harm to humans from GMOs is not yet fully understood; however, evidence strongly suggests health implications relative to CVD and obesity. Regarding government-based food subsidies, a foreseeable future for public health involves subsidizing the **farm-to-table** movement in the United States. Farm-to-table has the potential to become a population-level response to the growing problems posed by agribusiness.

A few of the final points made in this chapter shed further light on why millions of Americans continue to consume foods that exacerbate metabolic syndrome (i.e., **comfort eating**) and new research on the **inactivity physiology** created by chronic sitting. Ultimately, the public health approach that substantially averts both CVD and obesity begins in childhood and continues throughout life. The concept of **wellness** applies nicely to this point in that public health can and thus should constantly be a driver of more and more favorable numbers when it comes to metabolic syndrome indicators.

For Practice and Class Discussion

Practice Questions

1. Which one of the following is **least** relevant to metabolic syndrome?
   a. Built environments
   b. Triglycerides
   c. Body mass index
   d. Prevalence rates

2. Which term is the **least** consistent with the tenets of the farm-to-table movement?
   a. Organically grown
   b. Low to moderate use of mild antibiotics
   c. Smaller carbon footprint
   d. PBWF friendly

3. The concept of wellness implies all of the following **except**:
   a. Any given population will have relatively equal numbers of people at either extreme of a bell-shaped curve.
   b. **Normal** is represented by the entire area to the left of the mean in the bell-shaped curve.
   c. As a rule, lower numbers are always better when it comes to blood pressure, heart rate, and lipid levels.

4. In terms of METS, which statement is true?
   a. Even 1.5 METS is enough to qualify as moderate to vigorous physical activity (MVPA).
   b. METS must exceed 4.0 to truly count movement as a benefit to health.
   c. METS of 1.5 to 3.0 represent healthy movement and qualify as MVPA.
   d. METS are a measure of sodium intake and do not relate to movement or exercise.

5. Arnold is currently overweight but not yet obese. He is 15 years old and consumes a heavily animal-based diet. Barring public health intervention or independent behavior change, how likely is Arnold to become an obese adult?
   a. Extremely likely
   b. Somewhat likely
   c. It is unpredictable.
   d. Not likely because most teens grow out of this overweight phase

6. Which food is **least** likely to lead to chronic hypertension?
   a. Commercially canned tomatoes
   b. A GMO-free product used to make cornbread
   c. A sodium-free hamburger
   d. Red beans and rice made from scratch

7. Which example **best** illustrates the concept of a built environment?
   a. A city closes off entire downtown streets to all vehicles between 8:00 a.m. and 6:00 p.m. every weekday. Only pedestrians and cyclists are allowed to enter and use these streets.
   b. A workplace begins to offer all employees a 30-minute break between their lunch hour and the end of the shift at 5:00 p.m. Management constantly posts reminders that this added time should be used for vigorous movement.

8. Which term/phrase is **least** related to the concept of wellness as applied to CVD?
   a. Subsidizing corn
   b. Subsidizing farm-to-table movements
   c. Food labeling laws
   d. Regulating the fast-food industry

9. *The China Study* pertains to all of the following **except**:
   a. Metabolic syndrome
   b. Cholesterol
   c. Triglycerides
   d. Sustained daily movement

10. Which factor of metabolic syndrome tends to be socially contagious?
    a. Comfort eating
    b. Obesity
    c. Hypertension
    d. Inactivity physiology

For Discussion (in class or small groups, or online)

11. Among the most prominent sources of sodium in the American diet are fast-food chains such as Burger King, McDonald's, and Wendy's. Go online to find the sodium content of items at these chain stores, such as milkshakes, hamburgers, chicken filet sandwiches, and desserts. Using this information, construct a table similar to Table 5.1 in this chapter. Comparing tables with other students in the class, determine the **top five offenders** at fast-food chains in terms of sodium content.

12. Find at least one other student to work with, and go online to the landing page for the Food and Drug Administration. The FDA provides a mountain of information about countless topics. Your shared task is to sift through the FDA regulations relative to recent (since 2020) policies that control the use of growth hormones and/or antibiotics in animals that are subsequently consumed by people. Try to organize a one-page summary of your findings using these headings:

   - New FDA regulations pertaining to dairy cows

   - New FDA regulation pertaining to beef cattle

   - New FDA regulation pertaining to poultry

   - New FDA regulation pertaining to swine (pork)

13. If you were personally affected by the part of this chapter on the health advantages of eating a PBWF diet, you may enjoy reading *The China Study*. Specifically, read parts of the study about evidence suggesting that a PBWF diet may reverse CVD in some people. Then, to challenge yourself, try to answer a few key questions:

   a. Is the evidence clear, or is it simply anecdotal (i.e., based on a few case studies)?
   b. Can the level of plaque buildup in artery walls be substantially reduced through diet alone?
   c. How many years does an average person need to maintain a PBWF diet before any significant improvement in CVD occurs?

References

Harvard Health Publishing. (2016). The heart attack gender gap. https://www.health.harvard.edu/heart-health/the-heart-attack-gender-gap

Campbell, T. C., & Campbell, T. M. (2005). *The China study*. Bella Books: Belfast, Maine.

CDC. (2021). Adult obesity prevalence maps. https://www.cdc.gov/obesity/data/prevalence-maps.html#overall

Christakis, N. A., & Fowler, J. H. (2007). The spread of obesity in a large social network over 30 years. *New England Journal of Medicine, 357*, 370–379.

Farm Aid. (2018). Dairy: Family farmers in crisis. https://www.farmaid.org/blog/fact-sheet/dairy-family-farmers-in-crisis/

Illades, C. (2021). 10 high-sodium foods to avoid. Everyday Health. https://www.everydayhealth.com/heart-health-pictures/10-sneaky-sodium-bombs.aspx

Liu, K., Davigius, M. L., & Lorie, C. M. (2012). Healthy lifestyle through young adulthood and the presence of low cardiovascular disease risk profile in middle age. *Circulation, 125*, 996–1004.

Pollan, M. (2007). *The omnivore's dilemma: A natural history of four meals*. Penguin Books.

CHAPTER 6

PREVENTING DIABETES: A PUBLIC HEALTH PRIORITY

LEARNING OBJECTIVES

1. Understand the biological process of glucose metabolism, the role of insulin, and the conditions that lead to Type 2 diabetes.

2. Understand what is meant by the phrase "diabetes develops day by day."

3. Appreciate the magnitude of the U.S. diabetes epidemic, and know the associated statistics pertaining to incidence and prevalence.

4. Explain the role of refined carbohydrates in America's diabetes epidemic.

5. Give examples of how sugar consumption could be reduced on a population-level basis.

6. Describe public health practices and policies that can be applied to reducing the number of newly diagnosed cases of diabetes.

7. Differentiate between the medical approach to diabetes and the public health approach.

8. Learn about the long-term consequences of diabetes and the collective burden on the U.S. medical system.

If a frog is placed into a pot of boiling water, it will immediately try to jump out; but if it's placed into a pot of cool water that's gradually heated until boiling, it will stay put and never try to jump out.

—Richard Beckham II

Overview

Human nature is sometimes not in sync with reality. For example, the idea of a deadly disease – one that is chronic and requires daily attention – should be of great concern to people who care about their health and overall wellbeing. But each year in the United States, about 1.5 million new cases of Type 2 diabetes are diagnosed (CDC, 2018). Like a frog placed in cool water that is gradually heated, this staggering number of new cases could easily be avoided by "jumping out of the cooking pot." In essence, Type 2 diabetes occurs slowly – over many years – without warning and in a way that is unnoticeable. This gradual (day-by-day) overworking of the **pancreas** typically leads to a lack of **insulin**:—a hormone that serves as a type of valet to let glucose (the most elementary form of food) into the cells to be burned as energy. Sadly, like the frog in the pot when the water boils, the damage to the pancreas is irreversible and therefore permanent.

After presenting some of the basic biology of diabetes, this chapter will take you into the labyrinth of public practices and policies behind the staggering 1.5 million new cases each year, with an estimated 2018 total of 88 million Americans being in a stage known as **prediabetes** (CDC, 2020). Building on what you know from studying **Chapter 5**, you will learn extensive information about the refined foods that form the majority of the American diet and cause this epidemic to continue without signs of a decrease. More importantly, you will learn about the public health response, which is in the early stages of application but has a great potential to be amplified and ultimately mitigate America's diabetes epidemic. The majority of what you will learn is centered on the American preponderance of sugars and wheat in the daily diet. As you read this chapter, remember that elevated blood sugar levels (A1c) are a key factor in metabolic syndrome. As part of a syndrome, A1c levels are also linked to other factors you learned about in **Chapter 5**. For instance, over the past 20 years, evidence has rapidly accumulated to establish a

Understanding the Science and Practice of Public Health, First Edition. Richard Crosby.
© 2023 John Wiley & Sons, Inc. Published 2023 by John Wiley & Sons, Inc.

causal link between obesity and the onset of Type 2 diabetes. Also, as you might suspect, evidence strongly points to the protective effect of moderate to vigorous physical activity (MVPA) against the development of Type 2 diabetes. Therefore, it is fair to say that you have a head start – from **Chapter 5** – in learning about diabetes in this chapter.

As you study this chapter, keep in mind that public health is about primary prevention at a population level rather than simply ramping up the medical system to more effectively engage in tertiary prevention. This chapter serves as a great example of how upstream actions are superior to downstream actions, given the average cost of treating diabetes: the American Diabetes Association placing the 2017 estimated direct medical costs of diabetes at $237 billion per year (American Diabetes Association, 2018) This annual cost estimate will only increase, because the trend is clear: the annual incidence of diabetes in the United States is dramatically rising. Based on a modeling study projecting trends to the year 2050 (Boyle et al., 2010), the CDC has stated, "If current trends continue, 1 in 3 Americans will develop diabetes sometime in their lifetime" (CDC, 2021). Clearly, diabetes is a public health issue that warrants urgent and intensive intervention!

To better illustrate how adding a public health approach to the existing system of tertiary care can help save a faltering U.S. medical economy, this chapter will also provide you with an understanding of the long-term outcomes of diabetes.

Glucose Metabolism, Insulin, and the Pancreas

glucose is the most elementary form of food

As you begin reading this section of the chapter, set a goal for yourself of completely understanding the term **glycemic load**. To help you with this goal, let's begin with a few basic points. First, all energy in the body is derived from **glucose**. Thus, as noted previously, glucose is the most elementary form of food. Any food – carbohydrates, proteins, fats, or alcohol – is ultimately converted to glucose and used for energy, temporarily stored (in the liver), or stored for a long period (as fat). To be used for energy, glucose has to enter cells in the body. It cannot do this without insulin (insulin is the key that unlocks the cell to let glucose in). Insulin is produced by the pancreas, an organ that is part of the human endocrine system (the system that regulates all body functions via hormones). When the pancreas cannot produce enough insulin to meet the current need of the body to use newly consumed foods – especially those that burn quickly, such as refined sugars – the blood sugar level stays high for protracted periods. Alternately, a condition known as **insulin resistance** may occur. In this scenario, insulin is available, but the cells respond poorly. Either way, the result is elevated blood sugar levels. This ongoing sugar load in the blood can cause vascular damage to the vital organs (again, like turning up the heat slowly under the frog in the pot, this happens slowly and often without clear symptoms). Primary organs affected are the kidneys, heart, and retinas of the eyes, along with the central nervous system.

Another way to think about this is by using a metaphor. Imagine spending a cold winter day in a house heated only by a woodstove. The heat from the stove can be so intense that the house's temperature rises to 90 degrees or more. Conversely, the heat output may be so low that it produces little noticeable warmth. Your self-assigned task for that cold winter day is to regulate the type of wood and the amount of wood you place in the stove. You might be tempted to burn less-dense wood that is rapidly consumed by the fire and puts out intense heat. The problem is that this intense heat (like a candy bar or energy drink) burns hot and then quickly burns out, leaving you back in the cold. As the day goes on, you learn to tightly regulate the heat by adding wood only one or two pieces at a time, holding other supplies of wood in reserve. This tight regulation of burning calories characterizes the non-diabetic body. While some calories (fuel for the fire) are burned, other calories are stored in the liver (glucose stored in the liver is known as **glycogen**). Other calories that are consumed but not needed soon are stored as body fat (for later conversion to glucose if the fuel supply runs low).

To add to this metaphor, consider the term **slow burning**, which is often applied to food. Like a large piece of firewood that is very dense/heavy, a slow-burning food requires an active, complex set of metabolic actions before glucose is rendered. This means slow food cannot produce quick energy, but it can produce reliable amounts of long-lasting energy. Think of this as a slow and steady fire. In contrast, refined carbohydrates give a fast fire; in terms of blood sugar, this is a spike in blood sugar levels. The spike is soon followed by a precipitous drop in blood sugar, which may be severe enough to leave the person with a feeling of fatigue.

Ideally, a population-level approach to reducing the American epidemic of diabetes would be characterized by making slow foods affordable, accessible, and acceptable. Slow foods include meats, fish, dairy products, nuts, and complex carbohydrates such as broccoli, cauliflower, carrots, and oats. The slow foods are the ones that public health efforts must subsidize, promote, and bring – literally – to the table.

Diabetes Develops Day By Day

The Role of Sugars

Let's begin with a question that has likely been on your mind since you began reading this chapter: "Why is it called Type 2 diabetes – are there other types?" The answer is yes, there is also Type 1 diabetes. Type 1 used to be known as **juvenile-onset diabetes**, and Type 2 was formerly known as **adult-onset diabetes**. (This chapter does not discuss Type 1 because its origin is inherited, and thus public health implications for population-level prevention are non-existent.) Sadly, the term **adult-onset** was dropped in favor of the less descriptive name **Type 2** because Type 2 was increasingly being diagnosed in young people, even those not yet classified as teenagers. Indeed, recent statistics from the CDC demonstrate that Type 2 diabetes is occurring in progressively younger age groups (CDC, 2020). Consequently – and unlike CVD – diabetes prevention for school children is a relatively urgent public health concern, given that many of them may be diagnosed with Type 2 before the age of 20.

Estimates suggest that nearly one of every five teens and preteens (i.e., persons 12 to 18 years of age) can be classified with **prediabetes** (Andes et al., 2020). This condition is signaled by elevated A1c levels that are not yet high enough to constitute Type 2 diabetes. Most prediabetic youth do not know their condition, and most typically develop diabetes in subsequent years. It is also estimated that one-third of all U.S. adults have prediabetes, with only about 10% aware of their condition (Andes et al., 2020). An important review study of people with prediabetes concluded that lifestyle changes (i.e., improving dietary and exercise behaviors) are more likely to reverse this condition than medical treatment (Haw et al., 2017).

Now, let's take a very close look at **sugars**. The word is used in plural form on purpose, because sugars come in many forms. During your childhood, you most likely had an image of refined white granular sugar in mind when the term **sugar** was used. As this white sugar earned a poor reputation in terms of health, food companies came up with clever surrogates intended to sway buyers. The surrogates are nonetheless still sugar.

For a moment, let's glance at the structure of carbohydrates (see **Figure 6.1**). What is classically known as **sugar** (i.e., refined white or brown

Type 2 was increasingly being diagnosed in young people, even those not yet classified as teenagers

Estimates suggest that nearly one of every five teens and preteens (i.e., persons 12 to 18 years of age) can be classified with **prediabetes**

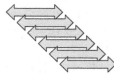

Monosaccharide (only 1 molecule)

Disaccharide (only 2 molecules)

Oligosaccharide (3 to 10 molecules)

Polysaccharide (11 or more molecules)

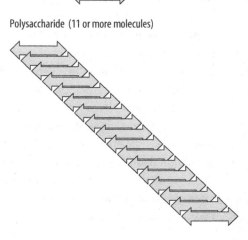

Figure 6.1   A simplified diagram of carbohydrates

sugar) is called a **disaccharide**, meaning that two monosaccharides are bonded to form a double sugar. A **monosaccharide** is a single molecule. For example, in the case of table sugar, the monosaccharides are **glucose** and **fructose**. Glucose is (as you already know) the most elementary form of energy for the body. Its digestion and absorption are not a cause of diabetes. Fructose, however, is handled differently by the body. To be used, it must be converted to glucose by the liver – a metabolic process that raises the level of triglycerides in the blood and may also contribute to obesity (recall from **Chapter 5** that triglycerides are a cause of metabolic syndrome). Thus, while fructose is not implicated as a direct cause of diabetes, it is part of the same syndrome that includes diabetes.

while fructose is not implicated as a direct cause of diabetes, it is part of the same syndrome that includes diabetes

The real problem lies with the digestion and metabolism of the disaccharide known as **sucrose** (this is what the public calls sugar). Sucrose is mostly to blame for the U.S. diabetes epidemic. It is typically refined from either sugar beets or cane sugar; however, it is also in foods like honey, agave, and maple syrup. Rather than memorizing lists of these offenders, a simple rule is that refined foods that taste sweet most likely have at least some sucrose and thus contribute to the diabetes epidemic.

The more complex carbohydrates are oligosaccharides and polysaccharides. As shown in **Figure 6.1**, these are far more complex in their molecular structures, and thus it takes the body longer to metabolize (i.e., break down) these carbohydrates into glucose and energy.

In addition to what you already know from reading this far in the chapter (i.e., that the overconsumption of sugars is the leading risk factor for Type 2 diabetes), other risk factors are obesity, physical inactivity, and genetics. Because both obesity and physical inactivity were topics of **Chapter 5**, we will now focus solely on refined foods. However, important side notes about genetics are relevant here (see **Box 6.1**).

BOX 6.1. WHY GENETIC FACTORS DO NOT MATTER

As you have been reading this chapter, you may have thought of a person in your family who should have developed diabetes but has not yet done so. You may have thought about the copious amounts of sugar in that person's daily diet, and perhaps his/her near complete lack of physical activity. It is indeed easy to wonder whether genetic factors play a major role in protecting some people against diabetes. In fact, genetic predispositions toward diabetes do exist, as do genetic "protections" against diabetes. So, why is this not important in the context of public health practice?

The answer to this question is simply a reminder that public health is about entire populations. For many students, this is a difficult shift in thinking about disease. Applied to diabetes, this population-level paradigm means the focal point of public health is a massive reduction in sugar consumption throughout the United States, accompanied by population-level increases in MVPA. Remember that the goal is to change the mean of the population. This goal is therefore not about any one person or even about understanding more about the role of genetics in the development of Type 2 diabetes. By reducing the mean level of U.S. sugar consumption, for example, a corresponding decrease in newly diagnosed cases of Type 2 diabetes will follow, in time. This higher level of thinking makes genetic factors a moot point in terms of intervention.

By contrast, a medical perspective would view diabetes risk as at least a partial consequence of a family history of diabetes. But this does not necessarily imply a genetic role, because families typically share much more than genes; they share te cultural habits involved with diet and exercise. Under the medical paradigm, a young person with a family history of diabetes might be counseled to avoid sugars and other refined carbohydrates in hopes of postponing or averting Type 2 diabetes. Although this is certainly a valuable approach, such one-to-one education has yet to have an impact on the rising rates of Type 2 diabetes.

To help you think at more personal level about refined foods and sugars, take the following quiz:

1. Which food option from this breakfast menu has the **least** added sugar?

    a. "A warm 4-ounce bowl of instant oatmeal sprinkled with cinnamon (no added fruit or sugar)"
    b. "Our famous French toast, made with fresh eggs and almond milk – no added sugar"
    c. "A generous 4-ounce serving of prepared tropical fruits, shipped from Costa Rica, served with a few spoonfuls of granola"
    d. "A favorite of health food addicts: our low-fat yogurt with a topping of marinated cherries"

2. Which food option from this lunch menu has the **least** added sugar?

    a. "A lunch portion of mushroom ravioli, served in a rich bed of marinara sauce"
    b. "A Southern favorite: mounds of coleslaw served over catfish filets coated with cornbread"
    c. "For the light eater, world-famous granola bars served with your choice of yogurt"
    d. "A delightful field green salad topped with walnuts, cheese, and balsamic vinegar dressing"

Let's see how you did! Starting with the breakfast options, you should have ruled out options C and D right away. With few exceptions, yogurt is loaded with hidden sugars (a typical serving has anywhere from 6 to 12 g of added sugar). Further, packaged fruits (usually canned) have large amounts of added sugars to enhance flavor and help preserve the fruit. From a sales and consumer perspective, think of granola as similar to yogurt in that the name creates (as intended by advertising) a **virtual halo** of goodness and health. Most commercially manufactured granolas are anything but wholesome, as they are loaded (like most breakfast cereals) with sugars. Food companies benefit by adding large amounts of sugars to their products – sugars are cheap to acquire and give consumers a feeling of satisfaction. So, think of the **prepared foods** as you look again at option A. On its surface, A seems like a healthy choice; however, the prepared instant oatmeal so often consumed in the United States is very high in sugars. This leaves option B as the correct answer. Bread does have some sugar, but a relatively modest amount. The egg in French toast has no sugar, and almond milk has very little sugar (cinnamon is a spice and thus sugar-free).

Now let's see how you did with the lunch menu. Hopefully you ruled out options B and C. As you now know, C is just two halo foods loaded with sugars. However, you might not think of coleslaw and catfish as high-sugar foods. A key to ruling out option B is the word "Southern." Southern-style coleslaw is typically high in added sugar, as is Southern-style cornbread (so, the breading on the catfish adds more sugar). This leaves options A and D. If you selected D, then pat yourself on the back – you are correct. But you may wonder why A has sugar. The idea of **hidden sugar** applies here. Tomatoes used for marinara sauce are a PBWF, but food companies stretch that expensive product by adding inexpensive, good-tasting fillers. Sugar is a corporate favorite as a cheap filler for sauces, creamy salad dressings, and even boxed juiced drinks marketed for children.

> Sugar is a corporate favorite as a cheap filler for sauces, creamy salad dressings, and even boxed juiced drinks marketed for children

The first take-home point from this two-question quiz is that sugars are ubiquitous in prepared foods as opposed to whole foods. A second take-home point is more subtle: marketing is blind to the health of the public, including children. In addition to children's juices, think about some of the energy drinks marketed to young people, and then look up their nutritional labels online – you will be surprised to see that the energy comes from a blast of sugar to the bloodstream with each swallow of the beverage.

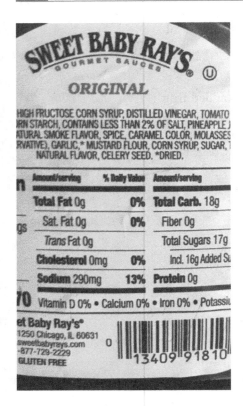

Photo 6.1   High fructose corn syrup is just another name for sugar!

acknowledge that food labeling laws do not protect us and that more aggressive regulation of the food industry is warranted

At this point in the chapter, think back to the public health approach to food labeling that you learned about in **Chapter 5**. These laws mandate that packaged products must display the number of grams of sugar per serving. But do people bother to look at the labels on foods that they do not associate with sugar? Consider, for example, an American favorite: barbecue sauce. Then look at **Photo 6.1**, and notice that just two tablespoons has 17 g of sugar! A frontier in public health is to acknowledge that food labeling laws do not protect us and that more aggressive regulation of the food industry is warranted.

The Role of Wheat

The overconsumption of refined carbohydrates (not just wheat products) creates a consistent challenge to the human body. The body tightly regulates blood sugar levels, keeping them as constant as possible. When foods close to their natural state (and thus loaded with fiber) enter the body, the metabolic process is slow and, therefore, easy to regulate. When highly refined foods – which are quickly and easily broken down into glucose – enter the body, a flood of quick energy occurs and challenges the body's attempt at regulation. Thus, people with prediabetes and diabetes are always counseled to avoid **refined carbohydrates**. Refined carbohydrates are simple sugars as opposed to complex sugars. Avoiding these also reduces the odds of developing metabolic syndrome.

Of all the refined food products adored by U.S. consumers, those with a wheat base are the cheapest to manufacture and thus dominate the market. Although evidence is still emerging, the role of wheat-based refined foods in the development of prediabetes and diabetes will certainly become a more prominent part of future public health research.

Examples of How U.S. Sugar Consumption Can Be Reduced

Up to this point in the chapter, you have learned a great deal about the problem of diabetes and its causes. All too often, public health research and even textbooks expound on the problem but offer very little in terms of actionable solutions at a population level. So, now that you have a more thorough understanding of why dietary changes are crucial to mitigating the diabetes epidemic, let's examine the relevant challenges to public health practice. The first involves eliminating a food subsidy. The second focuses on the foods available through government-sponsored public assistance programs. The third is to begin applying lessons learned from tobacco control (see **Chapter 4**) to changing the American diet. The final challenge, largely untapped by public health, centers on the U.S. school lunch program.

Food Subsidies

Recall that you have already learned about food subsidies. In essence, the federal government, via the Department of Agriculture, provides financial incentives to farmers who produce subsidized foods. Sugar has been one of those foods since 1981, when the U.S. Farm Bill was authorized by Congress. A 2018 editorial from the prestigious group known as Market Watch reported that only 4,500 U.S. farms produce sugar, each receiving an average of $700,000 annually in subsidies (Smith, 2018) This translates to a total yearly cost to taxpayers of approximately $4 billion. Ironically, about 50% of the sugar is harvested from sugar beets – a crop that grows in highly fertile soil capable of growing highly nutritious vegetables that would greatly benefit Americans.

Given that Congress has supported sugar farms since 1981, a logical and imperative question becomes, why aren't we fighting the diabetes epidemic by removing these subsidies? Of course, removing subsidies does not automatically translate into fewer new cases of Type 2 diabetes. However, removing subsidies would translate into significant price increases for sugar. In turn, the food industry's filler would be vastly more expensive and thus less appealing. As a result, at a minimum, consumers would buy less bagged sugar.

why aren't we fighting the diabetes epidemic by removing these subsidies?

An important principle applies here. When higher prices create less demand, or when lower prices create greater demand, the economic principle of **price elasticity** can be a useful asset to public health practice. Ultimately, this refers to how much the total price must increase before a significant decrease in consumption occurs. Retailers typically try to find a price point that is barely below the level at which demand would decline. In simplified terms, a product that is **inelastic** (i.e., low in price elasticity) is one that people will buy regardless of price. Examples of inelastic products are gasoline, milk, electricity, and health-care services. Other products, such as tobacco and sugar-sweetened beverages, are relatively **elastic** (meaning high in price elasticity). So, people will not keep buying sugar and sugar-based products as prices rise. In fact, as the price of sugar rises, the principle of price elasticity predicts a corresponding decline in consumption.

Supplemental Nutrition Programs

The U.S. government is heavily invested in feeding Americans through the program known by the acronym SNAP (**Supplemental Nutrition Assistance Program**). Although SNAP is federally funded, it is administered by the states. The question (and corresponding challenge) goes something like this: "Are SNAP benefits designed to promote slow foods (complex carbohydrates that require extensive metabolism)over refined carbohydrates/sugars?" Approached from a less positive standpoint, the question boils down to whether SNAP benefits may inadvertently promote diabetes and whether the taxpayers' money is allotted in a way that misses a public health opportunity to reduce the size and scope of the epidemic.

According to the SNAP website maintained by the U.S. Department of Agriculture, only five categories of products in a typical grocery store are not eligible to be purchased with SNAP debit cards (USDA, 2021):

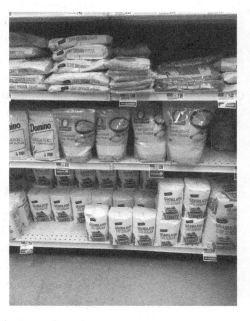

- All non-food items
- Any alcohol or tobacco product
- Vitamins and medications
- Any food consumed in the store
- Any hot foods sold in the store

Thus, it is entirely possible for a SNAP recipient to purchase large quantities of bagged and boxed sugars such as those shown in **Photo 6.2.** Recipients can buy the entire array of high-sugar foods, including breakfast cereal, packaged breakfast buns, cakes, pies, candy, granola bars, ice cream, popsicles, and yogurt.

Rather than simply lament the irony of the U.S. government paying for the foods that cause diabetes and paying huge medical bills for people with diabetes, a more useful response is to advocate for change. For instance, given that nearly all food items have a barcode (even fresh produce, as these products have barcodes keyed in by checkout workers), a reasonable policy

Photo 6.2   Foods loaded with sugar – and sugar itself – are eligible for purchase with SNAP benefits.

a reasonable policy change to the SNAP is to expand the categories of foods that are disallowed.

change to the SNAP is to expand the categories of foods that are disallowed. These might be, for example, categories such as

- Bagged or boxed sugars

- Frozen or deli-made cakes, pies, and desserts

- Ice cream, popsicles, and similar products

- Sodas and other sugar-sweetened beverages

- Boxed cake and cookie mixes, as well as readymade dough used for cookies, cinnamon rolls, biscuits, and so on

- Sauces, dressings, marinades, and ketchup that contain sugars

Remember from **Chapter 2** that the U.S. government is about "we the people." You may feel that any such public health effort to overhaul SNAP is beyond the control of citizens. But if that were truly the case, our society would not be a democracy. As a professor who has taught students for more than 30 years, I often enthusiastically wonder, "Who among my students will become a leader – a true agent for real change in the conditions that otherwise limit public health?" So, as a side note to this section of the chapter, let me implore you to think of yourself as a future leader!

In contrast to SNAP, the longstanding U.S. food program known as the **Women, Infants, and Children Nutrition Program (WIC)** has a relatively strict set of guidelines that each state must follow to receive federal funding that backs the program. For instance, one of the restrictions applies to breakfast cereals (a common source of sugar in the American diet). The guidelines specify that states can only include breakfast cereals with 6 g or less of sugar in a single serving. Consequently, when a state develops a list of WIC-approved cereals, it reflects products with very low sugar content (as cereals go). The guidelines apply to a wide assortment of foods, including milk products such as infant formula.

Given what you now know about WIC-approved foods, the logical question becomes, "Why doesn't the SNAP follow a similar method of state-by-state regulation to promote healthy eating and discourage the overconsumption of sugar?" This is a rhetorical question, as it does not have a straightforward answer. Again, you can see in this example that improving public health is often less about educating people and more about regulating government assistance programs. But the term **regulate** can inflame resistance. Throughout the full range of issues in public health – from state laws about helmet use for motorcycle riders to corporate policies about COVID vaccine requirements – a not-so-subtle undercurrent of individual freedom is constantly at odds with the concepts of primary prevention at the population-level. Upstream approaches, such as regulating the sugar industry and its products, are often unpopular because of perceived infringement on individual-level freedom. A valid plan B for this form of regulation is based on carefully planned media campaigns.

a not-so-subtle undercurrent of individual freedom is constantly at odds with the concepts of primary prevention at the population-level

Media Campaigns to Expose the Sugar Industry

Just as the California Tobacco Control Program made the truth known about the corrupt and deceptive practices of the tobacco industry (see **Chapter 4**), that lesson in public health practice can be applied to the sugar industry. Although sugar consumption is difficult to accurately assess without cooperation from the sugar industry, nearly all attempts at this task suggest that the trend is increasing and that about one-sixth of the average American diet consists of processed sugar. From a public health history perspective, it has been estimated that about 75% of all processed foods contain substantial amounts of excess sugars. Sugar is almost everywhere in a grocery store except in the produce, meat/fish, and shelf products in their unrefined state, such as nuts, seeds, and beans, and rice. With all of its profit from this overwhelming presence in the American shopping cart, it is clear that the sugar industry is well funded. Thus, a reasonable question becomes whether the sugar industry has been fair and conscientious relative to diabetes, as well as obesity and heart disease.

In 2016, Kearns, Schmidt, and Glantz published a stunning article in a prestigious medical journal. These authors obtained and reviewed nearly 50 years' worth of internal documents once held by the Sugar Research Foundation (SRF). The documents make it very clear that as early as 1965, the SRF was engaged in manipulating science to promote sugar as relatively harmless compared to fats and cholesterol-laden foods. This manipulation took the form of paying university professors of nutrition science to compose and publish a journal article (published in the *New England Journal of Medicine*) providing apparent evidence that heart disease was largely a result of dietary fats, with sugar **not** being implicated as a cause. The SRF supplied these professors with data and papers that the organization specified for use in the review. Further, the SRF participated in drafting the journal article. This level of tainting science is no longer easy because safeguards have been implemented that force authors of journal articles to disclose all funding sources and all potential conflicts of interest. Nonetheless, the "good food" image of its products perpetuated by the SRF seems to have become deeply embedded in American culture. Consider, for instance, the old saying "As American as apple pie and ice cream" (see **Box 6.2**).

the SRF was engaged in manipulating science to promote sugar as relatively harmless compared to fats

BOX 6.2. "AS AMERICAN AS APPLE PIE AND ICE CREAM"

Without question, culture is a very strong influence on the foods people eat. Cultural habits pass from one generation to the next, most often regardless of any negative consequences. In essence, the American diet is built more on habit and tradition than on health. Labeling a food as "American" makes it seem, by extension, like a good thing! But let's take a few minutes and see just how "good" this small part of American culture is for the health of the public.

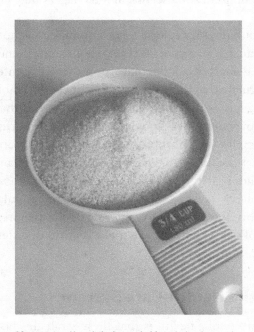

Photo 6.3   Your daily diet probably includes this much sugar or more.

Most reliable internet sources related to food and health publish data about the amount of sugar (sucrose) in common foods. The average estimate for a slice of apple pie (one-eighth of 12" pie) is 20 g. Also, the average estimate for a serving (1/2 cup) of regular ice cream is 14 g, with "premium" ice creams having as much as 20 g in that very small 1/2-cup serving. Barring larger servings, consider an average American dessert of apple pie and ice cream as providing 34 g of sugar – typically capping off a day when sugar was most likely consumed to levels far beyond the recommended 5 g per day for females and 10 g for males. One gram of sugar is approximately one-quarter of a teaspoon, so 35 g would equate with almost 9 teaspoons!

Now think also about the rest of a typical day on an American diet. For example, another American favorite is a donut for breakfast. Just by taking a quick look at the Dunkin Donuts website, you will see that an ordinary glazed jelly donut contains 34 g of sugar. Let's say you also have a vanilla latte at Starbucks – that adds another 16 g of sugar to your day. The American lunch typically contains less sugar than breakfast does, and let's assume you are typical! So, your lunch is a modest salad with French dressing. Although the salad is sugar free, dressings are typically laden with sugar. In the case of a serving of California French dressing, you would be consuming another 8 g of sugar. To go with your salad, let's say you have a glass of sweet tea – this adds another 48 g of sugar if it is the Lipton brand.

Assuming that your dinner on this hypothetical day is completely sugar free (other than the pie and ice cream for dessert) your day looks like this in terms of sugar:

- Breakfast = 50 g

- Lunch = 56 g

- Dessert = 34 g

The total is 140 g (again, assuming a sugar-free dinner and no snacking). At the conversion of 4 teaspoons per gram, you have consumed 35 teaspoons of sugar: approximately three-quarters of a cup (Photo 6.3).

The U.S. School Lunch Program and Sugar Consumption

You have already learned about prediabetes and the strong trend in our country for Type 2 diabetes to develop among young people. This trend implies a public health need to use our U.S. school lunch program (and breakfast programs) to encourage the consumption of low-sugar foods and discourage the consumption of sugar-laden foods.

The **National School Lunch Program** (NSLP) is a federally funded effort to provide free or reduced-cost lunches to school children. The program serves more than 30 million children per school year. Although the level of federal regulation for this program is significant, these regulations fail to limit the number of grams of sugar that can be included in a federally reimbursed school breakfast or lunch. High-sugar foods with a strong halo effect, such as ice cream for its calcium, orange juice for its vitamins, and canned fruit for its wholesome goodness, have a strong foothold in most schools that receive these funds. But as you know, halo foods are often heavy perpetrators of the sugar habit that children, adolescents, and teenagers may not be able to break.

policy – leveraged by political will and popular public support – can easily and definitively improve the problem

Sadly, sugar remains a low-cost method of bumping up calorie counts to make a school lunch meet federal or state requirements. For instance, a survey of 900 U.S. school lunch menus found that about 20% of all menus include a daily dessert of cake, cookies, or brownies (Center for Investigative Reporting, 2013). It is fair to speculate that these desserts help meet the whole grain requirements of the lunch, despite providing more grams of sugar in a single serving than people should eat during an entire day. Desserts, of course, are an obvious example of ignoring the long-term health of youth. Less-obvious examples (e.g., cornbread, processed meats, and sauces/condiments such as sugar glazing on sweet potatoes and ketchup on hamburgers and fries) predominate the landscape of America's school cafeterias. The silver lining within these dark clouds of school foods in America is that policy – leveraged by political will and popular public support – can easily and definitively improve the problem. Again, as noted in the preface to this textbook, a well-informed electorate of voting citizens can make a world of difference when it comes to public health – please stay informed!

The Burden of Type 2 Diabetes on the Health-Care System

A common problem with upstream approaches to public health is that these strategies take many years to make a tangible difference in rates of disease and death.

A common problem with upstream approaches to public health is that these strategies take many years to make a tangible difference in rates of disease and death. But it is a tremendous mistake to believe that adding funds to downstream approaches will solve issues such as a rising tide of Type 2 diabetics in the United States. Funds are nonetheless expended liberally for downstream approaches and sparingly for the more progressive upstream solutions to this problem.

Figure 6.2 provides you with a somewhat eye-opening representation of just how quickly the medical care costs of diabetes in the United States can double. In 2007, the estimated direct medical costs incurred for treating diabetes in the United States were $116 billion. By 2012, that cost was estimated to have risen to $176 billion – a 53% increase! By 2017, the cost was $237 billion – a greater than twofold increase compared to the cost just 10 years earlier (Riddle & Herman, 2018).

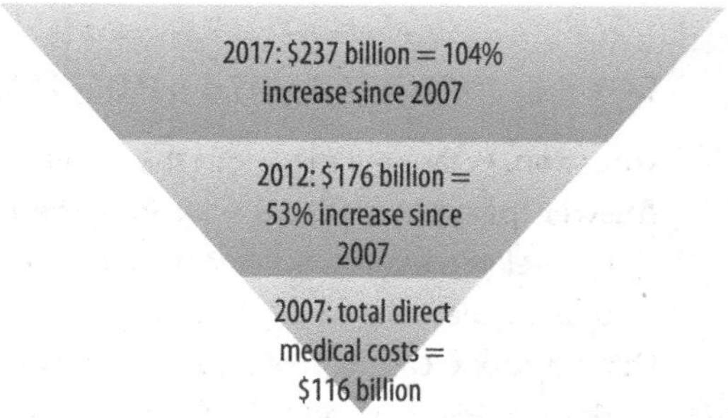

To place the numbers in a more human perspective, the 2017 estimate translated to an average direct medical expenditure of $16,752 per person (Riddle & Herman, 2018). Keep in mind that other estimates that take into account costs such as lost workdays, loss of overall (lifetime) productivity, and so on are typically about 50% higher than the estimates based only on direct medical costs. Now, to take a much broader view of the diabetes epidemic, consider the estimate that one of every four healthcare dollars is spent on diabetes patients (Riddle & Herman, 2018).

With the diabetes epidemic consistently expanding and thus consuming an ever-larger portion of the U.S. healthcare dollar, the question becomes when federal actions will begin to take this problem to heart. As you have already learned in this chapter, the federal government actually promotes the problem by subsidizing sugar farmers and by not regulating sugar content as part of the NSLP. This clear lack of an upstream response to the problem has only been met by more intensive downstream approaches. For instance, The Diabetes Prevention Program Research Group (2012) reported findings from a randomized trial of more than 3,000 people at high risk of developing diabetes. Based on these findings, it was estimated that an intensive and individualized lifestyle change program could reduce the odds of developing diabetes by 58%. Two key terms are important here: (a) **people at high risk** and (b) **intensive and individualized**. The first term should make you think back to a key principle you learned about in **Chapter 3**: that true public health interventions do not target those only at very high risk. Instead, they target the entire population and are designed to shift the mean level of risk in a more favorable direction for everyone. The second term should take your mind back to **Chapter 2**, where you learned that public health is not a one-at-a-time (i.e., individual-level) approach to disease prevention.

At this point, it will be useful for you to become a bit more familiar with the concept of **lifestyle intervention**. Almost endless approaches to changing diet and exercise behaviors fall under this catch-all phrase. For example, most U.S. hospitals provide the counseling services of a registered dietician to patients who may benefit from this form of lifestyle intervention. **Box 6.3** gives you an in-depth look.

All lifestyle interventions are education-based, and thus they typically occur as one-to-one counseling sessions, although small group sessions may also be feasible. This one-person-at-a-time approach is very much oriented around the medical paradigm and is thus quite limited in its reach. This does not imply that the lifestyle intervention designed and reported by the Diabetes Prevention Program Research Group (2012) lacks value. The program could be prescribed by physicians to their high-risk patients. However, even in a highly idealistic scenario, if this became a common prescription, our nation would still have an ever-increasing number of young people mired in habits that lead to prediabetes and eventually diabetes. Further, it would not impact those millions of Americans without a physician who monitors their A1c levels and makes judgments about being at high risk for developing diabetes. In short, the medical approach only works on a small part of the public. Moreover, this approach does not acknowledge the sheer strength of cultural practices related to food and eating in the United States.

2017: $237 billion = 104% increase since 2007

2012: $176 billion = 53% increase since 2007

2007: total direct medical costs = $116 billion

Figure 6.2   The rising direct medical costs for diabetes care in the United States

the medical approach only works on a small part of the public

BOX 6.3. INTERVIEW WITH A HOSPITAL DIETICIAN

Question. Please tell me about the typical patient you see relative to their issues with nutrition.

Answer (paraphrased). I see all ages, from pediatric to people in their 80s. Most are outpatients who can see me for any diet-related reason, not just diabetes. Obesity is major presenting issue but most people have many other health issues that are diet related.

I have a strong caseload of people with morbid obesity. They typically have a long history of dieting that is based on negative experiences and failure – they often just want a meal plan to follow – a list of foods to eat and not to eat. Instead, what I do is take a complete history to give them skills that can last a lifetime.

Question. How do dieticians conceptualize health and eating?

Answer (paraphrased). Health is a spectrum – it's about the things people choose to do most often. The idea is to help people learn to moderate any excess in their intake of unhealthy foods. People can and should broaden their food repertoire – eating new and healthy alternatives to the current diet is encouraged. The idea is that by helping people add dozens of new foods to their diet, the old reliance of highly refined and processed foods begins to waver. Part of this is also about lifestyle and taking the time to plan, prepare, and eat nutrient-dense meals on a regular schedule. This helps people break the dysfunctional habit of skipping meals, for example, in favor of high-calorie drinks (including beverages from fast-food chains) used to substitute for a meal. It is common for people on a diet to starve themselves all day and then graze all night – this creates issues with binge eating.

Question. Please talk about the main issues related to food and public health.

Answer (paraphrased). The medical world has greatly stigmatized being overweight, let alone being obese. By contrast, the "health at every size" movement acknowledges that people come in all shapes and weights. The goal is often to help people rethink and relearn eating habits rather than maintain this undue focus on weight. Many people I see have a history of lacking exposure to healthy foods – they may, for example, have no idea what do with a rutabaga! For many of them, childhood included being required to eat vegetables they didn't like – this may have created a generalized dislike for some foods and led to a lack of experimentation with others. The other common problem is that many people have small food budgets. They can buy calories easily: it is cheap to buy a case of Coke and a case of ramen noodles – they cost almost nothing compared to healthy foods. An important aspect of my work is to help people learn how to find good food at affordable prices.

Question. What about addictive foods, such as those loaded with sugar?

Answer (paraphrased). Some people have addictive behaviors because of the way they view food – as a reward or liberty they have earned. In trying to break these food addictions, too many people try to go all out and "be good" and then give into their cravings and revert back to their addictions. Generally speaking, people need to eat more of everything to, by extension, eat less of the junky things. The focus is not on demonizing sugar; instead, the goal is take sugar off its pedestal. Also, it is important to recognize that people do self-medicate with food. Food and psychology are welded together. New evidence about the microbiome also suggests that food may be linked to depression, anxiety, and mood disorders. In my experience working with patients, as nutrition improves, so does everything else.

Question. From a population-level standpoint, what needs to occur to avert new cases of adult-onset diabetes?

Answer (paraphrased). We need a paradigm shift that addresses the true underlying issues. Part of the solution is to stop the stigma relative to overweight/obesity – we miss people early in life because of this stigma. By the time they present for care/treatment/counseling, it may be from an admission to the emergency room. In short, we need to move way from a BMI-driven approach to health care to promote food as treatment. This new paradigm must also include the ethic of intervening in a non-stigmatized way much earlier in life. We can give young people produce and teach them why they need to add it to their diet, but cooking classes are needed. Schools can do better – too many programs have been cut, but cooking classes and farm-to-school remains very important to a more holistic approach to averting diabetes, obesity, and cardiovascular disease. Additionally, the medical world should stop treating food like a drug. In essence, the medical world is often in search a few foods that "heal everything." Food is far more than a substance (similar to drugs) that solves diagnosed problems or averts disease onset. Each person's best diet will be unique. Just as there is no magic pill, magic foods do not exist.

Changing people's diets in isolation from changing what their family members and friends consume is likely to fail in the long run. Foods are often a sacred part of people's lives, and many of the loved foods are loaded with sugar (see **Box 6.4**).

All this probably leaves you with the possibly unsettling question of what can be done. Here, a final term applies to this chapter: **behavioral economics**. In a highly simplified form, this is a field of research that has great potential to inform public health practice. A behavioral economic approach to sugar reduction would be centered on raising prices. For instance, think back to **Chapter 2** and what you learned about the sugar-sweetened beverage tax in Philadelphia, PA. Then recall a previous section of this chapter where you learned about the principle of price elasticity. Given the alarming trends in the incidence and costs of diabetes, a behavioral economic approach to diabetes prevention may someday no longer be overly radical for policymakers and legislators. When that time arrives, sugar subsidies will likely end, the sugar

BOX 6.4. THE HUMAN SIDE: THE HUMAN SIDE: LOVE, ROMANCE, AND CHOCOLATE

Have you ever wondered how Valentine's Day became a chocolate lover's favorite time of year? Growing evidence suggests that cocoa is a natural stimulator of four important neurotransmitters (**neurotransmitters** are chemicals in the brain responsible for rapid communication within a complex system of tissues that collectively direct our thoughts, feelings, emotions, and motivations). One of these four is oxytocin, which triggers feelings of attachment, happiness, security, and even love! Primary among the other three neurotransmitters are the endorphins. Endorphins provide a natural "high" that is not much different from drug-induced feelings of being high. The other two are serotonin and dopamine, both of which also trigger a state of happiness and may thus be part of the romance and love implied by a Valentine's Day date or outing. The main point here, of course, is about cocoa. In its pure form (i.e., 100% cocoa) this food has an optimal ability to stimulate production of the four neurotransmitters. Yet humans have eschewed the consumption of this pure form and, instead, gravitated to chocolate that contains a large percentage of sugar. The weight in grams of a typical Hersey's milk chocolate bar, for example, consists of nearly 50% sugar. Thus, despite the huge boost to happiness provided by cocoa, people opt to replace large amounts of the cocoa with sugar in their chocolate desserts, bars, drinks, and other delectables.

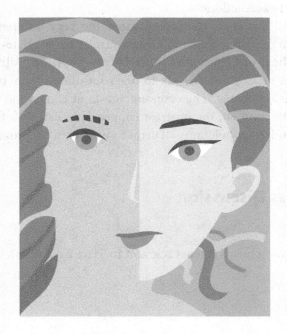
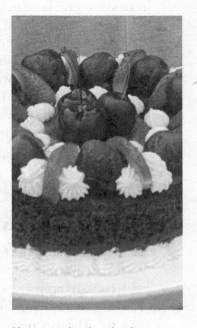

Photo 6.4 Somehow chocolate is culturally linked to love and romance.

content of subsidized meals will be tightly regulated, and cities – even entire states – will levy taxes on products such as sodas. Our nation is not yet at this point. For example, since the passage of the sugar-sweetened beverage tax in Philadelphia, fewer than 10 U.S. cities have passed similar legislation. Are we like the frog in the water that warms up gradually?

Review and Key Terms

This chapter began by teaching you some basic biology relative to Type 2 diabetes. You should now understand that the **pancreas** produces a true key to how the body works: **insulin**. Further, you know that the body tightly regulates blood sugar via insulin and a storage system for the most elementary form of food: **glucose**. Glucose can be stored in the short term in the as **glycogen**. The goal of the body is to keep the blood sugar – known as **glycemic load** – at a relatively constant level.

Maintaining a consistent glycemic load is more difficult when **sucrose** (i.e., sugar) is consumed because this form of refined carbohydrate burns quickly and thus causes spikes in blood sugar levels. Ultimately, this form of stress on the metabolism may lead to inadequate insulin production or a compromised ability of the cells to respond to insulin (known as **insulin resistance**).

Armed with a reasonable understanding of Type 2 diabetes, you then learned about some possible public health approaches to altering the rising trajectory of this epidemic. The discussion began with the 1981 Farm Bill and its subsequent and ongoing support of sugar producers and proceeded through the need to exercise regulatory authority over sugar content in the **National School Lunch Program**. You learned about **price elasticity** and how that principle applies to reducing America's sugar habit. Although the concepts of raising taxes on sugar-based products and removing sugar subsidies to farmers may seem extreme, this chapter provided you with ample evidence that the extreme nature of the diabetes epidemic warrants urgent and equally extreme public health intervention. Applying **behavioral economics** to the overconsumption of sugar in the United States is a likely first move in what should become a series of coordinated public health actions.

The chapter closed with a section that accentuated the very different approaches of upstream versus downstream thinking regarding sugar control. Current state-of-the-art downstream approaches feature the broad concept of **lifestyle interventions**. Although perhaps of substantial value to individuals (i.e., patients), one-to-one education will not be enough to turn back the rising tide of Type 2 diabetes. The economic costs of clinging to the downstream approaches are staggering. In contrast, the upstream approaches can shift the mean level of sugar consumption for entire populations. Further, upstream approaches are highly cost-effective.

For Practice and Class Discussion

Practice Questions

1. Which one of the following terms is **least** relevant to Type 2 diabetes?
   a. Glycemic load
   b. Glycogen
   c. Neurotransmitters
   d. The pancreas

2. In general terms, the trajectory of the U.S. diabetes epidemic is:
   a. Doubling every 10 years
   b. Staying relatively stable

    c.   Increasing only slightly each year

    d.   Decreasing as a result of lifestyle interventions

3.   The concept of behavioral economics, applied to the prevention of diabetes, implies that:

    a.   Increasing taxes on sugar-laden foods and eliminating subsidies to sugar producers can greatly reduce sugar consumption.

    b.   Sugar can become an inelastic market product.

    c.   The National School Lunch Program should be significantly revised.

4.   Regarding the Sugar Research Foundation (SRF), which statement is true?

    a.   The research produced by the SRF is vital to public health.

    b.   The SRF has engaged in practices designed to protect the "good food" image of sugar.

    c.   Supported by the U.S. Department of Agriculture, the SRF administers the WIC program.

    d.   The SRF has produced research supporting the role of sugar in the development of Type 2 diabetes.

5.   Which food item would be **allowed** for purchase using a SNAP debit card?

    a.   Hot baked chicken held in a roaster and ready to eat

    b.   Dry wine with no added sugar

    c.   An herb that curbs the appetite for refined carbohydrates

    d.   A marshmallow Easter bunny coated with milk chocolate

6.   Which statement about sugar subsidies is accurate?

    a.   These subsidies are a way to return funding to the states.

    b.   Subsidies only apply to producers of organic sugar.

    c.   These subsidies no longer exist. Congress has repealed the 1981 Farm Bill.

    d.   Sugar subsidies go directly to the sugar producers.

7.   Which example **best** illustrates the concept of a downstream approach to controlling Type 2 diabetes?

    a.   Lifestyle interventions

    b.   Life insurance companies offering discounts on yearly premiums to people with test results indicating normal A1c levels

8.   The National School Lunch Program regulates:

    a.   Sugar content

    b.   Minimum calorie content

    c.   Maximum fiber content

    d.   Minimum sodium content

9.   The role of culture is important to consider relative to sugar consumption. Which one of the following examples is **least** illustrative of this principle?

    a.   Chocolate is often loaded with sugar even though its value as a way to stimulate endorphins is compromised by diluting the cocoa content.

    b.   Halo foods such as pie and ice cream continue to be American favorites.

    c.   Sugar is relatively price inelastic: people buy it no matter what.

10.   Which food has the **least** sugar per gram?

    a.   Organic ketchup

    b.   Commercially made baked beans

    c.   Canned tuna (in water rather than oil)

    d.   Canned fruit (not in water or its own juice)

For Discussion (in class or small groups, or online)

11. Among the most prominent sources of sugar in the American diet are fast-food chains such as Burger King, McDonald's, and Wendy's. Go online to find the sugar content of items at these chain stores such as milkshakes, fried apple pies, and other desserts. Using this information, identify the three fast foods that you would classify as the worst offenders relative to the overconsumption of sugar.

12. Textbooks, by nature, are not the most recent source of information. This is especially true for public health, given the rapidly changing landscapes of policy, regulation, and legislation related to public health practice and people's health behavior. Go online to learn whether (and if so, how) the National School Lunch Program now regulates the sugar content of student meals. Then, in a one-page summary, explain and judge this progress (or lack thereof).

13. The American Sugar Alliance is the political organization for U.S. sugar producers. Its website is fascinating in that the stories and news are highly focused on subsidies, global and domestic markets, and human interest stories about sugar farmers and their families. Take a look! As you explore the website, try to locate news about research on the health effects of sugar. Anything you find may or may not be legitimate, so send the link to at least one other student also taking this course, and work with that student (or students) to determine the legitimacy of the information.

References

American Diabetes Association. (2018). Economic costs of diabetes in the U.S. – in 2017. *Diabetes Care*, *14*(5), 917–921.

Andes, C. J., Cheng, Y. J., & Rolka, D. S. (2020). Prevention of prediabetes among adolescents and young adults in the United States, 2005-2016. *The Journal of the American Medical Association, Pediatrics*, *174*(2), e194498.

Boyle, J. P., Thompson, T. J., Gregg, E. W., Barker, L. E., & Williamson, D. F. (2010). Projection of the year 2050 burden of diabetes in the US adult population: dynamic modeling of incidence, mortality, and prediabetes prevalence. *Popular Health Metrics*, 8, 29.

CDC. (2020). National diabetes statistics report, 2020. https://www.cdc.gov/diabetes/data/statistics-report/index.html

CDC. (2021). Cost-effectiveness of diabetes interventions. https://www.cdc.gov/chronicdisease/programs-impact/pop/diabetes.htm

Center for Investigative Reporting. (2013, October 13). No limits on sugar in school lunches. *The San-Diego Union-Tribune*. https://www.sandiegouniontribune.com/news/watchdog/sdut-cir-sugar-school-lunches-no-limits-2013oct03-story.html

Diabetes Prevention Program Research Group. (2012). The 10-year cost-effectiveness of lifestyle intervention or Metformin for diabetes prevention. *Diabetes Care*, *35*(4), 723–730.

Haw, J. S., Galaviz, K. I., Straus, A. N., Kowalski, A. J., Magee, M. J., Weber, M. B., Wei, J., Narayan, K. M., & Ali, M. K. (2017). Long-term sustainability of diabetes prevention approaches: A systematic review and meta-analysis of randomized clinical trials. *Journal of the American Medical Association, Internal Medicine*, *177*(12), 1808–1817.

Kearns, C. E., Schmidt, L. A., & Glantz, S. A. (2016). Sugar industry research and coronary heart disease research – a historical analysis. *The Journal of the American Medical Association: Internal Medicine*, *176*(11), 1680–1685.

Riddle, M. C., & Herman, W. H. (2018). The cost of diabetes care – an elephant in the room. *Diabetes Care*, 41(5), 929–932.

Smith, V. H. (2018). The U.S. spends $4 billion a year subsidizing 'Stalinist-style' domestic sugar production. Market Watch. https://www.marketwatch.com/story/the-us-spends-4-billion-a-year-subsidizing-stalinist-style-domestic-sugar-production-2018-06-25

USDA Food and Nutrition Service. (2021). Supplemental Nutrition Assistance Program: Facts about SNAP. https://www.fns.usda.gov/snap/facts

CHAPTER 7

AVERTING CANCER RATHER THAN WAITING TO TREAT IT

An ounce of prevention is worth a pound of cure.

—*Benjamin Franklin*

Overview

America would be well advised to begin heeding the famous words of Benjamin Franklin. His well-known quip is often repeated in family settings; however, its real value is at the level of government and commerce related to public health. The single best example of applying these words of wisdom to public health resides in cancer prevention. In 2021, nearly 2 million new cases of cancer occurred, with nearly one-third of those people (just over 600,000) dying from cancer. The number 600,000 has a context in the COVID-19 pandemic: approximately 1.5 years into the U.S. COVID-19 epidemic, this was the number of deaths recorded. Yet the 50% greater death rate from cancer goes unnoticed by news outlets and becomes normal in our society. Social responses typically center on runs and walks designed to raise awareness and funding to promote finding a cure. This idea of a cure places cancer in the wrong context.

As you will learn by reading this chapter, most cancers develop slowly and progress under physical conditions that could be altered by daily actions. Unfortunately, the required ounce of prevention regarding cancer is perceived by millions of Americans as far more than an ounce and not worth the effort. Thus, perceptions favoring the pound of cure become dominant, and people invest their hopes in the medical approach to solve the cancer epidemics. This is an easy way for people to opt out of the daily, weekly, and even annual or longer actions that must become commonplace to truly cure cancer. The fact that people trust their doctors and hospitals to take care of them if they develop cancer is an achievement by those who benefit from the large sums of money that undergird every step of the arduous process of treating cancer. Hence, one function of this chapter is to introduce you to the concept of the **medical-industrial complex**.

To keep this chapter modest in scope, it will focus on three common cancers: (a) cancer of the colon, (b) cervical cancer, and (c) breast cancer. Due largely to a rapidly advancing body of science, each of these cancers can now be considered largely preventable, placing the onus on public health practice to apply Benjamin Franklin's immortal words. Also, to keep this chapter fully in the context of public health, it will emphasize new research showing the full spectrum of primary

LEARNING OBJECTIVES

1. Broadly apply the concept of a Hygeia-based philosophy to cancer control in the United States.

2. Understand the current public health opportunities for the prevention of colorectal cancer.

3. Understand the current public health opportunities for the prevention of breast cancer.

4. Understand the current public health opportunities for the prevention of cervical cancer.

5. Explain the integration of public health with medical care relative to the secondary prevention of cancer.

Understanding the Science and Practice of Public Health, First Edition. Richard Crosby.
© 2023 John Wiley & Sons, Inc. Published 2023 by John Wiley & Sons, Inc.

prevention opportunities that exist for these three cancers. As a reminder from **Chapter 2**, *primary prevention* means the disease or health-compromising condition is avoided entirely. The application of primary prevention to cancer is a relatively new development in public health. The more traditional public health response to cancer has been tightly focused on secondary prevention. Again, as a reminder from **Chapter 2**, *secondary prevention* means the disease process is diagnosed early. Applied to cancer, secondary prevention entails screening tests designed to diagnose the early signs of cancer, thereby greatly tipping the odds of survival in favor of those fortunate enough to receive these healthcare services. But the key term in that last sentence is *healthcare services*, which implies an interface between public health and medical care.

Much like the previous two chapters, this chapter opens with a brief section that provides some basic biology about cancer and how it begins. Once you understand that the three cancers discussed in this chapter are relatively "forgiving," you will quickly grasp the concepts of primary prevention being applied at the population level to greatly reduce the need for a reliance on tertiary prevention applied to cancer (also recall from **Chapter 2** that tertiary prevention equates with medical treatments designed to lessen the damage of a disease process).

Finally, it is important to understand that the three examples in this chapter are being used to illustrate larger issues and public health solutions relative to cancer. For instance, when you learn about the cancer-protective value of phytochemicals (presented in conjunction with colorectal cancer), you will understand their value in preventing nearly all cancers. The selection of the three examples for this chapter (cancers of the cervix, breast, and colon) was also based on the unique public health opportunities that each presents. This chapter is exciting because these public health opportunities are all newly emerging and may ultimately make a dramatic reduction in cancer cases and cancer deaths a realistic possibility rather than wishful thinking.

A Hygeia-Based Philosophy for Cancer Control

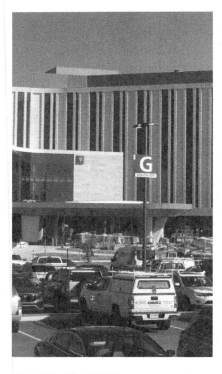

Photo 7.1   We still build huge monuments to Laso and Aceso.

The Greek god known as Hygeia served as icon for healthy living as a method of averting disease. Sadly, the absence of allegiance to Hygeia, then and now, creates a dependence of medical "gods." We spend far more of the gross domestic product on medical care than any other single commodity. The U.S. government spends far more on Medicaid and Medicare than even the lavish budget set aside for the Department of Defense. Let's take a look at **Photo 7.1**.

This is a 2021 photo of the yet-to-be-finished Indiana University Regional Academic Health Center. Built at a cost of more than half a billion dollars, the center is touted as a way to make Indiana residents among the healthiest people in the nation. The short name for this huge complex is *IU Health*. It is ironic that the name shamelessly borrows from Hygeia, while its services are very much based on medical care instead of primary prevention. As you may suspect from what you have learned by taking this course, this downstream approach to health lacks efficiency and fails to acknowledge that health is much more than the absence of clinically defined disease. In essence, the building in the photo is a type of monument to Laso and Aceso.

Applied to cancer control, the downstream thinking engendered by an allegiance to these two Greek gods tends to dominate U.S. culture, especially with respect to cancer. Indeed, the mindset that cancer is a matter of fate or bad luck, or is even just inevitable, creates a kind of resignation to healing. Sadly (and needlessly), this same resignation equates with a nearly complete lack of attention to the third goddess: Hygeia.

Cancer (as you know from reading the previous section of this chapter) is not just one disease. Barring those cancers that tend to be largely beyond primary and secondary prevention (e.g., Hodgkin's Lymphoma, pancreatic cancer, leukemia), the good news for current public health practice is that most cancers have an identifiable **etiology** (meaning the cause and co-factors are known). Even more exciting for public health practice is that most cancers also have an identified set of **protective factors**. A protective factor is much more than simply the absence of a risk factor: think of a protective factor as being a type of shield from harm. As a relatively simple example, consider the airbags in a car. These safety devices protect you in the event of a collision. Similarly, protective factors against cancer protect you in the event of a biological change in cellular reproduction. It's important to understand that risk factors and protective factors are not simply opposite sides of the same coin. When it comes to cancer, think about **risk factors** as either direct agents of cellular change or indirect agents in that a predisposition to cellular change occurs. **Figure 7.1** provides a visual illustration that distinguishes between risk and protective factors relative to the three cancers you are learning about in this chapter.

risk factors and protective factors are not simply opposite sides of the same coin.

As you study this figure, keep in mind that each day, a battle is occurring inside your body. The millions of cell divisions that occur will always produce mistakes! These mistakes (i.e., mutations) are constantly being cleaned up by the body's repair mechanisms. It is only when the mistakes become too overwhelming for the repair mechanisms that trouble begins. The protective factors keep the body optimally able to activate the repair system. Generally speaking, the science of cancer prevention has focused less on promoting protective factors and more on eliminating risk factors. As public health research advances, however, there is an increasing emphasis on factors that protect against cancer, with the ultimate goal being an equal focus on both sides of **Figure 7.1**.

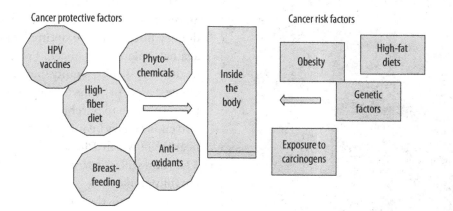

Figure 7.1   Risk factors are not the same as protective factors

Public Health Opportunities to Prevent Colorectal Cancer

It is somewhat arbitrary to think about cancers as isolated forms of the disease. This is because the protective factors (with a few notable exceptions, such as HPV vaccination) are broadly protective. Similarly, but to a lesser extent, the risk factors are typically not cancer-specific (a good example is obesity). So, with all this in mind, let's look at a specific cancer: **colorectal cancer**. Of the cancers with the greatest opportunity for prevention, colorectal is at the top of the list. Despite being nearly 100% preventable, this is a common cancer and a common cause of death from cancer. The cancer involves the lower section of the large intestine (the **colon**) and the final section (the **rectum**). It is highly preventable because of a "forgiveness factor." This is a forgiving cancer because it typically grows slowly, and the precancerous stages are well marked by growths called **adenomatous polyps**. A *polyp* is a precancerous growth inside the wall of the colon.

> This is a forgiving cancer because it typically grows slowly, and the precancerous stages are well marked by growths called **adenomatous polyps**.

The most important protective factors against the formation of polyps, and thus colorectal cancer, are found in foods. These broadly fall into two categories:

- Fiber

- Phytochemicals

The Role of Fiber

About two-thirds of all polyps found in the colon are of this type. Adenomatous polyps are far less likely to form and flourish in people who consume large amounts of **vegetable fiber** (Tantamango et al., 2011). This finding comes from a study population with many strict and long-term vegetarians. The study was based on more than 400 new cases of colon polyps, thus giving the conclusion strong rigor. In a nutshell, that conclusion was simple: people consuming the highest levels of vegetable fiber had the fewest polyps. However, this conclusion is worth a bit more explanation.

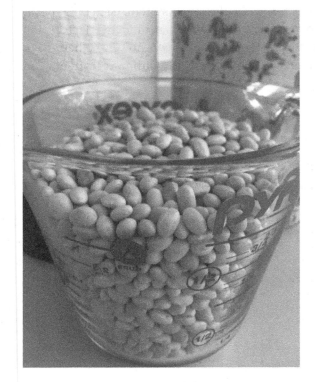

The vegetable fibers that were most protective in this study were those from legumes. This term is most likely unfamiliar to you, as it is to most Americans. A **legume** is any edible food that grows inside a pod (see **Box 7.1**). For example, peas are legumes. The most famous legumes are beans. Beans provide a huge amount of protein, and they are rich in dietary fibers that are optimally protective against colorectal cancer. From a public health and health equity perspective, the greatest asset of beans (of any variety) is that they are cheap to purchase. For instance, the two cups of navy beans (used to make baked beans) shown in **Photo 7.2** cost less than $2.00 and will fill a large pot when the beans are fully cooked).

> The most famous legumes are beans.

Photo 7.2   Beans are among the least expensive foods sold in stores, but they are one of the most valuable in terms of health.

Despite all the protective qualities of beans (which range far beyond colorectal cancer), it is unlikely that health-promotion programs could easily persuade people to begin replacing large portions of their diets

BOX 7.1. WHAT ARE LEGUMES?

Often overlooked due to their rock-solid texture, beans, chickpeas, and lentils are all legumes. The definition of a **legume** specifies that it must (a) grow in a pod that splits down the middle (lengthwise) into two sides and (b) **fix nitrogen** – meaning it draws protein from the soil into the plant and thus into the food we consume. All three of these foods (beans, chickpeas, and lentils) require extensive soaking before cooking and substantial cooking time. They do not fit the American ideal of being quick to prepare! However, they are inexpensive and a rich source of protein and fiber. They are underused in places such as nursing homes, schools, and workplace cafeterias, thus creating an opportunity for public health intervention. Given the typically large kitchens in such establishments, these otherwise difficult-to-cook legumes can become a staple.

Two other important legumes are peas and peanuts. These, of course, are much more user-friendly and therefore much more acceptable to consumers as quick foods. This is especially true of the very versatile peanut! However, peanuts and all the foods we make from them (e.g., peanut butter, peanut oil, and peanut cookies) are not superfoods like the other legumes. For instance, compared to red kidney beans, peanuts have two-thirds less fiber and more than 50 times the amount of saturated fat (which creates issues with heart disease and has been implicated as a potential risk factor for breast cancer).

(meats, for example) with a similarly large portion of beans and other legumes. This is because most people either do not know how to prepare beans from scratch (meaning the raw harvested bean) or are unwilling to engage in the relatively lengthy preparation process, which includes soaking the beans in water for several hours before boiling them for extended times. Cooking beans also requires a fair output of either electric or gas-based energy to heat the water used to boil the beans. So, is there a public health intervention opportunity here?

The answer to this question is a clear yes! The accessibility of beans to people of low income creates this public health opportunity. For example, a simple policy change to SNAP (see **Chapter 6**) could allow for the purchase of pressure cookers, thereby greatly reducing the preparation time for beans to as little as 30 minutes. This policy change could be made in a such a way that YouTube video links would be sent to SNAP recipients to (a) notify them of the opportunity to make this purchase, (b) teach them why beans are important relative to good health, and (c) teach them how to make dozens of good-tasting bean-based foods. Of course, countless other public health interventions are also possible relative to promoting a diet rich in vegetable fiber. The task for any of you who ultimately enter the workforce as a person positioned to make these ideas become a reality is to try!

The Role of Phytochemicals

Have you ever wondered why humans cannot just take a pill each day that automatically provides all the vitamins and minerals we need? The answer may be somewhat disheartening to you. The reason is that nutrition science is now advanced enough to inform us that vast numbers of other nutrients (not yet classified as vitamins or minerals) are essential to health. These other nutrients are collectively known as **phytochemicals**. The exciting news about phytochemicals relative to the prevention of colorectal cancer is that at least seven phytochemical compounds have been identified as having very strong **chemopreventive** action against the cellular changes preceding colorectal cancer, as well as the progression of this cancer (Li et al., 2015). **Table 7.1** displays these seven compounds by their source.

Given the relatively new evidence regarding the chemopreventive role of phytochemicals, the logical question becomes, "How can all this translate into more effective public health practice?" At least two possible answers to this question exist. The first involves the food industry. Just as the food industry was very quick to label products as gluten-free, consumer demand relative to cancer might also be elevated to the level of the demand pertaining to celiac

Table 7.1   Chemopreventive phytochemicals pertaining to colorectal cancer

Phytochemical	Source
Apples polysaccharides	Apples and cloudy apple cider/juice
Mushroom glucans	Most mushrooms
Curcumin	Turmeric
Ginsenosides	The ginseng plant
Soy saponins	Soy-based foods
Resveratrol	Berries, grapes, and peanuts[*]
Quercetin	Fruits, and drinks such as wine and tea

* Note that peanuts are legumes.

disease that triggered the massive gluten-free revolution in the industry. Products could be marketed and sold as containing, for instance, "5 phytochemicals with cancer prevention properties" (although the food industry would devise a way to shorten this to just a few words).

The second opportunity involves a much more aggressive public health agenda. As you know from reading the previous two chapters, a constant theme exists across the spectrum of chronic diseases regarding primary prevention. That theme is the outstanding value of a plant-based whole food (PBWF) diet (see **Chapter 5** for reminders). This is yet another point where public health greatly departs from medicine. While the medical approach seeks cures that are disease-specific, the public health approach seeks relatively simple preventive actions that apply broadly across several diseases. Because this is the third and final chapter of this book that includes the term *PBWF diet*, it is important for you to think about the myriad ways that foods that are part of this diet could be magnified to a higher level of desirability among massive numbers (i.e., millions) of people. Mushrooms, for instance (see **Table 7.1**), are a versatile food in cooking and a valuable part of a PBWF diet. Also important are apples, grapes, berries, and the other foods shown in the table. But the marketing of these foods as disease-fighters, for example, has not occurred on a large scale, even though restaurant menus could easily be devised and labeled to convey the complete item as a PBWF.

Although not a new approach to public health, a final method of promoting population-level consumption of phytochemicals is centered on health education. To illustrate, let's go back to resveratrol and quercetin from **Table 7.1**. These phytochemicals are found in wine, especially dark red wines.

Meat Consumption as a Primary Risk Factor

Shifting now from the protective factors for colorectal cancer (i.e., fiber and phytochemicals) to risk factors, this chapter will highlight the risk factor having the greatest potential for public health intervention: the consumption of meat and meat products. A recent study provides a succinct picture of just how strongly meat is implicated in the formation of polyps (Aykan, 2015). One key aspect of the study findings is that for every added 120 g of red meat per day a person consumes, the risk of colorectal cancer increases by about 20% (for reference, a Quarter Pounder from McDonald's weights 113 g). Further, for every added 30 g per day of processed meats (e.g., bologna, pepperoni, sausage, etc.), the risk of colorectal cancer increases by about 9%. Thus, for example, a person who eats one serving of red meat (i.e., 120 g) each day would have a seven times greater risk of developing colorectal cancer than a vegetarian or vegan.

The public health implication here lies in treating meat much like tobacco in terms of controlling its all-too-easy access. This point brings us back to the need for increased regulations on America's food industry. For instance, an economic analysis has shown that American consumers pay about two added dollars to cover the healthcare costs (and costs to the environment in terms of climate change) of our nation's meat-eating obsession for every $1 spent on meat products (Sewell, 2020). So, thinking in terms of simple math, the real cost of meat consumption in the United States is three times that of its annual sales value of about $250 billion. That $250 billion becomes $750 billion when you consider issues such as the resulting medical care needed due to diseases – especially colorectal cancer. But despite these rather shocking estimates, the U.S. meat industry is subsidized to the tune of about $38 billion per year! In contrast, U.S. subsidies for the entire fruit and vegetable industry are less than 1% of this annual $38 billion outlay of federal money (Sewell, 2020). All this begs the rhetorical question, "Are we using taxpayer dollars to support a product that clearly leads to overwhelming medical care costs?" Here again (as in **Chapters 5 and 6**), the public health intervention exists at the structural level: the policies set by the U.S. Department of Agriculture.

Of course, policy is difficult to alter, and people in the United States have grown accustomed to eating meat and meat-based products. This is a prime example of how culture profoundly influences public health practice. Consider, for example, the great American outdoor grill (see **Box 7.2**).

BOX 7.2. THE HUMAN SIDE

As a socio-cultural construction, gender is a strong influence on dietary behaviors. Most outdoor grills are typically used for grilling meat rather than vegetables, and U.S. culture has focused on men being the "masters of the grill." Masculinity seems to have become partly defined not only by grilling meat but also by the act of eating meat. This small bit of culture is magnified when we also consider a common myth: that meat is needed to make muscle tissue. Further, the power of advertising has contributed to a culture of "meat and masculinity." This concept of masculinity being partly defined by eating meat has

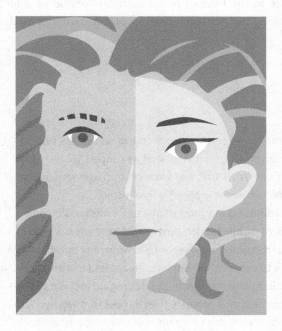

been well documented (Love & Sulikowski, 2018). This relationship has also been tested empirically by the author of this textbook. It turns out that the relationship between men, masculinity, and meat is firmly embedded in U.S. culture.

This study was conducted in 2018 (Crosby, unpublished data). The online survey of 300 men posed a number of questions, such as: "I would feel feminine having only a large salad (without meat) for lunch or dinner with friends," and "Men who **do not** eat meat are typically lacking in masculinity." The response options were provided on a seven-point scale and ranged from Strongly Agree to Strongly Disagree. The study found that scores on a measure of masculinity were correlated with two separate measures of attitudes toward eating meat. The findings were not a surprise: as scores on the measure of masculinity increased (meaning more masculine), scores on both sets of attitudinal measures also increased (meaning attitudes and behaviors were more favorable to meat eating). In turn, both measures of attitudes were strongly predictive of actual meat eating. In brief, this study found that masculinity was predictive of meat eating.

So, what is the take-home point for public health practice? The answer brings us back to culture and the sheer power of the food industry. Beef, for example, is marketed as manly! Until the food industry (via advertising) begins to take responsibility for protecting the health of the public, it is likely that "men and meat" will continue to be entwined. Ultimately, the "manly" habit of eating meat will become an important target for cultural change designed to promote public health and help reduce the pace of climate change (see **Chapter 13**).

Public Health Opportunities to Prevent Breast Cancer

The good news about breast cancer is that the overall (i.e., population-level) risk can be substantially reduced through daily changes in diet and exercise habits and by not smoking or drinking more than one serving of alcohol per day. Ironically, the bad news is that breast cancer risk can only be substantially reduced through these daily changes – there is no magic solution to prevention. The bad news part is centered on the myriad issues that so often preclude people from eating a PBWF diet and being engaged in daily exercise/movement routines. But as people become more public-health-aware and policies continue to favor improved dietary and exercise habits, it is notable that women can indeed play an active role in avoiding breast cancer (note that this is about primary prevention rather than the more traditional option of secondary prevention via mammography; see **Box 7.3** to learn more about mammography).

there is no magic solution to prevention.

The Possible Role of Antioxidants

To fully understand antioxidants, it is important to begin with the term **oxidation** (or "to oxidize"). Think about an ordinary apple. Once you cut into it, what happens? It turns brown on the inside. Similar to a car rusting from sitting out in the rain, the cut apple is affected by oxygen entering its molecules and removing mass (in the form of electrons). Oxidation in the human body also occurs on a fairly regular basis. One result is that some of the atoms in your body may wind up with an uneven number of electrons. These are called **free radicals**. So far, this science is like high-school biochemistry, but now comes the important part.

*Oxidation in the human body is broadly known as **oxidative stress**.*

Oxidation in the human body is broadly known as **oxidative stress**. This stress is reduced at a biochemical level by compounds known as **antioxidants**. Antioxidants can also bind to free radicals, thereby disabling their destructive abilities in the body. All this applies to the prevention of a broad base of chronic disease in the human body, with cancers being a large part of that base. As an example, let's consider the protective value of antioxidants against breast cancer.

BOX 7.3. WHAT IS MAMMOGRAPHY?

Mammography is a vital aspect of medical practice – a textbook example of secondary prevention. Annual mammograms can detect precancerous growths as well as cancers that are just beginning to form and spread. The value, of course, is that any excision of tissue required to remove the neoplasia (*neo* means new, and *plasia* means growth) is minimized.

Although not a public health practice, promoting mammography to women underserved by this life-saving technology is a vital aspect of **public health outreach**. Outreach is a type of crossover function between public health and medical care. The goal is to apply the approaches and people from the public health workforce to ensure that women can access (and are motivated to access) mammography services. Public health approaches in this regard include **social media campaigns** designed to promote awareness and enhance the chances that women will be receptive to being linked with a clinic or public health program that can successfully navigate them to a mammography service. However, the more important public health approach is to ensure access to mammography among women who are unable to pay for the service. As you can imagine, mammography is expensive, and women who are uninsured or under-insured typically may require financial assistance to obtain mammograms. The average price of a routine mammogram in the United States is about $300.

Sadly, the empirical question of whether (and, if so, how much) antioxidants provide significant protection against the development of breast cancer has not been adequately studied. This is, once again, due to an emphasis on treatment. Antioxidants have been studied for their potential role as an adjunct to treatment (e.g., in addition to chemotherapy) for breast cancer. In this medical approach, the concept of a PBWF diet rich in antioxidants was passed over in favor of a pill approach that provided selected antioxidants in their chemical form rather than as part of the foods in which they originated. Overall, these studies have yielded findings that suggest antioxidants may or may not be protective against the continued growth of breast cancer.

Let's take a minute to think about what is going on here. First, as you have already learned from reading this book, adding antioxidant supplements to a woman's diet after a breast cancer diagnosis is a downstream approach, despite its apparent appeal to improved nutrition. Second, the entire concept of an upstream approach is based on maintaining the body in a completely healthy condition to make it impervious to the unchecked cascade of cellular events that lead to cancer (of any kind). In essence, the medicalization of antioxidants in this example is too little, too late. Think of antioxidants as a long-term investment in a person's health – one that must build up over time and thus cannot be used as a quick way to reverse a disease process. This is a hard reality for people to accept if they have breast cancer or have a friend/family member who has breast cancer. It is also likely a hard reality for people working in the medical profession. But the reality is consistent with what is now known relative to how foods work to prevent disease: their action is based on years (if not decades) of consumption rather than a sudden influx after the disease has occurred. Third, the science of nutrition is still in its infancy. Thirty years ago, for example, we knew very little about phytochemicals or antioxidants. We still do not know about the absorption of these very tiny compounds into the bloodstream (via the small intestine) and ultimately into the cellular machinery. It is entirely possible that the absorption of any given antioxidant is reliant on the presence of one or several other compounds that have yet to be synthesized or even identified. Thus, studies based on pharmaceutically-prepared antioxidant supplements simply lack the insight that the protective value may be in the food-only version of any given antioxidant.

the medicalization of antioxidants in this example is too little, too late.

Although you are learning about antioxidants at this point in the book, it is important to understand that their value relative to an upstream approach to averting disease extends far beyond breast cancer. With that point firmly in mind, let's have a quick look at the foods supplying rich sources of antioxidants (see **Table 7.2**). Berries, in particular, are an excellent source of antioxidants (see **Photo 7.3**).

The Role of Obesity

In addition to the possible emerging role of antioxidants in preventing breast cancer, evidence suggesting the presence of a malleable risk factor – obesity – is also accumulating. This risk factor is one widely

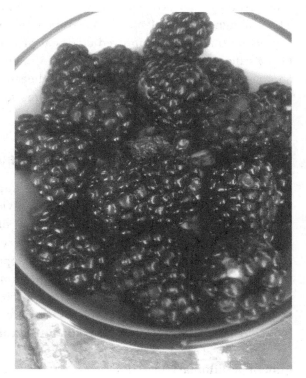

Photo 7.3   Fresh blackberries are a great way to enjoy your daily dose of antioxidants.

Table 7.2   Food sources of antioxidants

Leafy green vegetables	Root vegetables	Fruits
Broccoli	Potatoes	Cranberries
Spinach	Sweet potatoes	Raspberries
Kale	Beets	Blueberries
Swiss chard	Radishes	Apples
Lettuce	Onions	Grapes
Asparagus	Carrots	Strawberries

implicated in cardiovascular disease (**Chapter 5**), and it is part of metabolic syndrome. A review of studies on this factor yielded the following conclusion: "Excess body weight has been linked to an increased risk of postmenopausal breast cancer . . ." (Ligibel, 2011). The mechanisms for this cause-and-effect relationship appear related to four factors: (a) obesity triggers more estrogen production, which, in turn, may lead to breast cancer; (b) obesity also triggers more insulin production, which, in turn, may lead to breast cancer; (c) central obesity tends to be a greater cause of breast cancer compared to excess weight in the thighs and hips; and (d) the timing of obesity in life, with weight gain in the adult years being implicated as the causative factor.

Now that you understand a bit about the relationship between obesity and breast cancer, the next question becomes, "What are the implications for public health practice?" This question leaves us at a frontier, meaning that answers have yet to be devised. Of course, possibilities exist! For instance, many women are concerned about whether they have either the BRCA1 or BRCA2 gene in their genetic code. Both genes have been implicated as predisposing factors to breast cancer. Indeed, it is not unusual for women with BRCA1 or BRCA2 to undergo **bilateral mastectomy** (removal of both breasts) as a method of averting breast cancer (Alaofi et al., 2018). This willingness is emblematic of a strong underlying motivation to avert breast cancer, thus suggesting that greatly improved efforts at promoting weight loss as an effective method of breast cancer prevention may culminate in millions of women adopting this far less invasive approach to prevention. Such efforts would need to mobilize existing national resources such as the American Cancer Society, the Centers for Disease Control and Prevention, and the Susan G. Komen Foundation.

Public Health Opportunities to Prevent Cervical Cancer

Like colorectal cancer, cervical cancer is also "forgiving" in that it develops and grows slowly (in most cases). To understand this, think of cervical cancer as a process having three distinct phases, with only the third involving any type of cancerous growth. Let's first be sure you know where the **cervix** is and what it does. The cervix is simply the opening to the **uterus**. As such, it is located at the end of the vagina. The opening is known as the **os**. The tissue around the os (in adult females) is **squamous epithelium** (like the texture of the skin on your body). However, prior to adulthood, the os is not composed entirely of squamous epithelium, which creates a problem because the surface is far more susceptible to infections with a virus. These infections are known as **sexually transmitted infections** (STIs). During the teen years, and even into the early 20s, the os is a likely site of infection for a particular STI known as the **human papillomavirus** (HPV).

Phase One

It has been estimated that four of every five U.S. adults (80%) will be infected with HPV at least once in their lifetime. At least 18 variants of HPV are fully capable of initiating cancer development in the cervix. Because HPV is a virus, it cannot be treated/cured. Instead, the virus must be cleared by the immune system; a healthy immune system can do this in about 10 to 12 months.

So, this infection followed by clearance typically occurs among millions of women who are completely unaware that they have HPV. The problem is **persistent HPV infections**, meaning:

- The infection does not end on its own because of a weakened immune system.

- The infection does not end on its own because of co-factors such as having other sexually transmitted infections.

- Re-infection (with the same or different variants of HPV) keeps occurring.

Since about 2001, oncologists have widely agreed that persistent infections with variants of HPV are known to trigger cellular changes in the os and the cervix itself. These persistent infections are the prequel events of **cervical dysplasia**. Briefly, cervical dysplasia means "ill-formed" growth." It is the term used to denote cellular abnormalities in and around the cervix. This does not necessarily imply cancer; however, it does suggest that precancerous conditions are at least present.

Phase Two

The event of cervical dysplasia is fairly common among sexually active females, especially those having penile-vaginal sex with multiple partners (as each new male sex partner poses a new risk of transmitting HPV). The odds are that most cases of cervical dysplasia are never diagnosed. Among those diagnosed cases, the vast majority will not become cancerous (this is one reason it is said that cervical cancer is forgiving). One difference between cases that proceed to phase three and those that resolve naturally involves tobacco use. Decades of evidence implicate tobacco use as a risk factor for the progression of cervical dysplasia to cancer of the cervix.

The odds are that most cases of cervical dysplasia are never diagnosed.

Phase Three

Even in this phase, which involves cancer, a high degree of forgiveness exists because the cancer grows slowly. **Figure 7.2** provides a useful method of understanding this progression. The forgiveness refers to stages 1 and 2, which are considered localized: the cancer has yet to grow

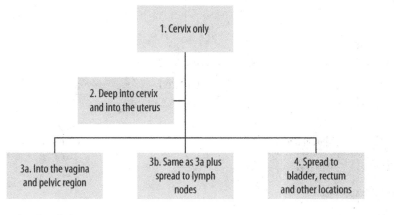

Figure 7.2   The progression of cervical cancer

into organs other than the cervix and uterus. Two medical options exist for tertiary prevention at these stages.

The first medical option is the **loop electrosurgical excision procedure (LEEP)**. In most cases, performing a LEEP does minimal damage to the cervix. The purpose of the LEEP is to remove dysplastic cells before they develop into cancerous cells. The second option is far more invasive, as it removes the entire cervix/uterus. This is known as a **hysterectomy**.

Primary Prevention Opportunities

In 2006, a historic event occurred in the United States. It was not heralded as such and garnered very little attention from the media or the public as a whole. It was the approval by the U.S. Food and Drug Administration of the first-ever vaccine against a cancer: specifically, cervical cancer. The current version of this vaccine provides acquired immunity against nine different variants of HPV.

In everyday language, the vaccine works by providing immunity against the variants of HPV most implicated in the formation of cervical dysplasia and invasive cervical cancer. The level of protection tends to be greater when the vaccine is given between the ages 9 and 14. It is vital to note that the vaccine is recommended for young males as well as females. The public health advantage lies in the simple fact that males transmit HPV to females. Unfortunately (and much like the vaccine against COVID-19), a lack of public health mandates regarding HPV vaccination led to sluggish uptake by the public. This problem is one beyond the scope of medical practice and clearly lies in the realm of public health.

The best practice public health approach to promoting the HPV vaccine begins with a fairly simple model. As shown in **Figure 7.3**, the ultimate goal of eventually vaccinating the entire population starting at age 9 (shown in the middle of the figure) is met through the mutual effort of three sources. At the top, you see the obvious source: the vaccine must continue to be developed with a top-rated safety record and a very high ranking in terms of efficacy (this is the role of industry). At bottom left, you see what is also obvious: healthcare settings must take part in the efforts to have a successful and ongoing vaccination campaign. At bottom right, you see what may not be obvious: the public – especially parents of young

> the vaccine is recommended for young males as well as females.

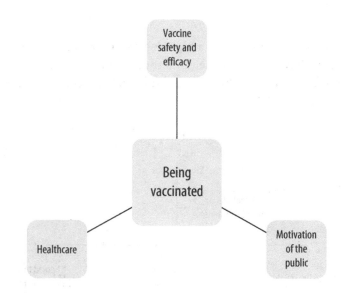

Figure 7.3   HPV vaccination model

1-2-3 Pap: Easy Steps to Prevent Cervical Cancer

PROGRAM SYNOPSIS | Designed to increase completion of the HPV vaccine series among 18- to 26-year-old women receiving their first dose of the vaccine, this intervention involves educating women on HPV with a DVD and fact sheet, scheduling follow-up vaccine appointments, conducting scripted reminder calls, and distributing appointment reminder cards. The study showed an increase in vaccine series completion.

Figure 7.4   Example of a research-tested intervention from the National Cancer Institute
Source: National Cancer Institute / Public Domain.

adolescents – must be willing to take the needed steps to be vaccinated. This last step (public motivation) has traditionally proven to be the weak point in most massive public health vaccination campaigns. Consider that after 13 years of having the HPV vaccine available, in 2019, only about 50% of teens had completed the vaccination series.

So, what can public health do to more fully achieve the goal of motivating the public? All too often, well-intentioned professionals (e.g., physicians, people working at the CDC, and news reporters) harbor the mistaken belief that simply telling the public about the vaccine is enough motivation. This has never been true! Instead, carefully crafted programs are tested and refined until they meet the standards needed to be a program that works. Consider just one example from an important public (government-funded) source: the National Cancer Institute (see **Figure 7.4**). This brief intervention program was implemented in everyday community settings such as Walmart stores and public gatherings such as fairs and festivals. It provided young women with a free first dose of the HPV vaccine, followed by having them view a 13-minute video produced by the research team (based on extensive research with the target audience). The video was designed to promote return for the required second and third doses of the vaccine. It was also designed to promote the lifelong habit in these young women of receiving periodic screenings to detect cervical dysplasia (known as Pap testing) (Rabarison et al. 2015).

One other primary prevention opportunity relative to cervical cancer warrants attention. Because HPV is sexually transmitted, it is possible to avert transmission through the consistent and correct use of **condoms**. This is very much a Hygeia-based approach! The caveat is that HPV spreads by genital-to-genital contact; this means condoms can only be partially effective because they do not cover the entire surface area of the male genitals (Winer et al., 2006). Further, even though the HPV vaccine is highly protective, it does not protect against all variants of the virus that can lead to cervical cancer. But partial protection, magnified to the level of entire populations, has the potential to substantially reduce the annual incidence of cervical cancer in the United States. Sadly, gynecologists and other healthcare providers who could counsel women at risk of persistent HPV infection are not encouraged by their professional organizations to spend time teaching about the potential value of condom use. This is an example of the clash between the medical and public health paradigms. Again, with the tight focus on the individual, the medical paradigm holds that partial protection is inadequate. This is fully logical and valid when the concern is the patient in the exam room. For instance, it would be less than compelling to explain to the patient that "condom use offers about a 30% reduction in risk of HPV acquisition." Conversely, with the population-level view of the public health paradigm, millions of partial protections add up to thousands of cases averted. The 30% is quite valuable in the larger picture: that is, the view of public health as opposed to medical care.

even though the HPV vaccine is highly protective, it does not protect against all variants of the virus that can lead to cervical cancer.

The Integration of Public Health and Medical Care

Of all the diseases and health-compromising conditions included in this textbook, cancer represents the ideal integration of public health and medical care. This integration particularly applies to colorectal cancer and cervical cancer (the forgiving cancers).

Beginning with colorectal cancer, a recent advance in laboratory technology now makes it possible to determine the presence of polyps in the colon or rectum using a simple at-home test kit. This test is known as the **fecal immunochemical test** (FIT). Unlike past tests that detected blood in stool specimens (i.e., solid waste from the rectum), FIT does not require dietary or drug restrictions, and sample collection involves less effort. Further, FIT has demonstrated a superior ability to detect the presence of polyps via antibodies to these polyps. FIT is now recommended for annual use by people 50 to 75 years of age. The challenge to public health involves the widespread diffusion of this innovation, preferably across entire states rather than merely isolated communities. It is not a medical challenge because far too many people at risk of developing colorectal cancer are not patients. More bluntly, the reach of medical care providers relative to promoting annual use of the FIT is very limited.

Since the approval of FIT, public health researchers have been devoted to devising approaches to promote its widespread – and annual – use. For instance, one study of rural residents at high risk of colorectal cancer included a full-scale outreach campaign (Crosby et al., 2021). The outreach efforts included flyers posted in prominent community locations and local health departments. Community outreach events were organized specifically to give project staff members a chance to talk with people about using FIT. These events included outdoor hog roasts, health fairs, and gatherings at senior centers. Additionally, project staff conducted presentations at senior citizen centers throughout an eight-county region. Collectively, these outreach efforts averted enough cases of advanced colorectal cancer to more than offset the costs of the public health campaign. The key to the success of this project (as well as its high benefits-to-cost ratio) was seamless coordination of services with local endoscopy providers (in this example, endoscopy is the use of a camera on a probe being inserted into the rectum and throughout the colon).

For people testing FIT-positive, endoscopy is the next step. This implies a movement from a public approach to a medical approach. To definitively diagnose (and remove) polyps, a procedure known as a **colonoscopy** must be performed by a skilled endoscopy specialist. Although colonoscopy is in the realm of medicine rather than public health, this is nonetheless a stellar example of primary prevention (in most cases) because most polyps are precancerous. Further, the opportunities created for secondary prevention as a result of colonoscopy are important. Even cancerous polyps tend to invade the walls of the colon slowly, so treatment options may be minimally invasive in contrast to the once common removal of the entire colon. As a rule, the earlier stages require far less surgical excision; thus, anyone who receives a diagnosis – followed by surgery – is highly likely to survive.

Moving to cervical cancer, the approach to secondary prevention (as mentioned previously) is known as Pap testing. This screening method for cancer of the cervix is performed in clinics and is often bundled with routine gynecological care. Compared to mammography, this is a simple procedure. Like colonoscopy, the role of public health in terms of Pap testing lies in outreach to at-risk women who are not medically engaged in their healthcare and thus are not being tested regularly. Public health outreach methods in this regard are well documented and highly successful. Again, seamless coordination between the two approaches (public health and medical care) is required to fully realize the potential of Pap testing to find women who are in the precancerous stage (i.e., cervical dysplasia) or the early stages (i.e., stages 1 or 2) of cervical cancer. In nearly all cases of dysplasia, stage 1 cancer, or stage 2 cancer, the treatment does

these outreach efforts averted enough cases of advanced colorectal cancer to more than offset the costs of the public health campaign.

Public health outreach methods in this regard are well documented and highly successful.

not involve hysterectomy, and the prognosis comes close to 100% survival. Thus, given adequate funding and support for public health outreach efforts, in today's world, it is no longer acceptable to have anyone die from cervical cancer.

in today's world, it is no longer acceptable to have anyone die from cervical cancer.

Review and Key Terms

You began this chapter by learning a bit more about a Hygeia-based approach to health as opposed to our nation's love affair with what is arguably a **medical-industrial complex**. By now, you may have concluded that the "ounce of prevention" suggested by Benjamin Franklin is much more than a small effort. The ounce is truly an underestimate in this metaphor. But Franklin's message remains clear: we have to ensure that the population can freely engage in the often daily protective behaviors that we now know avert cancers. This is less of an option or a good idea and more in line with a moral imperative to keep people healthy and cancer-free. A Hygeia-based approach to cancer prevention will not be easy, but it will address the root of the problem. The essence of this approach is a focus on **protective factors** instead of the now-dominant approach of screening for cancer and then treating it once it is diagnosed. Remember that protective factors are not simply the absence of **risk factors**. Instead, protective factors function as the level of **etiology**, meaning that the very start of the process leading to cancer is averted. Protective factors offer the human body a strong defense against the cellular alterations that may eventually lead to a cancerous growth.

A Hygeia-based approach to cancer prevention will not be easy, but it will address the root of the problem.

You began this chapter by learning about the **colon** and the **rectum**. As you now know, colorectal cancer is no longer an inevitable threat to health and life. A simple primary approach to averting colorectal cancers involves making high-fiber foods a socially normative and widely supported practice in the United States. This will involve replacing highly processed foods and animal-based foods with plant-based whole foods, particularly those found in the legume family (except peanuts), given their high concentration of **vegetable fiber**. Protecting the public will also involve creating conditions that fully support and encourage the consumption of **phytochemicals** for their **chemotherapeutic** value against this cancer.

Just as a PBWF diet must become part of the American food structure, meat-based diets will need to become a relic of the past. As perhaps the most significant risk factors for colorectal cancer, meat and meat products are well-established causes of **adenomas polyps**. Given the high potential of these polyps to become cancerous, America's future success against colorectal cancer will partly depend on the success of eliminating meat from the standard American diet. But the federal government stubbornly continues to subsidize meat production while providing less than 1% of the annual meat subsidy to vegetable farmers. Public health and government have yet to reach a marriage when it comes to working toward the goal of cancer prevention. This is not inevitable. As students earning a college degree, the people reading this textbook can someday begin to align government action with public health priorities.

the people reading this textbook can someday begin to align government action with public health priorities.

In the next section of the chapter, you learned about the primary and secondary prevention of breast cancer. You may have been somewhat surprised to learn how far the science has advanced relative to primary prevention. This is especially true regarding the potential role of **antioxidants** as a protective factor against breast cancer. The decay-like process of **oxidation** caused by **free radicals** is blocked by antioxidants. From a public health perspective, antioxidants are a freebie because they are abundant in a PBWF diet, and thus public health efforts targeting phytochemicals, for example, will automatically ensure ample antioxidants. Switching from a protective factor to a risk factor, you also learned that obesity is now a well-established risk factor for breast cancer. Again, the implications take us back to the overall public health value of diet and exercise to keep America thin.

In what is almost an obligatory part of any textbook devoted to public health practice, you learned about the value of mammography as a secondary prevention practice against breast cancer. Partnerships between public health and healthcare providers that use outreach functions are vital for screening women who may otherwise not have mammograms. Ultimately, a goal for public health practice should be to make advanced-stage breast cancer and **bilateral mastectomy** things of the past.

As the chapter continued, you may also have been surprised to learn that **cervical cancer** is an extension of a sexually transmitted infection: **persistent HPV**. Infecting first the **os of the cervix**, the **human papillomavirus** typically does not lead to abnormal cellular changes; however, this occurs frequently enough to lead to millions of women annually being diagnosed with **cervical dysplasia**. It is especially likely in younger women who lack a complete covering of **squamous epithelium** around the cervical os.

The final section of the chapter described how public health practice and medical care can and should interact synergistically to improve cancer prevention efforts in the United States. Using the **fecal immunochemical test** to detect polyps is emblematic of this synergy. Outreach by public health workers can promote the use of this life-saving test, while medical care can provide a safety net for colonoscopies to people testing FIT-positive who do not otherwise have a provider who can arrange for **colonoscopy**.

Regarding cervical cancer, you learned that the **LEEP** is a relatively less invasive treatment for cases that do not show signs of spreading to the entire **uterus**. Having a LEEP as opposed to a **hysterectomy** is a function of how early in the course of cancer the problem is diagnosed. This is an example of why routine **Pap testing** is so vital. Public health practice is well known for its ability to perform community outreach services designed to promote this routine testing.

For Practice and Class Discussion

Practice Questions

1. Which one of the following terms is *least* relevant to a Hygeia-based approach to cancer prevention?
   a. Protective factors
   b. Frequent cancer screenings
   c. Antioxidants
   d. The HPV vaccine

2. The standard American diet lacks this vital protective factor against colorectal cancer.
   a. Antioxidants
   b. Antibodies
   c. Vegetable fiber
   d. Iodine

3. The concept of primary prevention as applied to breast cancer is best represented by which term?
   a. A PBWF diet
   b. Removing sugar from the standard American diet
   c. The use of mammography
   d. Preventing BRCA1 from reproducing

4. Regarding breast cancer prevention, which statement is **false**?
   a. Obesity is only a potential risk factor; more research is needed.
   b. The consumption of berries is a protective factor.

   c.   Mammography is important because not all breast cancers grow slowly.

   d.   The presence of BRCA1 or BRCA2 is a known risk factor.

5.   Which term is most implicated in the etiology of cervical cancer?

   a.   Nicotine

   b.   Polysaccharides

   c.   Persistent HPV

   d.   Cellular deregulation

6.   Which statement about cervical cancer is accurate?

   a.   Virtually every case of this cancer is entirely preventable.

   b.   The HPV vaccine is 100% effective.

   c.   The cervix of middle-aged women is particularly susceptible to HPV.

   d.   Even stage 3 cervical cancer is relegated only to the os.

7.   Condom use does have a place in the prevention of cervical cancer. This is true more so from a public health perspective than the medical paradigm.

   a.   True

   b.   False

8.   Which screening test also serves as a method of primary prevention?

   a.   Pap testing

   b.   Mammography

   c.   Colonoscopy

   d.   Genetic testing for BRCA2

9.   The role of culture is important to consider relative to cancer prevention. Why is this true?

   a.   People do not want to invest in daily tasks to prevent something they believe can be fixed someday by a doctor.

   b.   Medical doctors are profit-driven and actively discourage prevention.

   c.   Most people are ready to change their diets; they just need guidance.

10.   Which general statement best summarizes this chapter?

   a.   Some cancers are highly preventable if public health practice creates the conditions that allow protective actions.

   b.   Thanks to chemoprevention, cancer is becoming a thing of the past.

   c.   A PBWF diet is the best defense against cervical cancer.

   d.   Mammography is an important form of primary prevention.

For Discussion (in class or small groups, or online)

11.   Take a piece of notebook paper and divide it in half lengthwise with a line. On the left side, use the heading "Hygeia-based approach," and on the right side, use the heading "Medical-based approach." Make entries under each heading so that the entry on the left is paired with its logical opposite on the right. For instance, the first entry on the left might be "Condoms to reduce HPV spread," and its opposite might be "Periodic Pap testing to detect signs of cervical cancer." Do this for all three cancers you learned about in this chapter until the page is full.

12.   Of the three cancers you learned about in this chapter, breast cancer has the most potential for new discoveries relative to primary prevention. Being sure you fully understand primary prevention, go online to find one outstanding example of a recent (e.g., in the past two years) study that suggests new types of protective factors against breast cancer.

Once you find an intriguing study in this respect, post it (using any platform your class is accustomed to) for others in this class to read and respond to.

13. Find five people in your life who you know consume meat at least once each day. As a type of study, ask each one this question: "What do you know about the connection between eating meat and the development of polyps that could lead to colorectal cancer?" Take brief notes as they answer. Compare these notes across the five interviews. Then, using no more than two double-spaced pages, create a document that answers these two questions: (a) What are the common themes you heard in these answers? and (b) What are the implications for public health practice?

References

Alaofi, R. K., Nassif, M. O., & Al-Hajeili, M. R. (2018). Prophylactic mastectomy for the prevention of breast cancer. *Avicenna Journal of Medicine, 8*(3), 67–77.

Aykan, N. E. (2015). Red meat and colorectal cancer. *Oncology Reviews, 9*(1), 288.

Crosby, R. A., Mamaril, C. B., & Collins, T. (2021). Cost of increasing years-of-life-gained (YLG) using fecal immunochemical testing as a population-level screening model in a rural Appalachian population. *The Journal of Rural Health, 37,* 576–574.

Li, Y., Niu, Y., Sun, Y., Zhang, F., Liu, C., Fan, L., & Mei, Q. (2015). Role of phytochemicals in colorectal cancer prevention. *World of Gastroenterology, 21*(31), 9262–9272.

Ligibel, J. (2011). Obesity and breast cancer. *Oncology, 25*(11), 994–1000.

Love, H. J., & Sulikowski, D. (2018). Of meat and men: Sex differences in implicit and explicit attitudes toward meat. *Frontiers in Psychology, 9,* 559.

Rabarison, K. M, Li, R., Bish, C. L., Vanderpool, R. C., Crosby, R. A., & Massoudi, M. S. (2015). A cost analysis of the 1-2-3 Pap intervention. *Frontiers in Public Health Service Systems Research, 4,* 45–50.

Sewell, C. (2020). Removing the meat subsidy: Our cognitive dissonance around animal agriculture. *Journal of International Affairs, 473*(2), 234–239.

Tantamango, Y. M., Knutsen, S. F., Beeson, L., Fraser, G., & Sabate, J. (2011). Association between dietary fiber and incident cases of colon polyps – the Adventist Health Study. *Gastrointestinal Cancer Research, 4*(5), 161–167.

Winer, R. L., Hughes, J. P., Feng, Q., O'Reilly, S., Kiviat, N. B., Holmes, K. K., & Koutsky, L. A. (2006). Condom use and risk of genital HPV infection in young women. *New England Journal of Medicine, 354,* 2645–2654.

CHAPTER 8

EXCESSIVE ALCOHOL USE: HOW CAN IT BE REDUCED AT A POPULATION LEVEL?

A clever person solves a problem. A wise person avoids it.

—*Albert Einstein*

Overview

As a legal way to become intoxicated, alcohol has enjoyed a unique level of social acceptance. Unlike tobacco (see **Chapter 4**), alcohol use has not been widely regulated to the point of placing the industry at risk of significant declines in sales. Indeed, a type of dimorphism exists, in that people (including those who work in public health) use phrases such as "drug *and* alcohol abuse," thereby separating alcohol from other substances that lead to intoxication. Some states still incarcerate (and attempt to rehabilitate) people who become intoxicated through the use of marijuana while providing no legal consequences for using alcohol to become intoxicated. This dimorphism is widely apparent in the United States; however, it is often masked by laws against drinking while driving and underage drinking. Government regulation against chronically using alcohol to become intoxicated simply does not exist. The chances are that you may not have ever thought about alcohol this way.

This chapter will not mimic other textbooks that include the topic of public health and alcohol use. Instead, this chapter will strictly focus on the fact that alcohol is ranked as the fourth leading cause of *actual death* in the United States (see **Chapter 3**), with the bulk of that morbidity stemming from chronic use as opposed to death from driving while drinking or from acts of homicide or suicide committed by drunk people. The chapter recognizes that chronic alcohol use has a profound and severe effect on relationships, families, and even worker productivity. Although these severe effects are important, the primary task for public health practice is to keep a tight focus on reducing the population prevalence of **chronic drinking** (meaning alcohol use that becomes an ingrained and **excessive behavior**).

In many ways, you can think of alcohol as the **new tobacco** in that the alcohol industry has yet to be challenged in the way that occurred through public health actions against the tobacco industry. This chapter will lead you through some of the possible public health actions that could be used to challenge and change the alcohol industry. At the same time, changing the social norms promoting alcohol use may ultimately become the most powerful tool in the public health quest to avert

LEARNING OBJECTIVES

1. Understand the U.S. burden of alcohol on premature death, the biological process of alcohol metabolism, and the consequences of excessive alcohol use on tissues, organs, and body functions.

2. List the chronic, alcohol-induced effects of excessive consumption on the human body.

3. Explain how excessive alcohol use impacts the liver and the cardiovascular system.

4. Understand what is meant by the phrase "alcohol is the new tobacco" in terms of possible strategies for regulation.

5. Identify regulatory approaches to reduce excessive alcohol use.

6. Apply the concept of reciprocal causation to the goal of changing social norms pertaining to alcohol.

7. Describe socially oriented intervention approaches to reduce the population-level consumption of alcohol use.

the premature death caused by excess drinking. As these norms change, a ripple effect may also permeate the lives of teens and others who do not drink excessively but engage in problem drinking based on binge use, drinking while driving, and alcohol-related violence.

This chapter will also feature an individual-level approach as a focal point. This implies that public health education about the long-term deleterious effects of alcohol on the human body will need to be intensified and delivered to adults of all ages as opposed to the past focus just on teens (as much of the effort to reduce teenage drinking is centered on the prevention of drinking and driving, which is **not** a major factor in the much larger alcohol-related toll of health).

Also, more than the previous chapters of this textbook, this chapter will have a somewhat early and heavy focus on the **pathophysiology** of excessive drinking. Pathophysiology is the study of how an agent (in this case, alcohol) changes the tissues, organs, and functions of the human body. As the chapter comes to a close, you will be introduced to the concept of **reciprocal causation** as it applies to socially normative behaviors such as drinking. This concept, of course, can be applied to a wide range of other health-compromising behaviors.

The U.S. Burden of Excessive Alcohol Use and the Biological Process of Alcohol Metabolism

To begin, keep in mind that alcohol is toxic to the body. This is something most of us never consider. We do not need to think about it because of an amazing vital organ: the human liver. As alcohol is being consumed, it triggers a series of chemical reactions that lead to detoxification. This entire process can be conceptualized as shown in **Figure 8.1**. It begins by converting the alcohol (known as **ethanol**) into an initial by-product known as **acetaldehyde**. Although you have probably never heard about acetaldehyde, you may have experienced its toxic effects because this initial by-product of alcohol metabolism causes a hangover. More importantly, this by-product is toxic to the liver and the upper sections of the small intestine (where a small amount of this conversion process occurs). Depending on the percent of body fat (low is more efficient), this conversion process takes longer in some people than others.

The conversion speed is particularly important for the next step: changing acetaldehyde to **acetate**. The quicker this second conversion occurs, the better, because acetate is not toxic. This is why people who want to drink responsibly are advised to combine alcoholic beverages with a meal. The food competes with the alcohol for absorption, thereby slowing the rate at which alcohol enters the liver (where most of these reactions occur). When the liver is suddenly given large doses of alcohol to metabolize, it takes longer to do so – leaving more time for acetaldehyde to create tissue damage. Once acetaldehyde becomes acetate, the dangers are gone, and eventually the acetate is converted to carbon dioxide and water.

The quicker this second conversion occurs, the better, because acetate is not toxic.

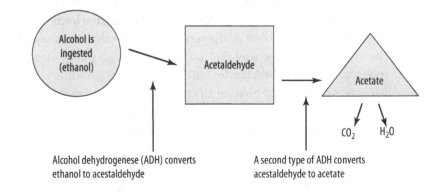

Alcohol dehydrogenese (ADH) converts
ethanol to acestaldehyde

A second type of ADH converts
acestaldehyde to acetate

Figure 8.1   A simplified illustration of alcohol metabolism
Source: U.S. Department of Health & Human Services.

Table 8.1   Examples of chronic conditions caused by excess drinking

Name of condition/disease	Brief description
Cardiomyopathy	The heart muscle becomes thin and weak.
Alcohol-induced pancreatitis	Chronic inflammation of the pancreas
Alcohol dependence syndrome	Physical and psychological addiction
Alcohol myopathy	Loss of muscle function throughout the body
Alcoholic gastritis	Irritation of the stomach lining
Nervous system degeneration	Loss of higher-level cognitive function
Cancers*	See the footnote at the bottom of this table.
Coronary heart disease	A weakened heart muscle works harder than it should, which leads to irregularities in rhythm and fluid accumulation.
Obesity	Alcohol has more calories per gram than protein or carbohydrates.
Hypertension	Disruption of the normal function of body enzymes, antioxidants, and steroids

* These include cancers of the stomach, pancreas, breast, esophagus, colon, larynx, and liver, as well as oral cancers.

Ultimately, chronic consumption of alcohol can wear down the body and lead to a host of long-term diseases. **Table 8.1** provides a summary of many of the better-known chronic conditions caused by excess drinking.

Despite alcohol's barrage of ill effects on the body, the human liver is a champion when it comes to detoxifying it! This is both a blessing and a curse, because while it keeps people relatively healthy for many years, the link between excessive drinking and poor health typically is not apparent even to those engaging in chronic, daily drinking. This lack of an obvious cause-and-effect relationship leads to a false sense of complacency relative to alcohol use, thereby precluding meaningful attempts to cut back or end the use of alcohol entirely.

the link between excessive drinking and poor health typically is not apparent even to those engaging in chronic, daily drinking.

Despite what any one person may believe about alcohol having a strong negative impact on health, it is important to understand that excess alcohol consumption is a leading cause of premature death in the United States. The CDC estimates that at least 95,000 premature deaths occur each year as a consequence of excess consumption (see **Photo 8.1**). As noted by the CDC (2022a),

> Excessive alcohol use is responsible for more than 95,000 deaths in the United States each year, or 261 deaths per day. These deaths shorten the lives of those who die by an average of almost 29 years, for a total of 2.8 million years of potential life lost. It is a leading cause of preventable death in the United States, and cost the nation $249 billion in 2010.

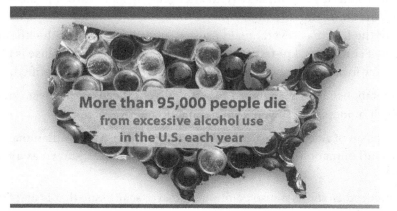

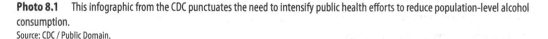

Photo 8.1   This infographic from the CDC punctuates the need to intensify public health efforts to reduce population-level alcohol consumption.
Source: CDC / Public Domain.

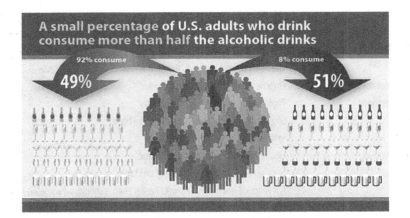

Photo 8.2   This infographic from the CDC (CDC, 2022b) provides a visual image pertaining to excess alcohol consumption in the United States.
Source: CDC / Public Domain.

At this juncture in the chapter, you may wonder whether your own alcohol use places you at risk of the premature death noted here by the CDC. The word *excess* has not been defined. However, to help place this into perspective, take a very close look at **Photo 8.2**.

After a careful look at this infographic, it may be easy to conclude that you are not in the 8% of the population that consumes 51% of the alcohol. However, and as a reminder, that is not a relevant question, because public health practice (as you know from **Chapters 2 and 3**) is about population-level health rather than person-level health. The public health goal is to decrease the overall consumption of alcohol in the United States. This goal will have an important impact on the 8% and help those who could someday fall into the 8% category avoid doing so. Also, remember that public health is about primary prevention! This means strategies such as Alcoholics Anonymous and other alcohol rehabilitation programs are not discussed in this chapter.

> The public health goal is to decrease the overall consumption of alcohol in the United States.

Alcohol Has Long-Term Effects on the Liver

As this is certainly not a textbook about medical care, there is no need to examine what it means to have **cirrhosis** of the liver. Instead, let's think about cells in the liver first inflaming and subsequently rupturing to produce scar tissue. To simplify that pathophysiology, think of the liver as the grand detoxification center of the body. Over-taxing this center leads to inflammation, which leads to scarring. This scar tissue becomes a permanent non-functional part of the liver. As this scar tissue accumulates (year after year), it begins to dominate the liver, thereby compromising the entire organ.

Scarring of the liver has several main causes, such as infection with either hepatitis B or hepatitis C and a chronic diet of fatty foods. An equally contributory cause is chronic alcohol use. Four primary forms of alcohol-induced liver damage have been identified:

> Four primary forms of alcohol-induced liver damage have been identified

- Alcohol metabolism has been linked to a buildup of fat cells in the liver (known as a **fatty liver**), which hinders the efficient functioning of this vital organ.

- The metabolism of alcohol can also lead to acute (sudden-onset) inflammation of the liver. When this inflammation resolves, scar tissue remains (this is known as **alcohol-induced hepatitis**).

- Alcohol-induced cirrhosis is also common. It leaves scar tissue that is non-functional (this is not a reversible condition).

- Alcohol-induced hepatocellular carcinoma is increasingly common – this is cancer of the liver caused by excessive drinking.

The Impact of Alcohol Use on the Cardiovascular System

Next, let's consider the cardiovascular system, especially the heart. This information is unknown to millions of Americans. The effects from chronic daily alcohol use include:

- Hypertension

- Irregular heartbeat

- Enlarged left ventricle (the chamber of the heart that pumps oxygenated blood out through a vast system of arteries throughout the body)

- Congestive heart failure (a condition that causes enlargement of the heart and ultimately leads to fluid accumulation that overworks the heart to the point of failure)

- A 40% increase in the risk of a heart attack

- Cardiac myopathy (a weak heart, meaning the muscle does not function well)

- Premature hardening of the arteries

These effects on the cardiovascular system are not apparent in younger people who use alcohol excessively. The effects take years –even decades – to develop. It is all too easy for a chronic heavy drinker to make assumptions regarding a lack of effect. When a cardiovascular disease finally becomes symptomatic and creates health issues, it is usually difficult to determine the cause, given ample other possible explanations such as metabolic syndrome, obesity, and excessive intake of saturated fats. But the extent to which alcohol shares in the blame for cardiovascular disease is a far less important question than its population-level counterpart: "What portion of the total U.S. burden imposed by cardiovascular disease could be averted by as little as a 20% reduction in total alcohol consumption for the population as a whole?"

> the extent to which alcohol shares in the blame for cardiovascular disease is a far less important question than its population-level counterpart

Population-Level Strategies to Reduce Overall Alcohol Consumption

As public health practice grows and matures into a progressively more viable alternative to medical care, the once-elusive goal of influencing policies will become less daunting. For example, taxes on alcohol sales have already been leveraged specifically to reduce population-level consumption. At this point in the chapter, we can finally come back to the opening quote! Einstein's insight applies wonderfully to the U.S. alcohol problem. At the very heart of this problem lies an industry that has yet to be regulated the way public health has regulated tobacco. The underlying (and unspoken) mission thus becomes something like "How can we realistically keep alcohol from being misused in a society that embraces it?" Solving this problem is a task that is yet to be fully attempted, and it misses the message of Einstein's quote. So, the second part of Einstein's quote sheds light here: *A wise person avoids it.* This concept of avoiding the problem implies that a more effective public health response is simply to make alcohol a far less prominent part of our culture. Herein lies the chasm of difference between the current approach to dealing with chronic disease caused by excessive alcohol use (i.e., improved medical treatments) and the approach advocated in this chapter (i.e., a population-level decline in alcohol consumption). As a nation, we need to drink far less than our current level of consumption.

> a more effective public health response is simply to make alcohol a far less prominent part of our culture.

Regulating the Alcohol Industry

A key aspect of regulating the tobacco industry centered on the *Master Settlement Agreement* (see **Chapter 4**), which was applied nationally. This national regulation is mostly lacking with respect to alcohol. The federal government does maintain some degree of control through the Bureau of Alcohol, Tobacco, Firearms, and Explosives. However, this control is largely limited to collecting federal tax on the sales of all alcoholic beverages. Instead of national regulation, it is very much the case that states have the freedom to regulate the sale of alcohol. This authority includes collecting state excise taxes on all alcoholic beverages, setting limits on hours of operation for sales outlets, setting the **minimum legal drinking age** (MLDA), and placing restrictions on advertising. Most states function in this capacity through a state-sponsored commission known as Alcoholic Beverage Control (ABC). State-level **ABC commissions**, in turn, typically control the permits relative to where a given tavern, bar, or liquor store can be located and how these outlets may or may not be integrated with restaurants, gas stations, convenience stores, and so on. Given the tremendous variation across the United States in terms of state laws pertaining to alcohol sales, our nation has a mosaic of loosely related policies rather than unifying policies. You may be wondering, "Why isn't this efficient?" The answer involves competing interests relative to the sale of alcohol versus the challenge of reducing its excessive consumption.

> our nation has a mosaic of loosely related policies rather than unifying policies.

Because the tax revenue (at both the federal and state levels) from alcohol sales is substantial, an inherent conflict of interest exists relative to the public health goal of reducing population-level consumption of alcoholic beverages. Consider that in 2020, total tax revenues (federal and state combined) on alcohol came to an estimated $9.49 billion, and this number increases each year. Because these tax revenues are spent at the discretion of the states and the federal government, the annual billions are used for hundreds of purposes. This, of course, raises suspicions relative to how seriously state and federal governments may intensify efforts to regulate such a lucrative product. At the federal level, these suspicions are augmented by the practice of the Small Business Administration providing low-interest loans to help open new bars, taverns, and liquor stores (Moore & Gerstein, 1981; O'Connor, 2021).

Added to the inherent conflict of interest relative to the taxation of alcohol, evidence is scant relative to the effectiveness of other regulator options (Blanchette et al., 2020). For instance, studies of how altering the MLDA influences key outcomes (such as driving under the influence of alcohol and alcohol sales) have yet to firmly demonstrate the utility of lowering the MLDA. Similarly, evidence is lacking relative to regulating the hours of operation for alcohol sales outlets and the zoning laws relative to places that serve and sell alcoholic beverages. However, two types of state-based regulatory actions are much more promising in terms of actual evidence: (a) increased taxation and (b) regulating the density of alcohol outlets.

Taxation of Alcoholic Beverages

This strategy relies on principles you have already learned about in this textbook: price elasticity and reducing access apply to the taxation of alcoholic beverages. The evidence in this regard is fairly clear – as tax increases inflate prices, consumption declines across the entire population in the purchasing area affected by the tax hikes (Chaloupka et al., 2019; Xu & Chaloupka, 2011). Thus, a fairly robust correlation exists between excise taxes on alcoholic beverages and sales (Naimi et al., 2016). This takes you back to previous chapters in this book that taught you about limiting access. If you are fond of thinking and have a bit of a skeptical nature, you may be asking, "Doesn't this added tax just discourage alcohol consumption in the lower class?" If you were thinking of this question, pat yourself on the back, because you are in great company. That very question has been a subject of much debate and research in the field of alcohol use and addiction. The question has been addressed to the point that a consensus has been achieved in the field that the answer is no. Known as the **distributive law**, the applicable principle is that even small increases in state and federal excise taxes on alcohol have an important impact on sales that traverses the entire spectrum of incomes. Keep in mind that those with higher incomes may still purchase products at a higher price; however, these people may then consume the product over a longer period, leading to less frequent purchases. As applied to the excise tax on alcohol, the distributive law states that the added tax burden will be equalized by income across the spectrum of classes in the United States. In other words, people with lower incomes who consume alcohol will experience proportionately the same level of the added tax burden as those in the middle class and upper class. Although studies do not find evidence that the distributive law would fail in the direction of lower-income consumers paying proportionally more of an added tax burden, a group of researchers from the CDC used a modeling study to suggest that the distributive law may be violated in that higher-income consumers pay a proportionally adjusted greater amount of the overall added excise tax on alcohol (Naimi et al., 2016).

> the distributive law states that the added tax burden will be equalized by income across the spectrum of classes

A key principle of population-level health involves the concept of access to products used in a way that creates health risk behaviors. This is especially applicable to products that carry an addictive quality (i.e., tobacco, alcohol, and opioids). Just as easy access to alcoholic beverages (such as very inexpensive beer that can be purchased almost anywhere) increases use, any regulatory actions that decrease access will positively affect public health. From a fairness perspective, such regulatory actions are easily justified. This is because the U.S. government bears a disproportionate burden of the healthcare costs associated with the broad spectrum of alcohol-induced chronic diseases that you have already learned about by reading this chapter. One estimate, for instance, suggested that the annual added healthcare costs incurred by alcohol consumption amounted to $249 billion. Calculated on a per-drink basis, this huge sum equates with healthcare costs of an estimated $2.05 per drink consumed, with state and federal government funds covering two-fifths of this cost (Sacks et al., 2015). From an economics perspective, the healthcare costs of alcohol consumption form what is known as a **negative externality**. In everyday language, this means the use of a product for its intended purpose carries a post-consumer cost that is substantial and ongoing. Of course, these post-consumer costs are not reimbursed by the industry producing the product. Instead, the costs are passed along to the public. Herein lies the ultimate non-health justification for greatly increasing state and federal excise taxes on alcoholic beverages: the added revenues are needed to pay for the disease burdens caused by excessive consumption.

> the annual added healthcare costs incurred by alcohol consumption amounted to $249 billion.

> the healthcare costs of alcohol consumption form what is known as a **negative externality**.

What Is Density, and Why Does It Matter?

One other set of emerging and promising public health strategies to reduce population-level alcohol consumption involves regulating the physical locations where alcohol can be sold. This body of evidence is less suggestive of zoning laws making a difference than it is of **density**. As applied to public health, the term **density** refers to the number of access points in a defined geographic area. In applying this concept specifically to alcohol, density represents the number of places licensed to sell alcohol or alcoholic beverages in a geographically bounded section of a city, town, or village. Dozens of studies have investigated the influence of density on alcohol sales, and these studies all support the original hypothesis that density functions through social norms. **Figure 8.2** simplifies this relationship.

> As applied to public health, the term **density** refers to the number of access points in a defined geographic area.

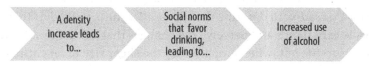

Figure 8.2   The mediating role of social norms on the relationship between density of alcohol sales outlets and alcohol consumption

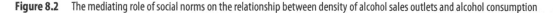

One of the first studies to provide rigorous evidence for the effect depicted in **Figure 8.2** was published in 2006. Using 24 census tracts, this study teased out individual effects from neighborhood effects to show that "the effect of alcohol outlet density on alcohol consumption functions through an effect at the neighborhood level" (Scribner et al., 2000, p. 188). This implies that the age-old adage "birds of a feather flock together" applies to drinking. It is consistent with the idea of social contagion, meaning people have a mutual influence on one another's health behaviors, including health-related behaviors (Christakis & Fowler, 2013). Thus, the next section of this chapter explains how social ties can be a strong determinant of health behaviors, including alcohol consumption.

The neighborhood effect is part of what is now widely termed the **alcohol environment**. In a nutshell, this refers to how much (or how little) immediate social settings (proximal to people who drink) encourage the consumption of alcohol. For example, consider the long-standing problem faced by university and college presidents across the United States of how to best control campus-based drinking problems. A study of college campuses found that social marketing programs designed to reduce alcohol use were only effective when applied to campus environments characterized as having alcohol environments that did not favor use (Scribner et al., 2011). In essence, behavioral and social science solutions to excessive drinking may only work in alcohol environments that are not highly supportive of drinking. This leads us back to previously described solutions, such as taxation and regulating density.

Beyond the concepts of taxation and regulating density, other examples of effectively regulating alcohol sales to produce substantial declines in consumption are not yet apparent. However, this does not imply that your generation should simply accept the status quo.

Socially Oriented Intervention Approaches

At this point, you will need to refer back to what you learned in **Chapter 3** about shifting the mean. The concept is relatively simple. When thinking about any given health behavior plotted on a graph for an entire population, the curve will take on a bell-shaped appearance. **Figure 8.3** shows what this looks like relative to alcohol consumption in the United States. Looking first across the horizontal axis (the abscissa) of this graph, you can see that this hypothetical figure shows the average number of drinks per week consumed by all U.S. adults. Looking at the vertical axis (the ordinate), you can imagine the percentage of adults indicating various averages in terms of the approximate number of drinks consumed in a typical week. The exact percentages are not shown because what matters here is the height of each curve and the length of its right-hand tail. Letting the curve indicated with black represent current use, the curve shown with a dotted line represents shifting the mean to the left (implying that the entire population shifts to the left). An interesting thing occurs when such a shift takes place: the length of the right-hand tail shrinks, and its size diminishes. It is vital to understand this because it is the essence of much of the modern-day thinking applied to public health practice. The concept is not new; rather, public health is just now beginning to embrace a way of thinking that was first proposed by a professor in London, Sir Geoffrey Rose, in 1985. Thus, the two curves in **Figure 8.3** represent what is known as the **Rose curve**.

The rose curve is often difficult for students (and the public) to comprehend fully because of its subtleties. Let's begin with that seemingly small shift of the mean to the left. Rose coined the term **prevention paradox** to describe the substantial shifts to the left that appear small in terms of how people experience and perceive the changes that led to the shift. In essence, even relatively small shifts to the left, when amplified by the sheer size of an entire population, create large benefits to public health. The paradox is that these benefits may not be correctly attributed to the seemingly modest changes in the overall population. In applied form, think of

when such a shift takes place: the length of the right-hand tail shrinks, and its size diminishes.

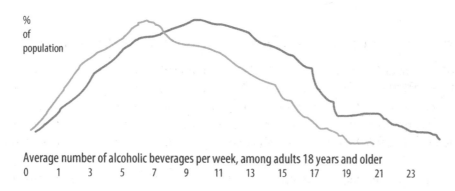
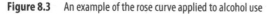

Average number of alcoholic beverages per week, among adults 18 years and older

0   1   3   5   7   9   11   13   15   17   19   21   23

Figure 8.3   An example of the rose curve applied to alcohol use

the mean shifting left by as little as two drinks per week. From the standpoint of one household, this hardly seems significant. Conversely, from the standpoint of the entire nation, this small change can have a dramatic long-term effect of reducing alcohol-related deaths and disease.

The other subtle point of the rose curve involves the right-hand tail. The medical approach to reducing alcohol-related death and disease involves intervening only at the extreme end of this right-hand tail (i.e., people who have developed clinically observable disease). For the sake of argument, let's assume that by the magic of medicine, all those seeking treatment for an alcohol-induced disease are cured and thus spared an early death. Does this mean the problem ends? If you remember a basic lesson from **Chapter 4**, you know the answer is no. Just as a bevy of new heavy smokers will regrow the right-hand tail after thousands die each day, the same phenomenon occurs with heavy drinkers. Now, let's mentally reverse this by thinking about the contrast between the dotted and black lines of the right-hand tails in **Figure 8.3**. By shifting the entire population curve to the left, the prevalence of clinically observable alcohol-related disease will decline significantly. This means the risky end of the curve drops off because everybody is drinking a bit less than they used to (again, even a change as small as two fewer drinks per week can have large effects).

By shifting the entire population curve to the left, the prevalence of clinically observable alcohol-related disease will decline significantly.

Bringing all this back to social norms, the intervention goal is a population-level shift in how people view alcohol. Currently, alcohol is considered a way to celebrate, commiserate, deal with problems, and party. Historically, alcohol has been a mainstay of public life, with its use being continued or even increased during times of national crisis. For instance, sales data indicate a substantial increase in alcohol sales at the height of the U.S. COVID-19 epidemic in 2020 (see **Box 8.1**). Its widespread acceptance as a way to relax (one that does not carry the stigma of using a drug) is deeply ingrained in the social fabric of our society. Consider, for example, how a bar or tavern can become an important meeting place for friends and neighbors (**Photo 8.3**). The neighborhood bar is often the place to be social! The question then becomes, "Can this change?" The answer involves the concept of **reciprocal causation**.

Used as part of what is widely known as **social cognitive theory**, the concept underlying reciprocal causation (as applied to the social acceptance of alcohol and its widespread use) is that each person's alcohol-related attitudes and behaviors collectively shape what becomes a type of unwritten set of social standards pertaining to

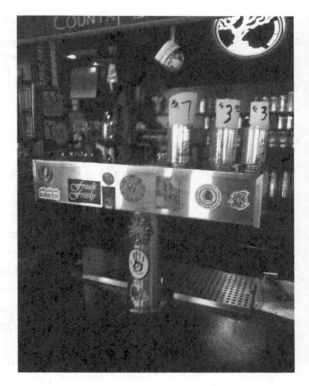

Photo 8.3   Neighborhood bars feature local taps and serve beer and other drinks to local customers in a way that reinforces the social norm of daily alcohol use.

BOX 8.1. NATIONAL INCREASE IN ALCOHOL CONSUMPTION DURING THE U.S. COVID-19 EPIDEMIC

In 2021, a well-designed study of sales data for beer, wine, and liquor was published in the journal known as *Alcohol* (Castaldelli-Maia, Segura, & Martins, 2021). This U.S. sales data was used to compare alcohol consumption during two distinct time periods: March through September of 2019 (prior to the COVID-19 pandemic) and the same months in 2020 (a period of heightened case rates and deaths from the COVID-19 pandemic). The data strongly suggested a 20% increase in alcohol consumption as a consequence of COVID-19. This increase equated with an estimated $41.9 billion in sales during that six-month period of 2020.

This increase appears to be a response to anxiety caused by COVID-19 and the associated safety precautions, restrictions, and social isolation experienced by millions of Americans. For instance, a study by Grossman and colleagues found that COVID-19–related stress was significantly associated with drinking during a greater number of days, with about 60% of the sample indicating an increase in overall alcohol consumption (Grossman, Neelan, & Sonnenschein, 2020). That same study found that people reported consuming approximately 27 drinks during an average of 12 days within the most recent 30-day period of completing the survey. More than one-third of the sample reported binge drinking at this time of the COVID-19 pandemic, with another 7% reporting "extreme binge drinking."

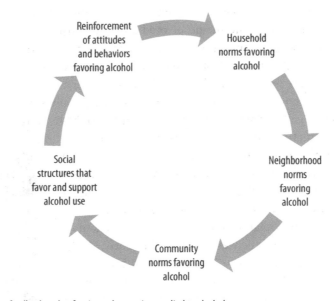

Figure 8.4   The positive feedback cycle of reciprocal causation applied to alcohol

reinforcement serves to intensify currently held attitudes and encourage the corresponding behaviors.

alcohol use. In turn, these social standards reinforce each person's alcohol-related attitudes and behaviors (see **Figure 8.4**). This reinforcement serves to intensify currently held attitudes and encourage the corresponding behaviors. As shown in the figure, social norms occur in units of people as small as a household and ultimately become embodied by large social structures (e.g., highly popular taverns, pubs, and bars – even annual citywide events that feature beer and wine consumption).

Now, let's reverse **Figure 8.4**. Without condemning alcohol, what if enough households, neighborhoods, and communities began to favor the norm "Be your best – drink less" in place of the previously held (more favorable) norms? Much like any social movement, this replacement norm could become socially contagious! Indeed, the social contagion of health behaviors is a well-documented phenomenon (see Christakis & Fowler, 2013). Given this possibility, the public health practice challenge becomes how to spark the social movement.

As an example, an intervention study of nearly 500 college students used print media displayed in residence halls to shift alcohol-related social norms toward less use (Mattern Clayton Neighbors, 2004). The intervention was particularly successful for students who experienced a significant decrease in norms favoring alcohol use, with these students reporting substantially less alcohol consumption compared to those less affected by the print media campaign. Of course, with the advent of social media since that study, social scientists are still highly engaged in learning how to most effectively use popular social media platforms to substantially alter social norms to leverage a significant decrease in alcohol use. In your lifetime, it will most likely be the case that social science will eventually prevail in changing the social norms that currently support alcohol use among adults.

social science will eventually prevail in changing the social norms that currently support alcohol use among adults.

Review and Key Terms

This chapter had a rather strict focus on the all-too-urgent public health need to reduce excessive alcohol consumption in the United States. Think of **chronic drinking** as leading to chronic disease. This topic of chronic (i.e., excessive) drinking led the chapter into a fairly lengthy section describing the **pathophysiology** that follows excess use. You first learned about **acetaldehyde**: the toxic by-product of alcohol metabolism. You learned that this toxic product accounts for a great deal of long-term damage to the vital organs of the body, including the heart, liver, and brain. Once acetaldehyde is converted to **acetate**, the body is protected from further damage until (of course) drinking begins again and more acetaldehyde is produced. The liver is an especially important organ that is not discussed or described elsewhere in this textbook. Among numerous damaging effects of alcohol on the liver, you learned about the condition of permanent scarring known as **cirrhosis**. You also learned about conditions such as **alcohol-induced hepatitis**.

Of course, the real challenge of this chapter lies in understanding how public health practice can be used to reduce excessive alcohol consumption. You learned that regulatory functions such as the **minimum legal drinking age** and the actions of state-level **ABC commissions** have had somewhat limited effects on the problem. Conversely, you learned about the **distributive law**, which suggests that added taxes on alcoholic beverages will reduce consumption across the spectrum of income classes in the United States. As you continued to learn about the prospects of intensified regulation of alcohol sales, it should have become apparent that the costs incurred as a result of excess consumption are not subsumed by the alcohol industry. These **negative externalities** are costs that have been absorbed by taxpayers since the founding of our country. Additionally, you learned about the zoning-related concept of **density**. Specifically, the density of outlets for alcohol sales appears to be tied to the social norms surrounding drinking in neighborhoods, communities, villages, and so on. Hopefully, you understood the concept of **reciprocal causation** as applied to the point that social norms pertaining to alcohol use are shaped by collective behaviors of individuals; in turn, these social norms reinforce and may intensify the strength of attitudes and behaviors that favor excess use. Changing these norms to create a preponderance of attitudes and individual behaviors supporting the non-use of alcohol is an important public health challenge for this century.

negative externalities are costs that have been absorbed by taxpayers since the founding of our country.

The chapter then employed the concept of shifting the mean to the challenge of creating a population-level reduction in the amount of alcohol consumption. This reduction applies to everyone and has its greatest benefits for those who previously consumed excessive amounts of alcohol. Based on the **Rose curve**, you should now understand that even small reductions, when magnified to the level of an entire population, can have profoundly meaningful advantages for the health of the public. Once you have grasped this somewhat difficult concept, you can be assured that you will not fall into the trap of what is known as the **prevention paradox** (i.e., the hidden way that small changes can amount to considerable benefits to the health of a population).

For Practice and Class Discussion

Practice Questions

1. Joe, a big drinker, is also an athlete. Joe read this chapter and now knows that acetaldehyde is probably negatively impacting his cardiovascular endurance. What advice is best for Joe (who will not abstain or reduce his consumption)?
   a. To minimize the time it takes to convert acetaldehyde to acetate, Joe should drink very slowly.
   b. To minimize the time it takes to convert acetaldehyde to acetate, Joe should only drink when eating a decent-sized meal.
   c. To minimize the time it takes to convert acetaldehyde to acetate, Joe should drink very slowly, and he should only drink when eating a decent-size meal.
   d. Joe should be screened for cirrhosis and alcohol-induced myopathy.

2. On a rose curve, about what percent of the U.S. population would be located at the far-right end in terms of alcohol consumption levels?
   a. Nearly 30%
   b. About 50% of all adults
   c. Less than 10%
   d. Between 30% and 50%

3. "Alcohol is the new tobacco" implies that:
   a. State and federal government-based regulations have not yet reduced the sales capacity of the alcohol industry.
   b. ABC commissions are functioning well; therefore, alcohol use will soon decline (just as occurred for tobacco).
   c. Science is just now learning about the negative effects of alcohol on the body.

4. Manufactures of whiskey may or may not be fully aware of the billions of U.S. dollars needed every year to pay for the large share of medical costs resulting from alcohol-induced chronic diseases such as cardiomyopathy, alcohol-induced hepatitis, and cirrhosis. This taxpayer-absorbed cost is known as:
   a. A form of reciprocal causation
   b. A negative externality
   c. The distributive law
   d. The density principle

5. After several decades of research, it is now known that a highly effective strategy to reduce overall (population-level) alcohol consumption is to increase the MLDA in all 50 states.
   a. True
   b. False

6. Alcohol sales in the United States increased at the height of the COVID-19 pandemic.
   a. True
   b. False

7. Which effect of excess alcohol use is also a risk factor for adult-onset diabetes?
    a. Hypertension
    b. Obesity
    c. Congestive heart failure
    d. Cardiac myopathy

8. As a long-time heavy drinker, Juan often finds himself feeling weak and lethargic. He complains that he "has no strength left in his body." This is most likely a consequence of:
    a. Alcohol-induced hepatitis
    b. Deregulation of acetate
    c. Myopathy
    d. Neurological deterioration

9. Of the following possible public health strategies, which one has the **least** chance of reducing population-level alcohol consumption?
    a. Warning labels on all alcoholic beverage containers
    b. Large increases in state excise taxes on alcohol
    c. Creating zoning regulations to reduce the density of sales outlets
    d. Social movements that support reduced consumption

10. The concept of social contagion relates to:
    a. Density of alcohol sales outlets
    b. The distributive law
    c. Reciprocal causation
    d. Social cognitive theory

For Discussion (in class or small groups, or online)

11. Go online to search for updated costs relative to the medical care provided to people with alcohol-induced chronic disease. How much have these costs increased compared to the estimates provided in this chapter?

12. For any state of your choosing, locate the current rate of excise tax on the sales of alcoholic beverages. Then, determine whether this rate has increased or decreased in the past 10 years, and, if so, whether the rise or fall was linked to consumption. If you can answer all three of these questions, post the answers in a way that lets other students taking this class know what you found.

13. Make a list of 7 to 10 chronic diseases you learned about in reading this chapter. Turn this list into a series of True/False questions by typing an opening question, such as "Excess consumption of alcohol causes _____." Then ask 10 people who are not taking this course to quickly complete the alcohol knowledge quiz you have created. After each person completes the quiz, go over the correct answers with them (all the answers will be True); for each question to which they responded False, use what you learned in this chapter to explain why True is correct. This exercise, by the way, is a great way to help truly learn the content of this chapter.

References

Blanchette, J. G., Lira, M. C., Heeren, T. C., & Niami, T. S. (2020). Alcohol policies in the United States, 1999–2018. *Journal of Studies on Alcohol and Drugs, 81*(1), 58–67.

Castaldelli-Maia, J. M., Segura, L. E., & Martins, S. S. (2021). The concerning increasing trend of alcohol sale in the U.S. during the COVID-19 pandemic. *Alcohol, 96*, 37–42.

CDC (2022a). Alcohol-related disease impact (ARDI) international classification of diseases (ICD) codes and alcohol-attributable fraction (AAF) sources. https://www.cdc.gov/alcohol/ardi/alcohol-related-icd-codes.html

CDC (2022b). Deaths from excessive alcohol use in the United States. https://www.cdc.gov/alcohol/features/excessive-alcohol-deaths.html

Chaloupka, F. J., Powell, L. M., & Warner, K. E. (2019). The use of excise taxes to reduce tobacco, alcohol, and sugary beverage consumption. *Annual Review of Public Health, 40*, 187–201.

Christakis, N. A., & Fowler, J. H. (2013). Social contagion theory: examining dynamic networks and human behavior. *Statistical Medicine, 32*(4), 10.1002.

Grossman, E. R., Neelan, S. E., & Sonnenschein, S. (2020). Alcohol consumption during the COVID-19 pandemic: A cross-sectional survey of U.S. adults. *International Journal of Environmental Research and Public Health, 17*, 91189.

Mattern Clayton Neighbors, J. L. (2004). Social norm campaigns: examining the relationship between changes in perceived norms and changes in alcohol drinking levels. *Journal of Studies of Alcohol, 65*(4), 489–493.

Moore, M. H., & Gerstein, D. R. (1981). *Alcohol and public policy: Beyond the shadow of prohibition.* National Academy Press.

Naimi, T. S., Daley, J. T., & Xuan, Z. (2016). Who would pay for state alcohol tax increases in the United States? *Preventing Chronic Disease, 13*, 150450.

O'Connor, B. (2021). How to get funding for a bar and open the venue of your dreams. *https://www.fundera.com/business-loans/guides/how-to-get-funding-for-a-bar*

Sacks, J. J., Gonzales, K. R., Bouchery, E. E., Tomedi, L. E., & Brewer, R. D. (2015). National and state costs of excessive alcohol consumption. *The American Journal of Preventive Medicine, 49*(5), e73–79.

Scribner, R. A., Cohen, D. A., & Fisher, W. (2000). Evidence of a structural effect for alcohol outlet density: a multisite analysis. *Journal of Clinical Alcohol and Experimental Research, 24*(2), 188–195.

Scribner, R. A., Theall, K. P., & Mason, K. (2011). Alcohol prevention on college campuses: the moderating effect of the alcohol environment on the effectiveness of social norms marketing campaigns. *Journal of Studies of Alcohol, 72*(2), 232–239.

Xu, X., & Chaloupka, F. J. (2011). The effects of price on alcohol use and its consequences. *Alcohol Research and Health, 34(2)*, 236–245.

CHAPTER 9

SOLVING THE U.S. OPIOID CRISIS: A PUBLIC HEALTH CHALLENGE

I hear you're feeling down
well I can ease your pain
get you on your feet again
Relax . . .
Can you show me where it hurts?

—*Pink Floyd, "Comfortably Numb"*

Overview

On the night of March 1, 2022, President Joe Biden outlined four national priorities as part of his State of the Union address. The first was to take action to stem the rising tide of the U.S. opioid epidemic. He stated, "There is so much we can do. Increase funding for prevention, treatment, harm reduction, and recovery" (https://www.cnn.com/interactive/2022/03/politics/state-of-union-annotated/).

The President's directive to prioritize a massive public health effort to reduce the national opioid epidemic came at a time in history when deaths from overdose have recently increased to record high levels due to the COVID-19 pandemic, with 93,000 deaths from opioid overdose reported to the CDC in 2020 (Vasquez, 2021).

Sadly, the opioid epidemic is far better referred to as the **opioid crisis**. This term transcends the ordinary meaning of an epidemic by raising its level of urgency as a national priority. On an upward trend that does not seem to have an end, the crisis is increasingly claiming lives, causing morbidity, costing people their life savings, bankrupting the healthcare system, and disproportionately impacting young people, those who live in poverty, and persons of color.

From a more nuanced point of view, the opioid crisis has actually become a **fentanyl crisis**. Published in 2019, a fascinating book known as *Fentanyl Inc.* describes the evolution of a pain management crisis into a deadly epidemic of drugs mixed with all-too-affordable fentanyl (Westhoff, 2019). The pain management crisis was spawned by a drug called ***OxyContin***. As this prescription drug found its way into the lives of people using it to get high at a low cost, OxyContin became as much of a street drug as any previous pill-based substance in U.S. history. Sadly, the eventual federal controls placed on OxyContin led millions of addicted users to turn to heroin, with fentanyl being used to cut the heroin to keep the price affordable to nearly anyone. Adding to the crisis, drug dealers (working on a massive

Understanding the Science and Practice of Public Health, First Edition. Richard Crosby.
© 2023 John Wiley & Sons, Inc. Published 2023 by John Wiley & Sons, Inc.

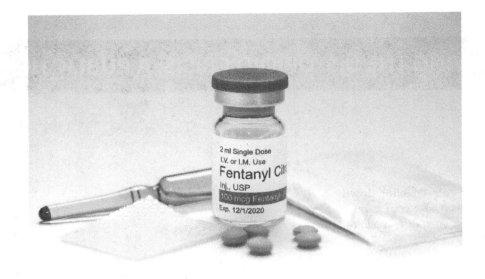

Photo 9.1   Within two years after his untimely death, it was determined that Prince died of an opioid overdose, most likely fentanyl.
Source: Sherry Young/Adobe stock.

scale) began to home-manufacture imposter OxyContin pills made from fentanyl. This prescription drug epidemic thus soon escalated to a street-drug epidemic, and wildly unpredictable amounts of fentanyl were used as a filler to keep the price of heroin low and thus easily affordable. Because of its extreme potency, the unpredictably high levels of fentanyl that were cut into heroin or sold as imposter OxyContin pills began to claim thousands of lives due to overdose. Perhaps one of the most notable among these was music superstar Prince (Francis, 2016) (see **Photo 9.1**).

Given that fentanyl is also an opioid and is widely implicated as the cause of death from drug overdose, you can understand why the opioid crisis is a bit more nuanced than merely its origin as prescription drug crisis. Thus, as you read this chapter, keep in mind that the term *opioid* is a classification name for drugs derived from opioid-based poppy plants (including heroin, OxyContin, and fentanyl).

A Brief History of the Crisis: Why Did It Happen?

In many ways, any form of drug addiction in the United States can be traced back to our medical system and its paradigm of using medication to fight pain. For many Americans, the idea that pain can always be alleviated through medication has become part of their inherited culture. Using a pill to cure pain is a health behavior that we as a society often take for granted. This historical context is important to fully understand the opioid crisis. The crisis can be traced back to medical practice and what is known as **The Joint Commission**, which was something of an accomplice in the initial abuse of opioids. In 2001, this commission created standards that encouraged pain management for patients and relieved physicians of liability in the event of patient addiction to medications such as opioids. The commission coined the term **fifth vital sign**. This sign is pain (the other four are temperature, pulse rate, rate of respiration, and blood pressure). As more than one decade went by without much attention paid to the harm triggered by the Joint Commission relieving physicians of liability for pain management, the crisis grew in scope. By 2016, a group of physicians known as Physicians for Responsible Opioid Prescribing and health officials from several U.S. states sent a letter to the chairperson of the Joint Commission, stating that "Pain is a symptom, not a vital sign" (Flore, 2016). This letter served as an initial objection to the idea that all pain should be medically managed.

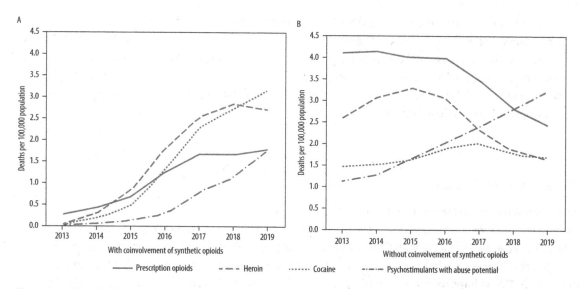

Figure 9.1   The role of fentanyl in the rapid escalation of overdose death rates
Source: Mattson, C. L. et al., 2021 / U.S. Department of Health & Human Services / Public domain.

By that time, however, the drug OxyContin had become a staple in the medical world, and most people who became addicted while managing pain symptoms could usually find a way to keep their prescriptions filled or find surrogate sources that were not pharmacy-based.

The problem with this fifth vital sign is that patients did become addicted to the drugs that now seemed to be an inalienable right of medical care. Compounding the original crisis, recipients of medical care gave their prescription pain pills to non-patients. Thus, regardless of engagement in medical care, a cycle of addiction to prescription medication began to spiral upward. As a result of both prescribed and street use of opioids, the United States experienced a skyrocketing increase in drug overdose deaths. **Figure 9.1** shows the magnitude of this increase between the years 2013 and 2019.

> The problem with this fifth vital sign is that patients did become addicted to the drugs that now seemed to be an inalienable right of medical care.

To understand this figure, it is important to know that "co-involvement of synthetic opioids" refers primarily to fentanyl. With this point in mind, look at graph A: you can see dramatic increases in overdose death rates involving fentanyl. The CDC reported that the increase corresponding to this graph is over 1,000% (Mattson et al., 2021). As shown in graph B, taking fentanyl out of the calculations results in an actual decline in overdose death rates. So, as this chapter proceeds, it is correct to think about the opioid crisis as being driven by fentanyl. Worth knowing at this juncture is that fentanyl is a synthetic opioid that is both legally and illegally produced. It is approximately 50 to 100 times stronger than morphine (Cooper et al., 2020).

> it is correct to think about the opioid crisis as being driven by fentanyl.

The Crisis Is More Than Just Overdose

Death from overdose makes the local and (frequently) national news, especially when celebrities such as Prince and Tom Petty are the victims and when new peaks of overdose deaths are observed by the CDC. However, these deaths are just the tip of the iceberg regarding morbidity and mortality. Underlying the overdose epidemic is a plethora of threats to our public health infrastructure. For instance, it has been estimated that for every death from overdose, 10 other people survived but required hospitalization to recover. Similarly, for every death from overdose, at least 30 more people were admitted to an emergency room. Even worse, it is estimated that for every overdose death, more than 800 other people are actively using illegally obtained opioids; it is as though a never-ending stream of potential new overdose victims exists in the

United States. In the age of COVID-19 and rampant gunshot violence, the added burden on ambulance crews, paramedics, urgent care centers, and hospitals cripples these systems. As described in an interview conducted for this chapter, paramedics often feel a type of burnout known as **compassion fatigue** (see Box 9.1). This represents an endpoint in what began as a caring profession but morphed over time into a loss of caring due to the seemingly endless flow of people who overdose on opioids.

BOX 9.1. INTERVIEW WITH A PARAMEDIC REGARDING "OPIOID RUNS"

Interviewer: Please tell me about the use of Narcan by paramedics.

Paramedic: The truth is that Narcan is over-utilized. A patient who has overdosed can just as easily be taken care of with a nasal spray or oral airway. We can also use an IV with fluids running just enough to keep the veins open, and supplemental oxygen. These courses of treatment are faster, cheaper, and just as effective but without the issues that Narcan cause (e.g., anger, irritability, etc.). This is important because the psych issues caused by Narcan can all be dangers to first responders (especially if you're in the back of the ambulance by yourself with the patient).

Interviewer: Do most of your overdose runs involve people who have Narcan at home and just do not know how to use it?

Paramedic: The thing about Narcan is that by time a victim of overdose needs it, they cannot use it on their own. This is because they have lost consciousness. Someone else has to "Narcan you" – it is usually done via a device that sprays a dosage up the nostrils of the patient. The layperson most likely gives the whole bottle, (which is over three times the recommended amount). This dose can cause both irritation and aggression when they wake up. To put it in perspective, imagine having drinks at a bar – are you going to get buzzed by having two to four shots? Most likely, depending on your weight/gender. But what if you had three times that amount? Six to eight shots? You'd most definitely be drunk, if not extremely buzzed. More is not always better, as is the case with Narcan.

Interviewer: Do the people you pick up deny using opioids?

Paramedic: Most patients will wake up and deny using opioids. Instead, they blame another drug (like Xanax or Valium). What these people, I am sure, do not get is that Narcan **only** works on opioids and their receptors. So their very logic is flawed, and I always make sure to remind them of that, not always very nicely – because the mere fact that you can save someone's life, and then their first words to you are a lie, does not sit well with many first responders. We are fed up with it, and we all are showing signs of compassion fatigue.

Interviewer: What happens with the typical ambulance ride once you pick up an OD victim? Do they try to "escape" once they have had the Narcan?

Paramedic: It's about a 50/50 chance that they try to escape after Narcan. On a typical OD call there will be cops, fireman, and EMS; so if they do try to run, there are many people there to stop that from happening. On the ambulance we also can utilize soft restraints if needed for safety of the crew or the patient. The ones who "come back" violent are often the ones who got too much Narcan. A typical dose is approximately .4 mg, but often 2 mg is slammed all at once by uneducated responders or the uneducated layperson.

Interviewer: Do they show remorse or a will to enter a treatment program to end their addiction?

Paramedic: Depends on the person. I have mentioned rehab to multiple people and usually get met with a stream of cuss words – but then again, I have had a handful of patients who have woken up and thanked me, apologized profusely, and sworn to never do it again. The angry ones far outweigh the latter, though.

Interviewer: As a paramedic, what are two policy actions that you feel should be used to reduce the opioid problem in America?

Paramedic: Heroin laws need to be enforced, and there needs to be a zero tolerance policy on it. Also, patients who overdose on opioids need to be arrested after they are healthy enough to go to jail, and then questioned thoroughly about the drugs – followed by harsh punishments.

Interviewer: Do you support the idea of providing Narcan to family members of opioid users?

Paramedic: No. If we're going to provide drug addicts with free Narcan then we need to provide diabetics with free insulin. Being a drug addict is a choice – it's a chosen lifestyle; being a diabetic is not. While it is true that some diabetes cases are a result of bad diet or lack of exercise, it is also true that most cases are heredity/poor pancreatic cells. My point is this: one of these health issues is **not** something you can change, and the other is. Why are we giving free medication to the issue that is fixable with rehab and better decision-making?

Interviewer: What are your thoughts about paramedics teaching users about using new needles/syringes to reduce the spread of blood-borne infections such as a hepatitis C?

Paramedic: I would rather focus my efforts elsewhere. The very essence of a drug addict is that they don't care about their health, their body, or their toll on anyone else in the world. In healthcare there are so many other people that would benefit from education (that would actually listen and make efforts to try and change). I think the needle exchange program was a failed attempt to fix an issue that the users don't want fixed. The program itself seems to encourage drug usage (with the flawed overtone that it is okay if you use a "fresh needle"). I have very little sympathy for drug addicts. I do not believe they want to change until it's far too late. Movies and television shows that glamorize drug use don't get that the those of us who have helped addicts breathe with a bag valve mask are often thanked by being lied to, hit, spit on, punched, cussed out, or bitten. Healthcare workers are tired, we have compassion fatigue, and our efforts are not going to be spent on people who do not even want to help themselves.

The epitome of public health threats stemming from the opioid crisis applies to people who use opioids by injection. Injecting carries some degree of risk even when a person has a constant supply of new needles and syringes. Paramount among these risks is a fairly common species of bacteria that typically inhabit the skin. Known as *staph aureus*, this species causes harm when it enters the bloodstream, with one result being an acute inflammation of the heart. Puncturing the skin with needles – often more than once daily – creates the risk of introducing this species of bacteria into the bloodstream. Moreover, the sheer number of puncture wounds can lead to the growth of other bacteria and ultimately create **soft tissue infections**. To give you a sense of how addicts who inject drugs can have a massive number of these unhealed puncture wounds, **Photo 9.2** shows needle tracks on an active user. And the unfortunate reality is that millions of people who inject opioids do not have access to a constant supply of new needles and syringes.

Barring access to new needles and syringes (bacteria and viruses can live for long periods in microscopic fissures and crevices in either the needle or the syringe), **persons who inject drugs (PWID)** and also share their needles and syringes with other PWID create a public health issue involving the rampant spread of life-threatening diseases, particularly **hepatitis B and C**, as well as the human immunodeficiency virus (HIV). To be clear about this spread, the terminology used to describe it is depicted in **Figure 9.2**.

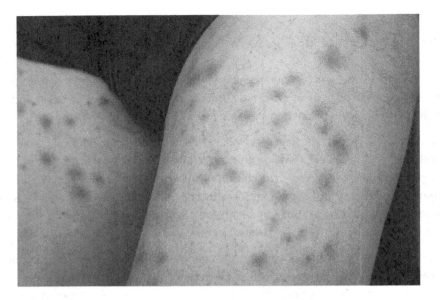

Photo 9.2   Known as **needle tracks**, these tell-tale marks are common among persons who inject drugs.
Source: Otto/Adobe stock.

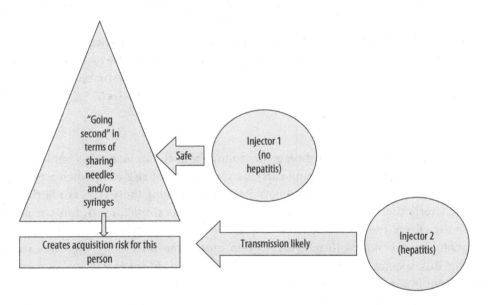

Figure 9.2   A graphic depiction of terminology relative to disease spread among people who inject drugs (PWID)

America's Hepatitis Epidemic

This chapter will describe why and how vaccines became a mainstay of highly effective public health practice. For now, it is worth knowing that since 1986, a safe and effective vaccine against hepatitis B has been widely available. As of the date of publication for this textbook, no such statements can be made relative to hepatitis C or HIV. Of course, like almost all vaccines, not all Americans have received even the first dose of this vaccine series. Thus, hepatitis B is also a concern for the transmission/acquisition of this virus by PWID. More importantly, it is hepatitis C that is rapidly proliferating as a consequence of the opioid crisis. HIV is an additional concern, but one of a very different nature regarding how it can be controlled by public health practice (see **Chapter 10**).

What Is Hepatitis?

In **Chapter 8**, you learned about the role of the liver in maintaining health. As a reminder, you know that this organ is constantly on duty to detoxify alcohol (as well as countless other toxins that enter the body as part of the daily diet). You also understand that the destruction of liver tissue is permanent, leaving only useless scar tissue. Now, as you learn more, you also need to understand the word **hepatitis**. The root (*hepa*) refers to the liver, and the suffix (*titis*) means inflammation. In the case of hepatitis, this inflammation is caused by a virus. Specifically, three types of the virus cause this inflammation of the liver: hepatitis A, hepatitis B, and hepatitis C (very easy to remember). Each virus differs from the other two in terms of effects on the liver and transmission routes. Fortunately, vaccines are widely available (and used) against types A and B. Vaccines for hepatitis C have not been developed, placing people who acquire the virus at risk of long-term chronic diseases, including cirrhosis of the liver and hepatocarcinoma (i.e., cancer of the liver).

Hepatitis C and the Opioid Crisis

For more than two decades, the CDC has been heavily engaged in a campaign promoting hepatitis C testing among Americans. The campaign features advertisements (**Photo 9.3**) that illuminate the crisis and let people know that anyone who has ever injected drugs should be tested. Putting aside the destruction of families, careers, and relationships, the opioid crisis has been directly responsible for a rapid rise in America's epidemic of hepatitis.

the opioid crisis has been directly responsible for a rapid rise in America's epidemic of hepatitis.

This rise is shown clearly in **Figure 9.3**. The CDC attributes this dramatic increase to the opioid crisis, an observation that is well supported by numerous epidemiology studies showing a direct correlation between the escalation of opioid use and the increase in the annual incidence of hepatitis C. Data indicate that about three-quarters of all new cases are the result of people sharing needles and syringes (even more so than HIV, this virus spreads efficiently through blood-to-blood transfer between people). The causal relationship can be changed. This relationship is based on the simple lack of access to new (meaning clean) needles and syringes among PWID. However, breaking this correlation between the injection of opioids and the spread of hepatitis C is well within reach of public health practice, given sufficient policy-based and legislative support for public health programs that provide PWID with easy access to free supplies of new needles and syringes. This evidence is nationwide and robust;

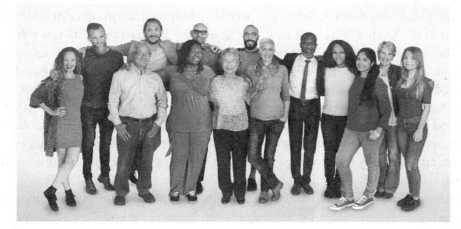

Photo 9.3 CDC campaigns to promote hepatitis C screening typically feature posters indicating who may be infected.
Source: Rawpixel.com / Adobe Stock.

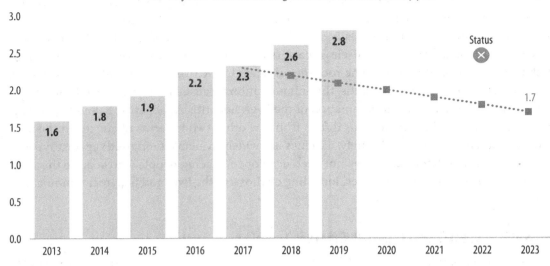

Figure 9.3 The rising tide of hepatitis C cases in the United States
Source: CDC (2021) / U.S. Department of Health & Human Services / Public domain.

however, it is often at odds with the personal experience of healthcare workers such as social workers, paramedics, and pharmacists. At this point in this textbook, you will learn about a tremendously important public health concept: **harm reduction**.

Harm Reduction Applied to the Opioid Crisis: Syringe Service Programs

During the Clinton Administration, politicians opposed to the idea of syringe and needle exchange programs added a provision in the proposed appropriations budget for the U.S. Department of Health and Human Services. The provision specifically prohibited the use of federal funds for these exchange programs until that department determined that the programs were safe and effective. To stymie any progress toward such a determination, the budget also eliminated funding for the research to investigate safety and effectiveness. Despite the fact that a liberal Democrat was president, this language remained in the budget, and thus initial government resistance to what had become a best practice in other developed nations was halted in the United States. By now, you have to be wondering "Why was this a controversy?" The answer lies in the common belief that people who use drugs are weak-willed and/or do not want to end their addiction. This is nothing more than a misguided belief, one possibly fueled by the White House administration preceding President Clinton. During the Reagan Administration, American began what is still known today as the War Against Drugs. Popularized by first lady Nancy Reagan, the war had a tagline message to the public: "Just say no." Of course, the problem with such a simplistic viewpoint on America's drug epidemic is that addiction is typically far beyond personal control; instead, it becomes an all-encompassing struggle to stay normal by maintaining the addicted state.

addiction is typically far beyond personal control

Realizing and accepting this reality, the concept of harm reduction is based on minimizing the damages of addiction rather than simply expecting people to end their addiction, typically without adequate support. Under this paradigm of harm reduction, it soon became apparent from the accumulating research evidence (coming first from other nations with more liberal outlooks) that providing addicts who inject with a constant supply of new needles and syringes would greatly aid in minimizing the damage occurring to PWID as a consequence of HIV. At this time in history (i.e., the 1990s), HIV was not well controlled; and until the later part of that decade, it was viewed as a terminal disease. At the turn of the millennium, combination therapies for HIV (see **Chapter 10**) advanced to the point of making life with HIV much more manageable, greatly postponing – at the population-level – the development of HIV into AIDS, leading to death. With this improved control over HIV, it was clear that needle and syringe exchange programs were still very important relative to averting the spread of hepatitis C.

The term **exchange** is important to understanding how this type of harm-reduction practice functions. To discourage sharing needles and syringes, these programs ask people to turn in their used equipment. By doing this, the local risks of hepatitis C transmission/acquisition among PWID drop dramatically. Then, by providing new needles and syringes, added prevention effects occur because addicts can inject safely. Also, in many exchange programs, the exchange ratio is greater than 1 to 1 (meaning for every used needle/syringe returned, more than one new set of works is distributed), simply because the added number of new needles and syringes creates an influx of safe injection equipment into the PWID community. This is an important feature because PWID usually remain hidden and thus will not take advantage of an exchange program. The exchange methods of a greater than 1-to-1 ratio were first known as **distribution programs**.

Abundant evidence strongly supports the very high potential of effectiveness for properly implemented needle and syringe exchange programs. The evidence further demonstrates that these programs **do not** lead to increased use of injectable drugs (Pitt, Humphreys, & Brandeau, 2018). The evidence further demonstrates that these programs, currently referred to as **syringe service programs (SSPs)**, on average promote a reduction in what is known as **injection-risk related behaviors** (IRBs). These behaviors include needle and syringe sharing, reuse of needles/syringes, sharing equipment used to prepare drugs into an injectable form, and sharing other injection paraphernalia. A review of U.S. programs found that SSPs had a significant and lasting impact, decreasing the occurrence of IRBs assessed at the population level (Vidourek, King, Yockey, et al., 2019). However, other reviews have found less encouraging evidence and offered conclusions that do not fully support the existence of SSPs. For instance, a review by Davis and colleagues (2017) concluded that SSPs are supported by evidence pertaining to a reduction of HIV incidence but not by evidence regarding hepatitis C.

In yet another review (one of 133 different studies), the results also supported the value of SSPs against IRBs, and HIV, but the evidence was mixed pertaining to hepatitis C (Fernandez et al., 2017). This latter review study, however, did provide valuable insight regarding the mixed evidence for reducing hepatitis C. Specifically, evidence suggests that more advanced and well-implemented SSPs do reduce the spread of hepatitis C; however, when reviewed in the aggregate (i.e., studies of all SSPs, regardless of program quality), the evidence becomes diluted. As stated in their conclusion, "Full harm reduction interventions provided at the structural-level and in multi-component programs, as well as a high level of coverage, are needed" (Fernandez et al., 2017, p. 309). The point made in this conclusion is consistent with what is known to be effective public health practice: intervention programs must be designed at the structural-level (see **Chapters 2 and 3**), and they must be widely implemented before we can expect to find population-level improvements in health. This concept of applying multiple forms of intervention simultaneously to solve the U.S. opioid crisis has been widely advocated and supported (Pitt, Humphreys, & Brandeau, 2018). As you will recall from reading **Chapter 4** of this textbook (which applied the framework for tobacco control to public health in general), it is indeed the case that successful public health interventions comprise an integrated and coordinated mass of actions and programs. The ultimate solution to the U.S. opioid crisis thus will not be a single approach. Instead, it will be a synchronized set of approaches to work synergistically.

intervention programs must be designed at the structural-level

The ultimate solution to the U.S. opioid crisis thus will not be a single approach.

In considering the quality of SSPs, it is widely agreed that the United Kingdom (UK) has been a leader in creating high-quality, structural-level SSPs that do far more than simply provide PWID with ample supplies of new needles/syringes. A modeling study (a type of public health study that relies on dozens of data-derived parameters to create a computer-based simulation of probable outcomes given changes in a given intervention program) of SSPs in three geographically distinct cities of the UK estimated that removing current SSPs in these three cities would lead to as much as a 64% increase in hepatitis C among PWID between the years 2016 and 2030 (Ward et al., 2018)

Given what appear to be advanced levels of success with SSPs in the UK, a key question for the United States involves how our SSPs can be significantly improved. One emerging option that is gaining a foothold is focused on pharmacies. Because pharmacies are typically a trusted source of healthcare for communities, the role of a pharmacist has greatly expanded throughout the opioid crisis. Pharmacists have the training to understand the severity of risks experienced by PWID who do not have consistent access to new needles/syringes. Further, it is increasingly the case that pharmacists are providing multiple prevention-oriented services to PWID (Meyerson et al., 2019a). Unfortunately, the sticking point in these multiple prevention-oriented services has been the provision of new needles/syringes. The main issue is whether state-based policies will allow pharmacists to freely engage in the provision of new needles/syringes to customers who inject drugs. This freedom for pharmacies to legally sell new needles/syringes to customers who inject drugs had been granted by at least 20 states. Quite different than an SSP, the pharmacy-based programs provide access at a cost – the new needles/syringes are sold to PWID just as they are sold to people who are diabetic and inject insulin. A problem, however (even in states with these supportive laws), is that a sizable percentage of pharmacists may harbor personal beliefs that preclude them from truly helping their PWID customers to inject safely. As the public health response to the U.S. opioid crisis escalates, it is likely that interventions will be developed and targeted toward pharmacists to help them more fully appreciate the value – and even the obligation – to become adept at creating a stigma-free relationship with their PWID customers: a relationship that leads to ease of purchase.

Beyond the concept of locating SSPs in pharmacies, the opioid crisis remains riddled with SSP-related issues such as legal barriers to implementation, limited funding, and a lack of synchrony between SSP locations and high-risk areas for the very dangerous practice of syringe/needle sharing. Throughout the United States, SSPs operate with greatly varying services, and they differ tremendously in quality and commitment to truly helping PWID. Thus, one key challenge to the future of public health is to rapidly expand the existence of uniformly high-quality SSPs in every state.

The Value of Methadone and Other Treatments

The one constant theme of the opioid crisis is best summarized by the term **dynamic change**. Regardless of when any given journal article or textbook chapter devoted to the crisis is published, it will almost certainly be outdated within a year. The long-standing use of methadone treatment programs, for example, has evolved tremendously. This rapid evolution is partly attributable to needs based on the escalation of the crisis; however, it also came about as a consequence of the COVID-19 pandemic. Restrictions imposed during the pandemic (see **Chapter 1**) broadly worked against the previously established systems for helping people with **opioid use disorder** (OUD) to overcome their addiction via **opioid substitution treatment** (OST). Of note, OST is a preferred and more generic term for the use of methadone and other drugs as agents to gradually help people with OUD withdrawal from the addiction. The previously described modeling study based on data derived from three geographically distinct cities

---

Margin notes:

Pharmacists have the training to understand the severity of risks experienced by PWID

one key challenge to the future of public health is to rapidly expand the existence of uniformly high-quality SSPs in every state.

in the UK concluded that OST was much more important than syringe/needle exchange to ultimately reducing the incidence of hepatitis C (Ward et al., 2018)

To solve the logistic barriers to OST treatment that arose from the COVID-19 pandemic, at least four strategies have been implemented:

- Policy-level change has been applied to loosen restrictions against pharmacists providing OST. Given their ease of developing a trusting relationship within the communities they serve, pharmacists are uniquely qualified to become frontline providers of OST to people suffering from OUD. In this regard, a key aspect of public health practice is to assist in the training of pharmacists to help them better understand OUD as a treatable disease and a social consequence of a massive epidemic related to pain management, as opposed to a personal choice. As the future of public health emerges, pharmacists will likely play a pivotal role in controlling the opioid crisis. With supportive state laws, pharmacists can provide a highly accessible and cost-effective means of reducing **blood-borne infections** (BBIs) among PWID. The inherent advantages of pharmacists playing a lead role in this public health effort include the point that pharmacies exist in every community, they are open for extended hours, syringe/needle sales are within the scope of pharmacy practice, and pharmacies have previously demonstrated an ability to effectively implement public health interventions.

- The COVID-19 pandemic served as a trigger to earnestly begin the widespread application of telemedicine (aka telehealth) to manage OUD via OST. Like so many other aspects of society during the COVID-19 pandemic, using web-based video-conferencing tools quickly and efficiently unites health care providers with OUD patients.

- Although previous conditions pertaining to the provision of OST included mandatory urine screening for opioids, this requirement was generally relaxed or removed entirely as a consequence of the pandemic. Even prior to COVID-19, many OST providers had argued that urine screens for stable OUD patients on OST were unnecessary.

- In response to the COVID-19 pandemic, the U.S. Office of Substance Abuse and Mental Health Services Administration (SAMHSA) allowed people being treated with OST to take home as many as 28 days' worth of medication. From a purely behavioral perceptive, this loosening of policy is a breakthrough because the seemingly simple act of constantly returning to a clinical setting for more OST-related medication is not simple for millions of people with OUD.

These four policy-level changes to OST are likely to be just the start of what will eventually become a much more consumer-driven approach to the following challenging tasks:

- Convincing people living with OUD to begin OST

- Ensuring that people who begin OST have a supportive social environment relative to maintaining their ongoing use of OST

- Developing behavioral and social science-based interventions designed to re-engage people with OUD who begin OST and then drop out of care

Despite this somewhat encouraging section of the chapter, it is vital to also understand a basic reality of OST: it functions only at the treatment end of the crisis. From a more comprehensive public health perspective, the other main goal is to prevent people from entering into opioid addiction. Working at the treatment end is a type of prevention (known as **tertiary prevention**). Working at the opposite end of the spectrum (**primary prevention**) will be infinitely more difficult. One –very daunting – approach to the primary prevention of opioid use lies in coming to grips with the massive social inequities that drive addiction. In many ways, it is entirely correct to think about the opioid epidemic as a problem that constantly highlights the myriad issues that separate the socioeconomic classes of our nation. In this regard, people often ask, "How do we know that this is really a problem of social class?" The answer brings us to an overarching principle in public health practice: place matters!

Why Does "Place" Matter?

One of the hallmark principles of public health is, indeed, "place matters." The term *place* is used here with respect to geographic location. For instance, notice in **Figure 9.4** that the southern states have a noticeably greater rate of giving out prescription drugs for pain control. In terms of illicit drugs, place matters regarding factors such as proximity to interstate highways, levels of local law enforcement, and even the degree of isolation from public view (for instance, the opioid crisis has taken an especially dramatic toll on rural Appalachia). As with many human behaviors, culture plays a prominent role in shaping drug use behaviors; thus, place also matters relative to the culture of the immediately surrounding social norms, beliefs, and practices.

Thinking now more specifically about the role of place in regard to controlling the opioid crisis, and looking again at **Figure 9.4**, a key question becomes, "Why are there place-based differences in policy and practice regarding pharmacies?" The answer comes back to local beliefs and local culture. Sadly, people holding key positions in public health (including pharmacists) may allow their personal convictions about right and wrong to interfere with implementing evidence-based public health practices.

As an example, consider the state of Arizona. Meyerson and colleagues (2019b) interviewed 37 PWID who had attempted (sometimes unsuccessfully) to legally purchase syringes and needles from pharmacies distributed throughout two urban locations and one rural location in Arizona. Although Arizona laws allow for the non-prescription sale of syringes and needles, all 37 people interviewed described at least one time when a pharmacist refused to make these sales to them. This study also found that 75% of pharmacists were asked about syringe/needle sales for injection drug use in the past two years; however, only 40% of these health professionals proceeded to sell the requested syringes/needles. The negative buying experiences of PWID, in turn, led to feelings of being stigmatized, fear of being reported to law

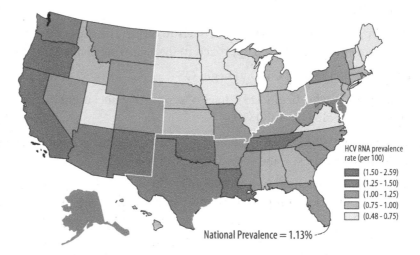

Figure 9.4   Case rates of hepatitis C are not equally distributed
Source: Adapted from CDC (2021).

officials as a drug user, a lack of trust in the use of pharmacies to obtain new syringes/needles, and, of course, the reuse of currently owned syringes/needles. So, at least in this one state, a law designed to protect public health was subtly subverted by the beliefs of professionals who were otherwise in a very strong position to promote this effective harm-reduction practice. This is a classic example of squandering a tremendously valuable public health opportunity. A quote from one of the 37 people interviewed provides a lasting impression of how some pharmacists have entirely placed people in harm's way: "What they don't know is that you usually have a syringe you've used many times in your pocket. It's all barbed up, and if you don't get a needle from them, you're gonna just use that one."

What Does the Future Look Like for the Opioid Crisis?

Beginning in 2017, the opioid crisis was partially mitigated through changes in prescription practices – this had an immediate and clear link to a similar decline in overdose deaths. This reversal of trends provided compelling evidence that policy changes can have a strong and live-saving effect. Tougher prescribing policies simply translated into less access. However, this success was short-lived.

Figure 9.5 provides you with a sense of the past in terms of how the opioid crisis has evolved, at least concerning deaths from overdose that were reported to the CDC. As shown, the crisis tailed off in terms of prescription opioid use and heroin use. But just as quickly as this success occurred, fentanyl and other synthetic opioids entered the drug market and sent overdose rates skyrocketing again. Whether synthetic opioids will continue to drive overdose death rates higher is an open question. The one forecast that can be made with a fair degree of certainty is that supply will always keep pace with demand. As long as people need to use an opioid-like drug, drug dealers will find a way to make and distribute a product that fills this need. So, yet another key challenge to public health practice lies in turning off the demand side of this equation.

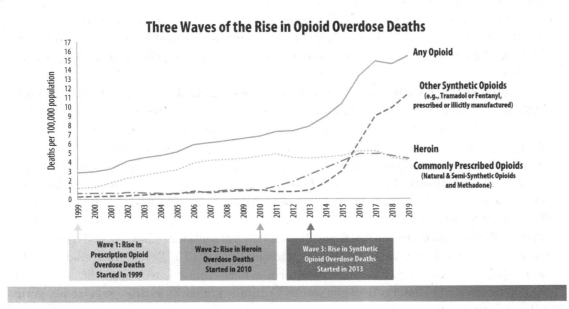

Figure 9.5 What will the next 10 years look like?
Source: CDC (2022) / U.S. Department of Health & Human Services / Public domain.

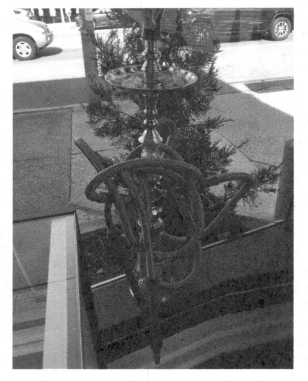

Photo 9.4   Once considered illegal drug paraphernalia, this bong gives a social aspect to the shared highs of marijuana use.

Although abundant evidence has not been collected, it is possible that one way to reduce the demand for illicit drugs such as synthetic opioids is to abandon the War on Drugs in favor of letting people have relatively safe methods of feeling high. Legalizing marijuana use (see **Photo 9.4**), for example, has been generally shown to provide users with a safe method of dealing with pain, finding relaxation, and experiencing controlled highs.

Unlike other chapters in this textbook, this chapter does not offer a clear direction for the future of public health practice relative to resolving the opioid crisis by reducing the demand side of the problem. The United States has been too far immersed in a culture of being "comfortably numb" when it comes to managing physical – and even mental – pain. As long as this culture continues to be sponsored and supported by the pharmaceutical industry, a parallel industry (one that is not legal) will likely continue to thrive. Thus, the ending to the story of the U.S. opioid crisis is completely unknown at this time in history. What is known is that population-level improvements will occur only in the presence of massive population-level awareness and action regarding evidence-based approaches to reducing the crisis. The past approaches of criminalizing (i.e., making drug possession a felony offense) and marginalizing drug users have not been effective and must be abandoned in favor of more positive intervention efforts.

> The United States has been too far immersed in a culture of being "comfortably numb" when it comes to managing physical – and even mental – pain.

Review and Key Terms

This chapter is a very broad overview of the U.S. opioid crisis, which is better described as a **fentanyl crisis**. Originating with a mandate from **The Joint Commission** that relieved physicians from liability over issues with patients' addictions to pain-management medication, the drug known as **OxyContin** quickly dominated this crisis until tougher prescribing laws were passed and enforced in 2017. Famously calling pain the **"fifth vital sign,"** this new mandate for physicians began the widespread medical practice of controlling pain through drugs such as OxyContin.

As opioids became somewhat less accessible, their synthetic counterparts (made mostly with fentanyl) began to drive an entire spectrum of public health problems steadily upward. As injectable drugs, opioids and their fentanyl-based twins led to a massive increase in unsafe injection practices (globally and in the United States). Even without reusing syringes/needles, **PWID** commonly develop soft tissue infections at injection sites, and they contract a host of **blood-borne infections** (BBIs) such as a fairly serious (and sometimes deadly) bacteria known as **staph aureus**. But because of laws and regulations that make purchasing new syringes/needles difficult for PWID, the sharing of used equipment spawned an exceptionally large increase in rates of **hepatitis C. Hepatitis B** and the human immunodeficiency virus (HIV) are also easily spread through the use of shared injection equipment. To alleviate the rapid spread of these BBIs, an increasingly valuable tool – a form of **harm reduction** – for public health practice is syringe/needle **distribution programs**. Currently known as **syringe service programs** (SSPs), the goal of these public health interventions is to foster safe injection practices as well as serve as a conduit to helping people with **opioid use disorder** (OUD) enter treatment programs based on **opioid substitution therapy** (OST). Accumulating evidence supports the value of SSPs relative to decreasing the risk of **injection-related risk behaviors** among PWID.

Emerging evidence also supports the concept of refining and improving SSPs to optimally impact this form of intervention against the rampant spread of hepatitis C.

As the fentanyl/opioid crisis evolves, it continues to become a seemingly intractable public health problem. Healthcare workers who handle a never-ending stream of overdose patients are experiencing **compassion fatigue**. Federal agencies such as **SAMHSA** are working hard to mitigate the crisis by engaging in **tertiary prevention** measures such as loosening regulations pertaining to Narcan use. Ultimately, however, the true public health challenge lies in **primary prevention**, meaning the demand-side of the equation has to change before the crisis can reasonably be resolved. This will involve large-scale efforts to change people and practices, including medical practice and the belief that pain must be recognized as a manageable problem that can be ideally controlled through opioid-based medication.

Ultimately, however, the true public health challenge lies in **primary prevention**, meaning the demand-side of the equation has to change before the crisis can reasonably be resolved.

For Practice and Discussion

Practice Questions

1. Harm reduction, as applied to the opioid crisis, is best described as:
   a. Changing the demand-side of the equation relative to the supply and demand of opioids
   b. Altering the strength of opioids by reducing potency with fentanyl
   c. Providing people with OUD with access to SSPs and OST

2. Which disease has become the largest epidemic of the opioid crisis?
   a. Hepatitis B
   b. Hepatitis C
   c. Human immunodeficiency virus
   d. Soft tissue infections

3. Tracing the history of the opioid crisis back to its origin, what term best captures the initial cause?
   a. The fifth vital sign
   b. Fentanyl
   c. Hepatitis
   d. The First Commission

4. Evidence supports the value of both SSPs and OST relative to harm reduction. Of these two options, however, the evidence is much stronger relative to OST.
   a. True
   b. False

5. Of the following professions, which one has the greatest potential to mitigate and resolve the opioid crisis?
   a. Police officers
   b. Parole officers
   c. Public health social workers
   d. Pharmacists

6. SSPs are also thought of as distribution programs for syringes and needles. This is particularly the case when:
   a. The exchange is greater than a 1 to 1 ratio
   b. These programs are co-located in pharmacies
   c. PWID can receive their injection equipment anonymously
   d. Law enforcement supports the exchange efforts

7. Which one of the following is not a BBI?
   a. Staph aureus
   b. Hepatitis B
   c. Needle tracks
   d. Hepatitis C

8. OxyContin is no longer the main driver of the opioid crisis. Instead, the more recent drivers are:
   a. Fentanyl and heroin
   b. Fentanyl and other synthetic opioids
   c. Heroin and methamphetamines
   d. Narcan and methadone

9. The public health response to the overdose death rates caused by the opioid crisis has largely been characterized by:
   a. An equal mix of tertiary and primary prevention
   b. Mostly tertiary prevention in the form of harm reduction
   c. Mostly tertiary prevention in the form of Narcan
   d. Mostly primary prevention based on the use of BBI inhibitors

10. One great public health success of the opioid crisis has been that SSPs are now implemented and conducted using a universal system overseen by the Joint Commission.
    a. True
    b. False

For Discussion (in class or small groups, or online)

11. Since the time this chapter was composed (2022), it is certainly true that state laws have continued to change and evolve relative to SSPs. Using a CDC or NIH (National Institutes of Health) website, find out how many states currently have laws allowing pharmacists to legally sell syringes and needles to PWID. Compare the number you obtain to the numbers obtained by other students taking this same course.

12. Fentanyl is often added to synthetic opioids in such large (uncontrolled) doses that overdose death may be inevitable. Go online to learn about fentanyl test strips. Summarize what you learn in a one-paragraph posting on your preferred form of social media. What did you learn from how people reacted to your post? For example, were they unaware of this overdose prevention option?

13. Following the election of Donald Trump in 2016, a wave of conservative legislation was passed across the United States. One aspect of this wave was ending harm-reduction programs relative to the opioid crisis. Learn as much as possible about how some states have either protected harm reduction or worked to make these programs inaccessible or non-existent. Compose a two- to three-page summary that your course instructor can critique and evaluate.

References

Abdul-Quader, A. S., Feelmeyer, J., & Modi, S. (2013). Effectiveness of structural-level needle/syringe programs to reduce HCV and HIV infection among people who inject drugs: A systematic review. *AIDS & Behavior, 17,* 2878–2892.

CDC (2020). *Vital Signs,* April. https://www.cdc.gov/hepatitis/hcv/vitalsigns/pdf/hepatitisc-vitalsigns april2020-H.pdf

CDC (2021a). National progress report 2025: Reduce reported rate of new hepatitis C virus infections among persons who inject drugs by > 25%. https://www.cdc.gov/hepatitis/policy/npr/2021/ NationalProgressReport-HepC-ReduceInfectionsPWID.htm

CDC (2021b). Viral hepatitis. https://www.cdc.gov/hepatitis/statistics/2017surveillance/TablesFigures-HepC.htm#tabs-1-6

CDC (2022). Understanding the epidemic. https://www.cdc.gov/drugoverdose/epidemic/index.html

Cooper, R., Thompson, J., & Edgerton, R. (2020). Modeling dynamics of fatal opioid overdose by state and across time. *Prev Med Rep. 20,* 101184. doi:10.1016/j.pmedr.2020.101184.

Davis, S. M., Daily, S., Kristhansson, A. L., Kelley, G. A., Zullig, K., Baus, A., Davideu, D., & Fisher, M. (2017). Needle exchange programs for the prevention of hepatitis C virus infection in people who inject drugs: A systematic review with meta-analysis. *Harm Reduction Journal, 14,* 25.

Fernandes, R. M., Cary, M., Duarte, G., & Jesus, G. (2017). Effectiveness of needle and syringe programmes in people who inject drugs – An overview of systematic reviews. *BMC Public Health, 17,* 309.

Flore, K. (2016). Opioid crisis: Scrap pain as the 5th vital sign? *Medpage Today; Public Health and Policy,* April 13. https://www.medpagetoday.com/publichealthpolicy/publichealth/57336

Francis, E. (2018). Police release findings into Prince's death, giving glimpse into his final days. ABC News, April 20. https://abcnews.go.com/US/police-release-findings-princes-death-giving-glimpse-final/story?id=54619334

Mattson, C. L., Tanz, L. J., Quinn, K., Kariisa, M., Patel, P., & Davis, N. L. (2021). Trends and geographic patterns in drug and synthetic opioid overdose deaths – United States, 2013-2019. *Morbidity and Mortality Weekly Report, 70*(6), 202–207.

Meyerson, B. E., Dinh, P. C., Agley, J. D., & Hill, B. J. (2019a). Predicting pharmacist dispensing practices and comfort related to pre-exposure prophylaxis for HIV prevention (PrEP). *AIDS and Behavior, 23*(7), 1925–1938.

Meyerson, B. E., Lawrence, C. A., Cope, S. D., Levin, S., & Thomas, C. (2019b). I could take the judgment if you could just prescribe the service: non-prescription syringe purchase experiences at Arizona pharmacies, 2018. *Harm Reduction Journal, 16,* 57.

Pitt, A. L., Humphreys, K., & Brandeau, M.L. (2018). Modeling health benefits and harms of public policy responses to the United States opioid epidemic. *The American Journal of Public Health, 108*(10), 1394–1399.

Ward, Z., Platt, L., Sweeney, S., Hope, V. D. & Maher, L. (2018). Impact of current and scaled-up levels of hepatitis C prevention and treatment interventions for people who inject drugs in three UK settings: What is required to achieve the WHO's hepatitis C virus elimination target? *Addiction, 113,* 1727–1738.

Vasquez, M. (2021). Biden administration grapples with American addiction as overdose death hits a record high. https://www.cnn.com/2021/09/30/politics/biden-administration-drug-epidemic/ index.html

Vidourek, R. A., King, K. A., Yockey, R. A., & Becker, K. J. (2019) Straight to the point: A systematic review of needle exchange programs in the United States. *Journal of Behavioral Health, 10.*

Westhoff, B. (2019). *Fentanyl Inc.* Grove Press: New York, NY.

CHAPTER 10

HIV IN THE UNITED STATES – WHAT ELSE CAN WE DO?

But touch my tears with your lips, touch my world with your fingertips . . . Who wants to live forever?

—*Queen, "Who Wants to Live Forever?"*

Overview

This chapter is unique to the textbook because HIV/AIDS is a disease that typically begins with the passion of sex and progresses through a series of stages that cause its victims severe life changes. Among the challenges faced by the victims are significant difficulties in managing sexual and love-based relationships with persons romantically involved in their lives. Although living for decades after infection has expanded these life challenges, this longer life span was only a dream back in the years when HIV/AIDS quickly became a global reality (approximately 1981 through 1996). At that time in history, when death occurred within just a few years following infection, this very tiny virus united communities, mobilized massive research efforts, and touched the hearts of millions. When Freddie Mercury, the famed singer for the rock group Queen, died of AIDS in 1991, the world was still five years away from the first generation of medications that would control the replication rate of HIV and ultimately allow people to live for decades rather than only years. However, this extension of life is not enjoyed equally around the world: far too many nations have been left behind to mourn the loss of those who die, most of whom are young.

Public health history has already shown that HIV/AIDS has taught (and continues to teach) humanity how to intervene more effectively and respond to a disease that has eluded vaccine development for over 40 years. The virus has also spotlighted the sweeping inequities that exist in the United States, other developed nations, and nearly all developing nations. Sadly, HIV/AIDS also carries a great deal of stigma, a form of discrimination that often precludes people from being tested and treated for HIV infection. As a species, we are slowly learning that people's social and economic marginalization creates fertile ground for the virus to spread and claim an ever-expanding number of human lives. The ultimate public health response to HIV/AIDS would be resolving the health disparities that allow the virus to continue despite great medical advances. However, this chapter will be

LEARNING OBJECTIVES

- Understand the basic disease process and terminology associated with HIV/AIDS.

- Explain the **Continuum of Care** as related to PLWH.

- Describe the actions, advantages, and issues related to PrEP.

- Define biological synergy relative to HIV transfer through sexual contact.

- Be able to articulate the public health advantages of treating bacterial STIs to reduce HIV transfer.

- Describe the primary principles that make social science–based intervention programs effective against the sexual transfer of HIV.

- Appreciate the value of stable housing for PLWH to the population-level control of HIV transfer.

- Understand the principles and practice of HIV prevention case management and harm reduction.

- Comprehend the delicate balance of power between HIV and humans.

Understanding the Science and Practice of Public Health, First Edition. Richard Crosby.
© 2023 John Wiley & Sons, Inc. Published 2023 by John Wiley & Sons, Inc.

grounded in the realities of our world: realities that, for now, preclude solving the crisis by addressing its true causes.

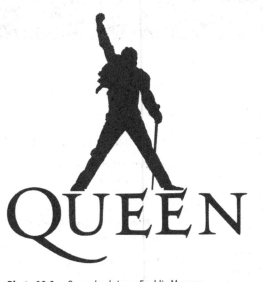

Photo 10.1   Queen lead singer Freddie Mercury.
Source: rayyan/Adobe stock.

Unlike so many hundreds of chapters about HIV/AIDS that scholars have written for college students, this chapter will not focus on the history, biology, or disease process involved with this ongoing U.S. epidemic. Resolving the epidemic is urgent and requires all of us (meaning all citizens living in the United States) to have a shared understanding of the best possible solutions to ending the epidemic (at least in the United States). Hence, this chapter is devoted to the population-level prevention of HIV: the virus that, left untreated, eventually leads to a state of immune decline classified as AIDS, with death from a host of possible diseases following that stage of infection. Before the advent of effective medication to slow viral replication, it was common for people to discover that a friend or family member was just diagnosed with HIV (or, in its advanced stages, AIDS) and for this news to be followed by learning that any of several diseases were present and eventually that the person had died. There was a time when **people living with HIV** (PLWH) did not expect (or even desire) to "live forever" (including Queen idol Freddie Mercury).

Fortunately (at least for now), the virus has been highly responsive to medication regimes that control (but do not cure) what is known as the **HIV viral load**. Although the medical world often "celebrates" this achievement, it is very much the case that this medical approach to resolving the epidemic has exacerbated health disparities between races and economic classes. This occurs due to what can be described as "holes" in the healthcare system that either keep people from entering HIV treatment in the first place or allow them to easily drop out of care.

The medical and pharmaceutical professions have also created various versions of a prophylactic medication known as **PrEP** (pre-exposure prophylaxis). The term **prophylactic** means that the strategy is preventive in nature. Thus, PrEP is unique in the medical and pharmaceutical world because it is used only for perfectly healthy people. This too (like the medications that lower viral load) leads to health disparities due to holes in the healthcare system.

To be fair to the medical and pharmaceutical professions, the holes in the healthcare system are not the only reasons these two drug-based approaches to ending the epidemic create large disparities. An equally important reason involves a lack of investment in the underlying and supportive social structures. For instance, making people at high-risk f HIV acquisition aware of PrEP is typically the domain of clinicians rather than social workers, community health workers, or educators. This general lack of awareness, combined with a lack of a **medical home** (a term used to denote a primary source of medical care for a given person), equates to a bias for PrEP use and PrEP-related care (which must be ongoing) that favors people with at least modest incomes and stable housing and who are not marginalized from a mainstream society based on race, ethnicity, sexual orientation, or gender expression. Sadly, these very types of marginalization typically lead people into social environments and sexual milieus that spawn greater levels of HIV risk behavior. In other words, PrEP may be used mostly by the people who need it the least.

PrEP may be used mostly by the people who need it the least

To date, the United States has yet to put its full weight into a true public health approach to ending HIV/AIDS. After this chapter reviews highlights of the medical approach, it will then focus solely on a public health approach. Specifically, the chapter will teach you about the use of four additional HIV prevention strategies that follow a public health approach (i.e., these are population-based approaches): 1) widespread treatment of bacterial sexually transmitted infections (STIs) as a method of removing these catalysts to HIV transfer from person to person during sex; 2) social science–based intervention programs that promote the consistent and correct use of latex condoms among persons at risk of **HIV acquisition**, as well those living with HIV who are therefore at risk of transmitting HIV; 3) providing stable housing for persons at risk of transmitting HIV; and 4) using intensive case-management practices for persons at risk of transmitting HIV.

As you study this chapter, it will be valuable for you to know that the very long time (measured in years or even decades) that **people living with HIV** (PLWH) can appear and function as being perfectly healthy has given the virus a tremendous advantage in its fight for person-to-person propagation. Indeed, it is useful to think of a virus such as HIV as a type of evolving entity – like all things, its goal is survival, which occurs as a consequence of successful propagation. Humans are also constantly engaged in a quest for survival. Thus, humans are constantly reacting to HIV such that its propagation can be halted. This all means that a great portion of the human effort (i.e., the public health response to HIV/AIDS) must be focused on PLWH. For example, if every single person PLWH posed no risk of propagating the virus, HIV/AIDS would soon end. Of course, this gross oversimplification is not grounded in the basic realities that constantly give HIV advantages over humans. While this chapter summarizes these realities, it also instructs you on how a public health approach can and should be tightly focused on PLWH. The idea of population-level protection achieved through person-level intervention is not unique to public health practice; however, your first introduction to the principles involved here will be in this one chapter of the textbook.

Finally, this chapter also provides a somewhat sobering vision of HIV/AIDS as it exists globally. This is vital to understand because all pathogens (especially HIV) "enjoy" residing for long periods in humans, as doing so provides them with ample opportunities to improve themselves. For a virus to improve in its quest for survival against the preventive measures of humans, it must constantly evolve via mutation. As the global HIV/AIDS pandemic rages (and may be exacerbated by the COVID-19 pandemic), some of these mutations will inevitably produce variants of HIV that are less responsive (or not at all responsive) to the current formulations of HIV medications. That occurrence will greatly alter the balance of power between HIV and humans, with the balance favoring the virus. The time to proactively plan for this inevitable occurrence is now.

> For a virus to improve in its quest for survival against the preventive measures of humans, it must constantly evolve via mutation.

Fundamental Aspects and Terminology of the Disease Process for HIV

First, be very sure you understand that HIV is the name of the virus and AIDS is the name of the syndrome. A **syndrome** is a collection of bodily issues that share a single cause. In the case of HIV, the syndrome is a severe loss of immune function (hence the name **Acquired Immunodeficiency Syndrome** – AIDS). Owing to the incredible resilience of the human body, the loss of immune function may not cross the threshold to severity for 3 to 30 years after a person is infected with HIV (the average for an untreated person is about 10 years). Once this threshold is crossed, a person is said to have AIDS; prior to AIDS, but after infection, the person is said to be living with HIV.

To be very clear about the syndrome, you must understand that a person does not die from AIDS. Although this seems confusing, it is more accurate to think about the syndrome as leading to multiple causes of death that would not normally occur if the person did not have AIDS. These multiple causes are known as **opportunistic illnesses**. The term **opportunistic** is informative because the illnesses take advantage of a greatly weakened immune system to thrive in a person with very few defenses. **Table 10.1** provides examples of CDC-classified opportunistic illnesses.

Table 10.1   Selected opportunistic illnesses that may lead to death

Disease	Brief explanation
Invasive cervical cancer	If not treated early, spreads to nearby organs
Cryptococcosis	A potentially fatal infection of the lungs
Cryptosporidiosis	A bacterial infection leading to chronic diarrhea/dehydration
Encephalopathy	Inflammation (swelling) of brain tissue
Histoplasmosis	An often fatal lung infection
Kaposi's sarcoma	An often fatal form of systemic cancer
Tuberculosis	A bacterial infection in the lungs that can spread to the body
Lymphoma	A cancer that destroys lymphocytes (a key part of immunity)
Mycobacterium avium	A bacterial infection in the lungs that can spread to the body
Pneumocystis pneumonia	A typically fatal condition of fluid filling the lungs
AIDS wasting syndrome	Chronic diarrheal disease leading to dramatic weight loss

Source: Adapted from Centers for Disease Control and Prevention.

The opportunistic infections displayed in **Table 10.1** are quite common globally. In the United States, however, they are increasingly rare because of the advances in treating HIV with **highly active antiretroviral therapy** (HAART). HAART is especially effective when it is started immediately after HIV infection occurs (this is one reason a public health focus on screening at-risk populations for HIV is so important). Beyond averting the onset of opportunistic illnesses, the primary goal of treating PLWH with HAART is twofold. First, from a medical perspective, the goal is to keep the person's total level of HIV in the body as low as possible – this is known as a **suppressed viral load**. Second, from a public health perspective, the goal is to keep everyone living with HIV virally suppressed to create a very low level of what is known as **community viral load**. Community viral load matters most in public health practice because this is the best predictor of how quickly (or slowly) HIV can be transferred through a geographically defined population of at-risk people. Much like COVID-19 (see **Chapter** 1), this principle is simply a matter of the odds/chance that any one person will encounter and then have the contact needed with an infected person for the virus to move from one host to the next. PLWH with very low viral loads are unlikely to transmit their infection to sex partners. Therefore, in a city (for instance) with an extremely successful public health program that keeps community viral load at extremely low levels, the odds of acquiring HIV from an HIV-infected sex partner are very small compared to an HIV-infected sex partner living in a city that has high levels of community viral load.

One last category of terms will be important for you to understand before reading the rest of this chapter. These terms revolve around the concept of HIV testing. HIV acquisition cannot be determined until the newly infected person develops antibodies to the HIV antigen (this is known as **seroconversion**). Seroconversion takes place on average two to six weeks after the virus enters the body. Because most HIV screening tests are designed to detect antibodies, these assays do not provide useful information until seroconversion occurs. However, a new method of testing for HIV detects a combination of HIV antibodies and the HIV antigen, thus making it possible to detect HIV acquisition in as little as two weeks after infection. Thus, a window of time exists between the suspected day of exposure to HIV and the time at which a negative result on a screening test can be trusted, with that **window period** being from about two weeks to two months. It is also important to understand that a positive test result is referred to as being **reactive** (meaning the assay indicates the presence of antibodies to HIV). Reactive results form the basis for more advanced methods known as **confirmatory** testing.

As a final note, in terms of HIV testing and seroconversion, a person newly infected with HIV typically will experience symptoms. This occurs when a person develops antibodies to HIV (i.e., during seroconversion). The symptoms are actually a physical response (think of them as side effects) to the newly activated immunity. This phase is known as **acute infection** – it is not yet AIDS.

Finally, it is far more appropriate to think about the behaviors that efficiently transfer HIV from person to person, rather than relying on labels such as gay, bisexual, drug users, prostitutes, etc. The virus spreads most readily when at least some blood-laden or otherwise compromised tissue is involved. Because rectal tissue is far less resistant to abrasions than vaginal tissue, the most common behavior for HIV acquisition is being the receptive partner (i.e., a "bottom partner") in anal sex; this is known as **receptive anal sex**. Although the **insertive partner** (i.e., a "top partner") may acquire HIV from an HIV-infected receptive partner, the deposit and pooling of ejaculated semen place receptive partners at much greater risk. This same principle applies to females having **penile-vaginal sex** with males – the pooling of ejaculated semen poses a prolonged exposure to the female as opposed to the male's transient exposure to her vaginal secretions (which may include blood from menses). Thus, in terms of sexual behaviors, the most common modes of transmission are receptive anal sex, insertive anal sex, and penile-vaginal sex for females, followed by penile-vaginal sex for males. Oral-genital sex is not a likely method of HIV transfer. Direct blood-to-blood transfer is also common among people who inject drugs with shared needles/syringes (see **Chapter** 9).

> The virus spreads most readily when at least some blood-laden or otherwise compromised tissue is involved

The Medical Approach to HIV/AIDS

American folklore, advertising, and even art often portray the physician-patient relationship as being a safe and comfortable haven for people who are sick or struggling with illness. The idea that medical doctors and the pills they give can cure all forms of disease is an alluring myth. The term **myth** is applicable here because of the growing number of diseases (many of which were unknown until the 1980s) that are simply not amenable to a reliable cure or may not be curable. HIV is indeed a viral infection that has yet to become listed as having a vaccine or a cure. The best medical defense against HIV becoming AIDS involves keeping the reproductive rate of the virus at an extremely low level.

The Continuum of Care as Related to HIV

As previously described in this chapter, at a population level, a primary goal of widespread HAART use is to decrease the amount of viral replication occurring in PLWH, thereby leading to a decline in community viral load. In turn, low levels of community viral load offer passive protection against HIV acquisition as the odds of the virus being transferred from person to person drop dramatically. The public health mission to create widespread initiatives that lower community viral load is known as **Treatment as Prevention** (TasP).

Although TasP is a viable solution to resolving the HIV crisis in the United States, its actual implementation has been far less than ideal. To understand this, it is first imperative that you learn about what is known as the **continuum of care**. **Figure 10.1** displays this continuum in visual form. Although the percentages in this figure are subject to fluctuations from year to year, the figure is instructive because it clearly portrays a cascading effect: that is, as the continuum progresses from left to right, you can see that the percentages drop somewhat dramatically at each successive step. To provide some added context and emphasis to each step, think of the entire process as being analogous to a person starting a new, long-term job. Using this metaphor, whether this person qualifies for the job is based on whether they have a confirmed

> low levels of community viral load offer passive protection against HIV acquisition

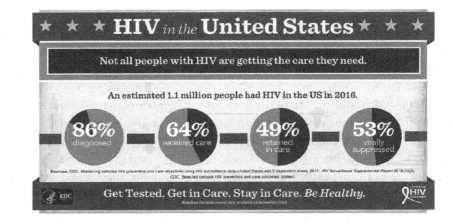

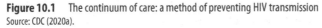

Figure 10.1   The continuum of care: a method of preventing HIV transmission
Source: CDC (2020a).

HIV-positive test result. This first step sounds very simple in words; but in practice, testing those most at risk and thus most likely to be HIV-infected is far from easy. This is why the CDC has estimated that about 15% of the PLWH in the United States are unaware of their infection. Because these people are very likely spreading the virus (albeit unknowingly), this is an extremely high proportion.

Moving to the next step in **Figure 10.1** and sticking with the job metaphor, once a person qualifies for a job, he/she is then formally enrolled as an employee. In the case of the continuum of care, the counterpart to enrollment is becoming an established patient of a clinic that will become the primary medical home for the person's ongoing and lifelong treatment with antiretroviral medications. This second step, known as **linkage to care**, requires the following:

* A trust relationship on the part of PLWH
* Ability of the clinic to accommodate people without health insurance
* Ability of patients to attend the clinic during its open hours
* A stable patient-provider relationship for each patient
* The support of clinic staff in helping new patients navigate the complex paperwork involved in HIV care

As you can easily imagine, many people who test positive for HIV fall through the cracks of the medical system and thus are not successfully linked to the ongoing care and regimes of antiretrovirals needed to better serve the goals of TasP. Again, barring complete abstinence from sex and shared needle/syringe use, the people dropping out of the continuum at the second step become sources of HIV transmission to others.

Moving to the third step, this is where the job metaphor can really help you understand the challenges. Most people are eager to begin a new job. They may make great plans for the money they expect to earn, move closer to the workplace, make friends on the job, etc. The real challenge, however, is staying with the job with each passing month and year while continuing to serve the role that was part of the initial job offer. The same applies to HIV care. Successful treatment implies taking daily medications (as directed), routine return visits to the clinic for monitoring, STI testing, and assessment of current viral load. While this may at first be an easy task, as time goes by, some patients miss taking days of medication and fail to attend routinely scheduled appointments. They may even drop out of care entirely. Similar to quitting a job, those who drop out of care may never be heard from again. This quitting, of course, allows for increased viral replication and thus adds to the total volume of community viral load. This third step determines whether the fourth step is achieved.

people dropping out of the continuum at the second step become sources of HIV transmission to others

The fourth step – optimal viral suppression – forms the ideal in TasP. Ideally, if every person living with HIV was diagnosed, linked to care, and retained in care, community viral loads would be universally minuscule, thereby dramatically reducing the odds of HIV transfer from person to person. But this ideal (as shown in **Figure 10.1**) is far from becoming a reality.

The CDC has established goals that are believed to be possible and would come very close to creating the low levels of community viral load needed to bring an end to new cases of HIV in the United States. The goals are to diagnose at least 90% of all people infected and link at least 85% of those people to care. The goal for those linked to care is to achieve optimal viral suppression in at least 80%. Whether these goals are reached is, naturally, a function of greatly expanded and revised efforts undertaken jointly by outreach workers (a key part of any public health program) and skilled HIV care providers.

Before moving into the next section of this chapter, one vital point about the HIV continuum of care must be clearly understood: minority members do not fare as well as whites across the continuum. For instance, a comprehensive study (Rosenberg, Millett, Sullivan, del Rio, & Curran, 2014) of differences in the HIV care continuum between Black men who have sex with men (MSM) and white MSM found that

- Although 84% of white MSM living with HIV were estimated to be diagnosed, this value dropped to only 75% among black MSM.

- Retention in care was low for white MSM (51%) but even lower for black MSM (33%).

- Viral suppression was more than twice as likely for white MSM (34%) compared to black MSM (16%).

This stark contrast between Black and white MSM is a poignant example of what so often plagues public health practice: health disparities that place racial and ethnic minorities at much greater risk of morbidity and mortality than their white counterparts. In this example, all the men were sexual minorities (i.e., gay, bisexual, or simply having sex with other males); but within that minority status, pronounced racial disparities were observed. A take-home point here is that TasP-related medical interventions, and public health interventions, must strive to eliminate all forms of disparity to ultimately make TasP an effective public health response to the HIV/AIDS crisis.

TasP-related medical interventions, and public health interventions, must strive to eliminate all forms of disparity

A Medical Form of HIV Prevention

As noted in the overview of this chapter, PrEP is a medical approach to resolving the HIV crisis. Using two of the three drugs comprising the antiretroviral therapy given to PLWH, PrEP works by blocking the ability of HIV to replicate once it does enter the body. Although this protective effect is remarkable, the underlying theme of this drug is somewhat of an anomaly because it is being used by people who are essentially healthy. Much like hormonal contraception, PrEP can be taken daily or delivered by periodic injections into muscle tissue. Unlike hormonal contraception, however, its use is predominately among males – a population that has not traditionally become accustomed to taking medications on a preventive basis. Thus, the challenge with PrEP has been less about its mechanism of action in the body than about the very basic issue of **adherence**.

Like the adherence issues for PLWH, PrEP presents similar issues to public health practice. Further, the same level of disparities previously noted for the continuum of care also exists relative to using PrEP. For instance, an Atlanta-based study compared the **PrEP cascade** (i.e., points in a continuum of PrEP-based HIV prevention where people drop out of care) between Black MSM and white MSM (Kelley, Kahle, & Sanchez, 2015). This study assessed men's responses to survey questions about PrEP. Of 260 Black MSM surveyed, 50% were sexually at risk of HIV acquisition. Of these men, 130 (50%) were unaware of PrEP as a prevention option. Of the 130 who were aware of PrEP, 99 (76%) believed they could access PrEP through a clinic. Of these 99, 63 (64%) indicated that they would begin to use PrEP. Of these 63, however, only 32 (51%) indicated that they would most likely adhere to PrEP over time. Thus, starting with the 130 who were at least aware of PrEP as a prevention option, the overall percentage of Black MSM who indicated they would most likely adhere to its use was less than 25%. In contrast, this value was 36% for the white MSM surveyed. So, again, it is the case that medical approaches tend to spawn health disparities. Resolving these disparities is a vital challenge to HIV prevention efforts as the United States continues to advance PrEP as a frontline solution to the HIV crisis.

Considering now both the continuum of care for PLWH and the PrEP cascade, it is clear that a key public health challenge lies in rectifying what has become a predictable pattern of people dropping out of care. In essence, people are not simply "on PrEP" or "on ART"; instead, they cycle in and out of care, and even those remaining in care may not be taking their medications (Rebeiro, Althoff, & Buchacz, 2013). The public health response to this problem includes the use of peer outreach workers, also known as community health workers. As accepted members of the same community they serve, these workers may effectively reach PLWH or people high at risk of HIV acquisition to help promote adherence to medications and provide basic services, such as quarterly testing for **sexually transmitted infections** (STIs) and condom use education (both of these services are recommended for people taking HIV-related medications).

> The public health response to this problem includes the use of peer outreach workers, also known as community health workers

Again, with PrEP becoming a type of medical prevention, a public health lesson learned from this novel approach involves a tremendous increase in the STIs occurring annually in the United States. **Figure 10.2** shows a CDC infographic that portrays the recent dramatic rise in U.S. rates of STIs. Although PrEP use is not the only likely cause of these dramatic increases in STIs, it is nonetheless one cause that can be addressed by improved public health practice.

The most likely reason for the surge in STIs occurring in conjunction with the widespread use of PrEP as an HIV prevention strategy involves a phenomenon known as **risk compensation** (which broadly applies to a host of health behaviors). This phenomenon occurs when perceived protection from one prevention method (such as PrEP) precludes or reduces the use of a second method (such as condoms). From a behavioral perspective, it is easy enough to imagine that a person taking a regime of prophylactic medication, along with the extensive clinical care involved in PrEP use, would feel empowered to then have sex unhampered by the use of condoms. From a public health perspective, it is plausible that many people taking PrEP occupy fairly central positions in their sexual networks (sexual networks are the defining function of how quickly and intensely STIs spread). Given risk compensation in the form of trading PrEP use for the past behavior of condom use, it is therefore possible that people taking PrEP who are centrally located in a sexual network may acquire and then repeatedly transmit STIs to others in the network. Thus, PrEP may serve as an amplification system that expands network-based rates of new STIs. This is precisely why the CDC recommends that all PrEP-related care be provided along with behavioral interventions designed to promote the simultaneous use of condoms and PrEP. This is known as **dual use**. However, this model of dual use has been a difficult sell for people going through the medical system to take PrEP – a medication regime frequently perceived to be an alternative to condoms.

> PrEP may serve as an amplification system that expands network-based rates of new STIs

Despite its medical appeal, PrEP has not been thoroughly embraced by populations at risk of HIV acquisition. Condom use has saved millions of people from HIV acquisition, and many recognize the value of making this their primary method of preventing infection. The effectiveness ratings of PrEP for typical use (meaning people are not always fully adherent) are about the same as the effectiveness ratings of condoms (Crosby, 2017) Clearly, not all people at

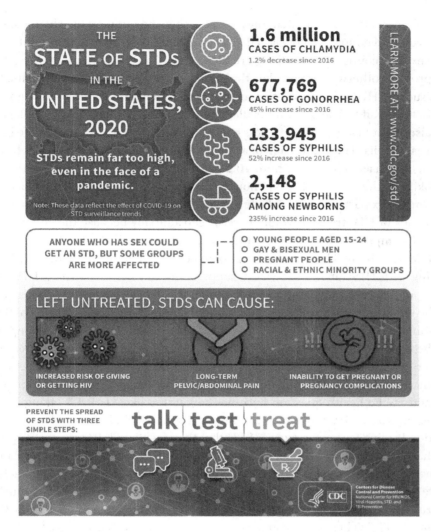

Figure 10.2 Increasing STI rates in the United States
Source: CDC (2020b).

risk of HIV acquisition desire to be on PrEP. Thus, public health has an important obligation to offer and encourage the more affordable and non-medical prevention option of consistent and correct condom use.

Clearly, not all people at risk of HIV acquisition desire to be on PrEP

What Is Biological Synergy with Respect to HIV Transfer?

In the previous section, you learned about the dual use of PrEP and condoms to efficiently respond to the growing public health crisis of STIs. At this juncture in the chapter, let's consider the relationship of STIs to HIV transfer. Again, as a reminder, the term **HIV transfer** is used to represent both HIV acquisition (i.e., a person becoming infected) and HIV transmission (i.e., infected people spreading HIV to others). So, the question is how HIV transfer is biologically changed by the presence of STIs. The answer to this question brings us to the concept of **biological synergy**. The concept is simply that HIV attaches to cells that are part of the body's reaction to invading microorganisms. Thus a rather common STI, such as the bacterial infection known as chlamydia, rallies an immune response by the same cells that have an affinity for HIV. For example, a person with an active chlamydia infection of the cervix has a dramatically greater risk of HIV acquisition through penile-vaginal sex with an HIV-infected

HIV attaches to cells that are part of the body's reaction to invading microorganisms

male who does not use a condom than they would if they did not have the chlamydia infection. Both chlamydia and gonorrhea are classified as **non-ulcerative STIs** that facilitate HIV transfer during sex. The counterparts to these are **ulcerative STIs**. As the term implies, these infections compromise otherwise intact skin that would normally be protective against invading pathogens such as HIV. The most common of these is genital herpes (a lifelong infection in about 25 to 30% of all U.S. adults). In its ulcerative stage, a seeping fluid is visible, emanating from the raised pustules. Although far less common than herpes, a good example involves the STI known as syphilis. The telltale sign of a new syphilis infection is the mark left by the invading bacteria, known as a **chancre**. **Photo 10.2** gives you an excellent example of this ulcerative sore. In looking at the photo, it is easy enough to understand that if this man placed his penis in contact with a sex partner's HIV-infected fluids (e.g., semen, fecal fluids, vaginal secretions, blood), the odds of HIV transfer would increase substantially because the chancre creates an open area of comprised skin that provides easy entry for HIV into the previously HIV-uninfected person's body. This entire scenario can be flipped in that if the man with chancre is already living with HIV (and is not virally suppressed) and has sex with an HIV-uninfected person, the odds of HIV transfer increase based on the ease with which blood (a good transmitter of the virus) can pass from the chancre into the mouth, rectum, or vagina of the partner.

Photo 10.2   This is a photo of a chancre caused by syphilis, located on the head of a penis. Source: CDC (2016).

Depending on whether the STI is non-ulcerative or ulcerative, and depending on the extent of the immune response to the STI, the synergy part comes down to increased odds of HIV transfer ranging from a risk 5 times greater to as much as 20 times greater. As you might imagine, since PrEP is a cause of nationwide, record-breaking increases in annual STI incidence, a valid public health question becomes something like, "Is PrEP taking us two steps forward (i.e., improved HIV prevention for those most at risk) and one step backward (i.e., risk compensation leading to greater rates of STIs that then facilitate HIV transfer)?"

Now that you have a basic understanding of biological synergy, this chapter can take you from the medical-level approach to HIV prevention into a population-level approach. The differences are not always distinct, with the medical and population levels sharing much in common. **Figure 10.3** provides you with a grand overview of both approaches. Notice that the figure shows "Control STIs" as being in a shared space between the two approaches. So, this raises the natural question of how STI control is applied to HIV prevention at the population level.

Long before TasP and PrEP became terms used in public health practice, global efforts to prevent HIV focused on massive (i.e., population-level) "test and treat" campaigns. The "test" was simply screening people in clinics and community settings. The "treat" was the immediate provision of antibiotics to cure chlamydia and/or gonorrhea among those screening positive

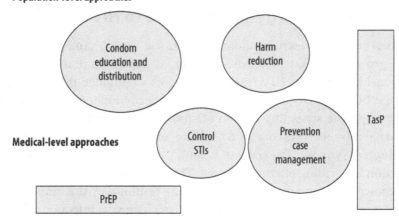

Figure 10.3   An overview of two complementary approaches to HIV prevention

(or those with clearly visible clinical signs). From an initial study of two African nations, epidemiologists were able to speculate that the massive test-and-treat programs did contribute to HIV prevention, but only when the population prevalence of STIs was relatively low (i.e., test-and-treat programs do not appear effective for HIV prevention in nations with ongoing high levels of STI prevalence) (Grosskurth, Gray, Hayes, Mabey, & Wawer, 2000). Fortunately for the United States, even with the recent increase in STIs, our nation still has a relatively low overall prevalence. Therefore, intensified efforts to test and treat can be a productive HIV prevention strategy.

Applying Social Science to HIV Intervention

Look at the upper-left area in **Figure 10.3**: you'll find that condom use education and distribution programs are considered population-level approaches. In this regard, these types of programs can be highly effective, especially when they are guided by the application of evidence-based practices developed and refined within the social sciences. By virtue of their roots in social science, these programs are typically tailored and therefore capable of serving vastly different needs of people at risk of HIV acquisition or HIV transmission.

Rather than review the hundreds of programs successfully applied to the promotion of condom use for HIV prevention, a better use of your time here will be learning about the principles (e.g., theories, models, and practices) that are foundational to all of the programs. Perhaps the best example is a behavioral theory (more appropriately referred to as a model – the term **model** is used when theories have been combined) that was specifically designed in response to HIV/AIDS. Known as the **information-motivation-behavioral skills** (IMB) model, this set of principles has been successfully applied to HIV prevention efforts since the 1990s. As implied by its name, IMB focuses on three targets of change:

* Providing HIV-prevention-relevant **information**

* Encouraging beliefs about positive outcomes when adopting HIV protective behaviors (thus enhancing **motivation**)

* Teaching a combination of task-specific self-confidence and skills needed to adopt and maintain HIV protective behaviors, such as the correct and consistent use of condoms

The IMB model is foundational to condom education and distribution programs. The model specifies the somewhat limited value of information and the potential value of enhancing the anticipated positive outcomes of a behavior (e.g., condom use with a hook-up sex partner). More importantly, IMB is designed to show that information and motivation each have an effect through the conduit of behavioral skills. The skills aspect of the model is the most critical and the most broadly defined. For instance, the skills needed to adopt and maintain the use of condoms against HIV transfer include

The skills aspect of the model is the most critical and the most broadly defined

* Being able to reliably obtain good-fitting condoms that fit the user and feel satisfactory for both sex partners

* Being able to reliably obtain water-based or silicone-based lubricants that can be added to the exterior of a condom after it is applied to the penis

* Having the self-regulatory skills to always use condoms from the start to the end of any one sexual act

* Having the confidence and the corresponding ability to discuss and negotiate condom use with sex partners who are reticent about their use

* Being able to apply and use condoms (to the self or a sex partner) regardless of being drunk or high

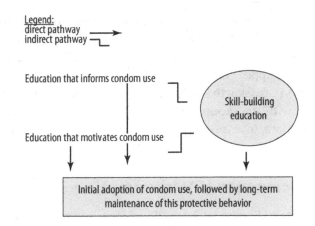

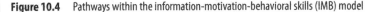

Figure 10.4   Pathways within the information-motivation-behavioral skills (IMB) model

So, now that you understand the broad-based nature of this third principle in the model, let's take a close look at the pathways within the IMB model shown in **Figure 10.4**. As you can see, information and motivation are separate and conceived of as equal in the model. Each of these aspects of a condom promotion program will most likely directly influence the ultimate outcome of condom use to prevent HIV transfer. Further, each of these aspects will have an indirect effect that primes people to acquire the requisite skills to become dedicated condom users. In turn, the skills-based aspect will directly affect the outcome of condom use.

To help better understand how the IMB model has been applied to promoting population-level increases in condom use, **Box 10.1** provides a summary of a social science-based program designed to protect young Black males against HIV transfer.

BOX 10.1. EXAMPLE OF AN EDUCATION- AND DISTRIBUTION-BASED HIV INTERVENTION PROGRAM

Focus on the Future (FOF) is a peer-delivered, clinic-based, single-session, individual-level behavioral intervention. **FOF** aims to educate and motivate clients to use condoms correctly and consistently in order to reduce the spread of HIV and other STDs.

FOF is based on the Information, Motivation, and Behavioral Skills (IMB) model, which states that people need information, motivation, and practice with a behavior in order to properly learn that behavior. It is also based on Bandura's Social Learning Theory, which states that people learn new behaviors through observational learning, imitation, and modeling.

Target Population: African American men, who have sex with women (MSW), ages 18-29 who are seeking care in an STD clinic due to reported symptoms of an STD or who have received an STD diagnosis, who have used a condom in the last three months, and who are not knowingly HIV-positive.

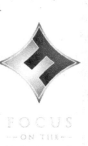

Because of its focus on promoting consistent and correct condom use and its adherence to the IMB model, this program is an example of an education-based method of HIV prevention. Further, because the program also provides (at no cost) an ongoing supply (based on a broad selection) of condoms and single-use vials of lubricants, it is also a form of condom distribution. As the social sciences increasingly inform public health practice, it has become clear that education alone is not enough – solid connections must be made between the target population and the recommended services or products (in this case, condoms and lubricants).

As the social sciences increasingly inform public health practice, it has become clear that education alone is not enough

Distinct from a medical approach, a defining characteristic of an education-based approach is that it is provided in community settings, schools, and even the context of online intervention efforts. A second defining characteristic is that such programs are adaptable to a wide variety of populations. Populations, in the case of HIV prevention, may be defined by serostatus (i.e., whether they are currently living with HIV), race, ethnicity, economic marginalization, and social marginalization. Again, as an example, the original application of **Focus on the Future** (see **Box 10.1**) was for young Black men having sex with women; a subsequently published version was adapted for use with two populations of young Black MSM: those who knew they were living with HIV, and those who recently tested non-reactive to HIV. The findings suggest a protective effect of the brief (1 hour) counseling-based condom education program, which included the provision of free condoms and lubricants (Crosby, Mena, Salazar, Hardin, Brown, & Vickers-Smith, 2018). Among HIV-infected MSM, the findings showed that those receiving this intervention were 64% more likely than those not receiving it to report the consistent use of latex condoms during anal receptive sex over a subsequent period of 12 months. Among HIV-uninfected MSM, the findings showed that those receiving this intervention were more than twice as likely than those not receiving it to report the consistent use of latex condoms during anal receptive sex over the next 12 months.

As an ongoing service to public health practice, the CDC has created, maintained, and regularly updated a collection of effective HIV prevention intervention programs. This collection is known as the **Compendium of Effective HIV Prevention Programs** and is coordinated through the CDC's **Prevention Research Synthesis** Project. **Photo 10.3** is a screenshot of the 2022 search page that can be easily used to locate information about population-specific options for HIV prevention programs.

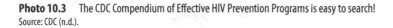

Photo 10.3   The CDC Compendium of Effective HIV Prevention Programs is easy to search!
Source: CDC (n.d.).

As the HIV epidemic continues in the United States, the public health approach to prevention must also evolve. At this juncture in learning about programs to promote condom use, it is important to understand that the average age of HIV acquisition is steadily declining. This, of course, means that progressively greater proportions of teens and persons in their early 20s are now PLWH. Because STIs are rampant in these age groups (about two-thirds of all STIs are diagnosed in people under the age of 25), and based on a need to avert unintended pregnancies, condom use is an especially valuable tool for public health practice. Conversely, thousands of U.S. school districts and even entire states actively discourage condom education programs and condom distribution programs. This clash between politics and public health is not new; however, its lack of resolution in favor of HIV prevention has been elusive.

For political factions that disfavor condom use education and distribution, an easy alternative is to simply turn the control of the U.S. epidemic over to the medical approaches (i.e., PrEP and TasP). However, this abdication of public responsibility is costly when we consider, for example, that the price of keeping one person on PrEP for one year is about $20,000. In contrast, even the most specialized condom brands (such as Trojan's Magnum Gold) can be purchased in bulk for less than $1 each. The obvious question that applies here is, when will the U.S. public health system stand up to conservative factions that have not been supportive of a condom-based public health response to one of the most devastating and socially inequitable diseases of our time? To get a sense of the beliefs and misconceptions that form the mindset of these conservative factions, read **Box 10.2**.

when will the U.S. public health system stand up to conservative factions that have not been supportive of a condom-based public health response

BOX 10.2. A UNIVERSITY REVIEW BOARD REARS ITS CONSERVATIVE HEAD ABOUT CONDOMS

This story is based on my own experience (i.e., the author of this textbook) when I first began receiving grant support from the National Institutes of Health to conduct trials of condom-based HIV prevention programs in the United States. In 2004, I was planning a recruitment strategy for use in the only publicly funded STI clinic in Louisville, KY. An in-house agency (one that was part of the University of Kentucky – my place of employment as a professor of public health) charged the grant approximately $5,000 to create a clever recruitment poster (see **Photo 10.4**).

As a matter of protocol and ethics, all university-based studies must undergo an ethics review by an accredited board (known as an **internal review board**). As part of this review, the board obtained the recruitment poster and included it in their ethics considerations. A scathing letter from the chairperson of that board informed me that the poster "suggests fornication" and that people would be offended by its imagery. The letter also stated that a revised poster would remove the two cars and only show condoms inside their packaging (i.e., the board found the images of condoms taken out of their packaging to also be offensive). Despite my written appeal stating that the poster was only to be used within the waiting room of an STI clinic, the board would not reverse their edit. Therefore, this $5,000 poster was never used for its intended purpose of study recruitment.

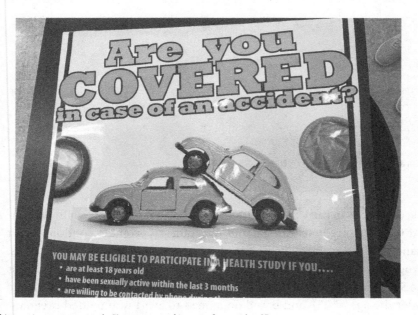

Photo 10.4   This recruitment poster reads, "Are you covered in case of an accident?"

Condom use is only one effective tool that is promoted as part of the effort to control the spread of HIV in a community. Thus, in addition to programs promoting condom use, a second breed of social science approach to HIV prevention is very important. This approach involves the sexual networks of people at risk of HIV transfer. Sexual networks are defined by their density (i.e., the number of people in the network), the existing connections among network members, and the interconnections between two or more sexual networks. Social scientists have developed specialized analytic techniques to better identify and understand the spread of HIV within a network and between two or more networks. The utility of sexual network analysis lies in its ability to predict the spread of HIV through a network once it is first introduced. This ability is a valuable public health tool relative to averting local outbreaks of HIV. Social network analysis also provides the basis for identifying persons who are highly sexually active and living with HIV – thus implying that they play a central role in HIV transfer. Identifying these people –referred to as **core transmitters** – provides an ideal opportunity to apply what is known as **prevention case management**.

> Social scientists have developed specialized analytic techniques to better identify and understand the spread of HIV within a network

What Is Prevention Case Management?

Looking again at **Figure 10.3**, note that prevention case management (PCM) is located partly within the medical approach and partly within a population-level approach. This shared location in the figure shows that PCM is a hybrid design for controlling HIV. It is a generalized approach to helping PLWH stay virally suppressed, avoid risk situations that may lead to unprotected sex or shared use of needles/syringes, and lead safe sex lives with partners who are spouses or considered to be primary partners in their lives.

Rather unique to public health practice, the ongoing nature of HIV is such that the level of threat to the person living with the virus is less than that posed by the significant potential for ongoing transmission to others. Thus, a PCM approach is based entirely on preventing HIV transmission. The goals of PCM are as follows:

- Provide stable housing for PLWH.

- Ensure that PLWH have a secure and trusted "medical home."

- Teach PLWH the skills needed to avoid risk-triggering situations.

- Teach PLWH the skills needed to have enjoyable sex that is fully protected by the correct use of latex condoms.

- Ensure that PLWH are virally suppressed and always adherent to their antiretroviral medications.

- For PLWH who have HIV-uninfected spouses or primary sex partners, PCM services include connecting these sex partners to PrEP-based care and related prevention services (such as condom use education and distribution).

As you study this list of PCM goals, you should already be familiar with most of the terms being used. The one exception is the very first bullet point. The idea of providing people with stable housing as a method of protecting public health is novel to HIV/AIDS. Although this idea may appear costly, a systematic review of evidence strongly supports the contention of the need and benefits associated with stable housing for PLWH (Aidala et al., 2016). The review included evidence from rather simple studies that correlated housing stability with outcomes such as engagement in HIV care. Stability was assessed based on a continuum ranging from complete homelessness to long-term (stable) housing. Engagement in care was also assessed based on a continuum, typically ranging from no care at all, to occasional care and low-level adherence to medication, to various levels of greater attendance to clinics that provide care for HIV and greater levels of adherence and thus viral suppression. These correlational studies robustly indicated the value of stable housing. Even more impressive, the authors also reviewed randomized, controlled trials of housing-based interventions for PLWH and found strong evidence supporting this structural-level intervention. Thus, providing stable housing, or at least some level of financial assistance toward that goal, for PLWH is a potential emergent form of intervention relative to averting 1) HIV transmission, 2) dropping out of the continuum of care by PLWH, and 3) maintaining low levels of community viral load.

Examples of Harm Reduction Applied to HIV/AIDS

Taking one final look at **Figure 10.3**, notice that harm reduction is fully a part of the population-level approach. You should recall learning about harm reduction in **Chapter 9**. In that chapter, harm reduction was relegated to needle and syringe exchange programs. In this chapter, harm reduction also includes needle and syringe exchange programs; however, it extends to a host of other prevention-oriented behaviors. The goal of hard-reduction practices is to mitigate the risk of HIV transfer rather than promote the exclusive ideas of sexual abstinence, complete monogamy, and avoiding sex with high-risk partners (such as PLWH who are not virally suppressed). For example, primary among harm-reduction practices is the goal of reducing the number of new sex partners. For many people in their 20s (or even in their teen years), hook-up sex and other forms of non-relational sex can easily result in having 10 or more different sex partners per year. Rather than judgmentally attempting to "convert" people to long-term monogamy, the harm-reduction approach simply attempts to have people cut back on the number of new sex partners in service of HIV prevention.

Among MSM, a set of somewhat effective harm-reduction practices can be identified. For instance, the practice of **serosorting** is fairly common among MSM. This term implies that both people in any one sex act are either HIV-infected or HIV-uninfected. Given that both people have full and accurate awareness (and disclosure) of whether they are living with HIV, serosorting occurs when two PLWH have sex. It also occurs when two people not living with HIV have sex. In either case, however, the practice of serosorting typically precludes the use of condoms. Thus, serosorting becomes a type of compromise safety measure for people who choose not to use condoms.

> serosorting becomes a type of compromise safety measure for people who choose not to use condoms

A related harm-reduction practice is known as **seropositioning**. The practice, also common among MSM, applies when one sex partner is living with HIV and the other is not infected. Based on the reality that being the receptive partner in anal sex is far more likely to transmit the virus from a "top to a bottom," the goal of seropositioning is to always have the HIV-uninfected person be the insertive sex partner (i.e., the top partner). Estimates of transmission from an HIV-infected insertive partner to an HIV-uninfected receptive partner place this risk at between 5-fold and 10-fold greater compared to the risk posed by an HIV-infected receptive partner to an HIV-uninfected insertive partner.

A Delicate Balance

Now that you have mastered the fundamentals of HIV prevention, it is time to think ahead regarding future threats. These threats all revolve around a single issue: the very likely possibility that predominate strains of HIV will eventually mutate to become partially or fully resistant to antiretroviral therapies. The term **resistance** implies that a given microorganism evolves in a way that allows it to elude the previously destructive effects of medication. In the case of HIV, resistance becomes increasingly likely when

- Persons who are on PREP (but who lack adherence) become infected with HIV

- Infants exposed to in utero antiretroviral medication later become infected through blood-to-blood contact or breastfeeding

- PLWH who drop out of care stop using antiretroviral medications

- PLWH use antiretroviral medications only occasionally

The overarching principle here is that exposure to antiretroviral medication, followed by discontinued use, sets the stage for what is known as **microbial resistance**. This same dynamic is common relative to ordinary infections such as strep throat. The odds are very high that you have been diagnosed with strep throat at least once. Do you remember the doctor, nurse, or pharmacist stressing the importance of taking every pill in the prescription? This instruction is mandatory for people being given antibiotics because the prescribed dose is designed to destroy all invading bacteria. When the dose is cut short (such as when people feel well again and stop taking their medication), the remaining bacteria have a chance to make a comeback. As this occurs, the new generations of bacteria may have the advantage of already outwitting the medications used previously. These "smarter" bacteria then become predominant. Although HIV is a virus rather than a bacteria, this same dynamic of using antiretroviral medication only sporadically or ending its use entirely leads to a smarter version of the virus that can then gain an advantage over its host.

Globally, the balance between HIV and its hosts is precarious. What happens, for instance, when a nation such as Russia invades a neighboring country such as Ukraine? Do you think the PLWH in Ukraine who have been fully adherent to antiretroviral medications manage to stay that way? What happens when a nation alters policies that have the effect of making antiretroviral medications more difficult to afford? Or, what happens when social movements convince followers living with HIV to stop using antiretroviral medications? Most importantly, and as you have already learned in this chapter, what happens when the public health system fails to respond to the challenge posed by PLWH dropping out of the continuum of care? Of course, you know the answers to all of these questions: each scenario will add to the ever-growing problem of resistance to antiretroviral medication.

> what happens when the public health system fails to respond to the challenge posed by PLWH dropping out of the continuum of care?

The often-unspoken threat behind the global HIV pandemic is the question of when (not if) medication resistance will become a reality that quickly drives up the annual rates of new cases. A type of precursor to this is gonorrhea. Currently, the CDC is closely monitoring the ever-growing presence of medication resistance against this bacterial STI. As of the time when this textbook was written, only one class of antibiotics remained effective against gonorrhea (all others had become ineffective due to microbial resistance). A CDC report stated, "Gonorrhea is skilled at outsmarting the antibiotics that are used to kill it" (CDC, 2022). This concept of "outsmarting" is appropriate, given that bacteria are living organisms. In many ways, our entire existence as the human species is a fragile balance, with competition from all other species, especially microorganisms. That balance can easily be disrupted, as has already occurred in the case of gonorrhea. So, one vital question for the future of public health is focused on how humans can avert the otherwise inevitable issue of HIV becoming resistant to the antiretroviral drugs that are so widely touted as a global success against HIV.

Much as with COVID-19 (see **Chapter 1**), it is imperative that you fully appreciate and understand that not all HIV/AIDS-related problems can be addressed by any one nation (including the United States). Microbial resistance that develops in the smallest African nation, for example, can lead to strains of HIV that end up in San Francisco or New York City within weeks or months. We should all be concerned about this rapid movement, which lets a mutated strain of HIV travel around the globe. Unless we as a species can outsmart HIV, current public health hopes of ending HIV will likely be replaced by hopes of simply controlling the rapid

public health practice must always have one eye on the present and the other on the future

growth of the pandemic. The larger take-home point here is that public health practice must always have one eye on the present and the other on the future.

Review and Key Terms

Overall, this chapter provides a roadmap for understanding how public health practice has so far responded to the U.S. epidemic of HIV/AIDS. You have learned about relatively straightforward concepts such as the difference between **HIV acquisition, HIV transmission,** and **HIV transfer**. In learning about the **window period** relative to HIV testing, you gained an understanding of **seroconversion**: a time when the immune system produces **antibodies** to HIV. A person producing these antibodies will have a **reactive** test result when screened for HIV. Reactive test results are a signal for further testing, known as **confirmatory testing**. Although screening is not always linked with possible infection, an event known as an **acute infection** is often taken as a warning sign of possible exposure and thus HIV acquisition.

Even more importantly, you learned about **HIV viral load** and the companion concept of viral suppression from using **HAART** or the lifetime use of **antiretroviral medications**. You also now understand that people with AIDS die of other causes known as **opportunistic illnesses**.

On a positive note, this chapter taught you about the **continuum of care** and its broad purpose of keeping PLWH virally suppressed for a lifetime. Improving the success rates across all four steps in this continuum is a major public health priority. The great advantage is known as **TasP** – a type of medical-based approach to prevention that greatly reduces the odds of HIV transfer. Of course, you also learned that a lack of HIV testing and dropping out of care are primary public health concerns with the idea of HIV prevention via the TasP model. Indeed, lack of **adherence** to medication regimes among PLWH is a problem that requires urgent attention, especially given that this lack of adherence may lead to HIV **medication resistance**. In a related approach, you also learned about **PrEP** and the adherence issues with this medication regime (which is thus yet another source of concern relative to medication resistance). As part of learning about PrEP, you should now understand the concept of **risk compensation**. Applied to "trading in condoms in favor of PrEP," the problem is that PrEP has been partly responsible for record numbers of annual STI cases in the United States.

From a social perspective, you learned that the term **people living with HIV (PLWH)** refers to those who have HIV but are not yet classified as having AIDS, as well as those who are classified as having AIDS. The great advantage of viral suppression is also relevant to a social perspective because a low level of **community viral load** can be highly protective for the people selecting sex partners in that community.

A key part of this chapter involved the concept of **biological synergy**. You learned that both **ulcerative** and **non-ulcerative** STIs facilitate HIV transfer. As a specific example, you learned that the primary symptom of syphilis – known as a **chancre** – acts as an open door to easily allow HIV to pass between sex partners. This synergistic effect of STIs magnifies the odds of HIV transfer from 5-fold to 20-fold greater risk. Mitigating local epidemics of STIs is thus a vital tool of HIV prevention. Unlike PrEP, condom use protects against many more common STIs as well as HIV.

Next, you then learned about the **information-motivation-behavioral skills model**. This model is an example of how behavioral and social science theories guide effective programs designed to promote the consistent and correct use of condoms among people at risk of HIV transfer. In addition to condom use, you were introduced to the social science methodology of **sexual network analysis** and the principle of identifying **core transmitters**. Although not a part of a social science approach, behavioral studies – primarily among MSM – have identified adaptive responses to HIV prevention. The two featured in the chapter are **serosorting** and **seropositioning**. These methods are of far less value than the consistent and correct use of condoms; however, they are of significant protective value when practiced diligently.

In reading this chapter, you should also recall that the practice of prevention case management has both a strong medical approach and a strong set of prevention implications for public health. An emerging practice within this approach involves providing assistance in obtaining stable housing for PLWH. The overarching concept here is that housing forms a basis for avoiding risk behaviors that further transmit the virus and the stability needed to stay fully engaged in the continuum of care.

As the chapter came to a close, you learned to look ahead to the future regarding **microbial resistance** of HIV against the medication used for viral suppression. This part of the chapter may ultimately be the most valuable because of the currently fragile balance between HIV and its human hosts – a balance that can be easily tipped in favor of the virus. This section also taught you to think globally, because medication resistance is a worldwide issue rather than being confined to any one nation. Until all nations can gain improved control over HIV/AIDS, the virus poses an ongoing threat to public health globally and domestically (i.e., the United States is not a privileged pocket of the world).

> Until all nations can gain improved control over HIV/AIDS, the virus poses an ongoing threat to public health globally and domestically

For Practice and Discussion

1. Which one of the following prevention options was developed and is intended primarily for people who are HIV-uninfected but at high risk of HIV acquisition?
   a. PrEP
   b. TasP
   c. The information-motivation-behavioral skills model
   d. HIV testing and counseling

2. The cascade regarding the continuum of care refers to:
   a. The event of seroconversion that happens soon after HIV acquisition
   b. "Falling out" of care, which results in only a small percentage of people having the full benefit of antiretroviral therapies
   c. A lack of medical attention to the condom use needs of PrEP users

3. In regard to PrEP, risk compensation refers to:
   a. People who begin using condoms after they acquire a sexually transmissible infection
   b. People giving up on condom use because they begin PrEP use
   c. The use of condoms in the context of seropositioning
   d. The use of condoms in the context of serosorting

4. In a monogamous male couple where one person is not living with HIV and the other is a PLWH, which sexual behavior of the HIV-uninfected partner is the most likely to lead to HIV transfer?
   a. Receiving oral sex (no condom)
   b. Receiving vaginal sex
   c. Being an insertive partner (top) in anal sex and not using a condom
   d. Being a receptive partner (bottom) in anal sex and not using a condom

5. The United States has experienced record levels of STI incidence in recent years. This may be partly attributable to PrEP.
   a. True
   b. False

6. Lowering community viral load, promoting adherence to ART, and averting the ART cascade are critical to:
   a. The CDC's compendium model of HIV prevention
   b. TasP
   c. Reducing racial and sexual minority HIV disparities
   d. PrEP

7. Which of the following does not apply to the concept of prevention case management?
   a. Counseling for PrEP
   b. Housing assistance
   c. Assistance with low literacy issues
   d. Education and distribution of condoms

8. PrEP is designed to avert the acquisition of HIV from an HIV-infected sex partner, whereas TasP is designed to avert HIV transmission for the person taking it.
   a. True
   b. False

9. Jerri is a male who has a chancre on his penis. He is also living with HIV. To avoid transmitting the virus to his male sex partner while still having a sex life with him, they determine that Jerri should be the bottom partner in anal receptive sex. What level of risk does this pose to his HIV-uninfected partner?
   a. The risk is the highest possible because of syphilis.
   b. As long as Jerri is the receptive partner only, there is no risk to his partner.
   c. This seropositioning only reduces the risk for the partner – risk still exists.

10. A potential harbinger of HIV medication resistance is:
    a. The rapid emergence of drug-resistant gonorrhea
    b. The fact that PrEP use is becoming far less protective than it used to be
    c. The observation that HIV seroconversion is happening before the window period

For Class Discussion

11. Using the CDC's HIV surveillance website, find a graph, table, or chart that you feel most dramatically illustrates the racial/ethnic disparities relative to the annual incidence rate of newly diagnosed HIV infections. Post it electronically so that others taking this course can react and comment.

12. The estimates relative to success rates at each of the four steps in the continuum of care are for the entire U.S. population of PLWH. Using Google Scholar as a search engine, go online to find a journal published within the past three years that provides estimates specific to only one minority population (this includes sexual minorities). Using these four estimates, create a side-by-side visual against the latest all-population estimates published on the CDC's website. What is the main difference, and why do differences exist? (A one-page response would be a great way to stimulate class discussion about health disparities and HIV.)

13. Pretend you are the parent of a 13-year-old. Using at least seven bolded terms from this chapter, what would you want to say about HIV/AIDS to this adolescent? Write this in no more than one page, and compare it to what others in the class wrote for this assignment.

References

Aidala, A., Wilson, M.G., Shubert, V., Gogolishvilli, D., Globerman, J., Rueda, S., & Bozeak, A. K. (2016). Housing status, medical care, and health outcomes among people living with HIV/AIDS: A systematic review. *The American Journal of Public Health, 106,* e1–e23.

CDC (n.d.). Prevention Research Synthesis (PRS) compendium intervention search. https://wwwn.cdc.gov/HIVCompendium/SearchInterventions

CDC (2016). Syphilis images. https://www.cdc.gov/std/syphilis/images.htm

CDC (2020a). HIV continuum of care. https://www.cdc.gov/hiv/policies/continuum.html

CDC (2020b). The state of STDs – infographic. https://www.cdc.gov/std/statistics/2020/infographic.htm

CDC (2021). Living with HIV. https://www.cdc.gov/hiv/basics/livingwithhiv/opportunisticinfections.html

CDC (2022). Gonorrhea. https://www.cdc.gov/std/gonorrhea/arg/basic.htm

Crosby, R. A. (2017) Dealing with pre-exposure prophylaxis-associated condom migration: Changing the paradigm for MSM. *Sexual Health, 14*(1), 106–110.

Crosby, R. A., Mena, L., Salazar, L. F., Hardin, J., Brown, T., & Vickers-Smith, R. (2018). Efficacy of a clinic-based safer sex program for HIV-uninfected and HIV-infected young Black MSM: A randomized controlled trial. *Sexually Transmitted Disease, 45,* 169–176.

Grosskurth, M. H., Gray, R., Hayes, R., Mabey, D., & Wawer, M. (2000). Control of sexually transmitted diseases for HIV-1 prevention: Understanding the Mwanza and Rakai trials. *The Lancet, 355,* 1981–1987.

Kelley, C. F, Kahle, E., & Sanchez, T. (2015). Applying a PrEP continuum of care for men who have sex with men in Atlanta, Georgia. *Clinical Infectious Disease, 61,* 1590–97.

Rebeiro, P., Althoff, KN., & Buchacz, K. (2013). Retention among North American HIV-infected persons in clinical care, 2000–2008. *Journal of the Acquired Immune Deficiency Syndromes, 62*(3), 356–362.

Rosenberg, E. S., Millett, G. A., Sullivan, P. S., de Rio, C., & Curran, J. W. (2014). Understanding the HIV disparities between black and white men who have sex with men in the USA, using the HIV care continuum: A modeling study. *The Lancet HIV, 1*(3), e112–e118.

PREVENTING GUN VIOLENCE AND PROMOTING HIGHWAY SAFETY: A STUDY OF STARK CONTRASTS

> Every country has violent, hateful, or mentally unstable people. What's different is that not every country is awash with easily accessible guns.
>
> —President Barack Obama, https://obamawhitehouse.archives.gov/ blog/2015/06/19/president-obama-addresses-us-conference-mayors

Overview

After reading the first 10 chapters in this textbook, one overarching theme may be apparent to you: that public health interventions are typically most effective when they follow an ecological model of development and implementation. Each of the public health challenges covered in **Chapters 4 through 10** is generally amenable to interventions at the individual level, the peer level, the community level, the level of societal changes, and the very important structural levels of change. Unlike the previous chapters, this chapter will be the first in the book to address two prominent public health challenges using only structural-level changes. The solutions to our national epidemics of gun violence and traffic deaths/injuries stem from policy-level changes rather than relying on interventions based on the behavioral and social sciences. Policy changes, by definition, are structural-level interventions. The eloquence of these interventions is their broad reach and long-term maintenance.

As you study this chapter, please keep in mind the larger mission of public health practice: "creating conditions that control and even reverse the tide and trajectory of any one nation's current epidemics" (see **Chapter 2**). With estimates suggesting that an average of 110 people are killed and another 200 are seriously injured by guns each day, you can quickly grasp the concept of a raging epidemic in America regarding gun violence (Everytown Research & Policy, 2020). Of course, homicide via gun violence is only one dimension of the much larger American problem of gun violence in general. This includes robberies, domestic abuse, suicide, and long-term disabilities that people sustain when surviving gunshot wounds. You may, however, be less inclined to describe a similar epidemic of deaths from driving cars and other on-the-road vehicles. This is because of massive structural-level interventions that have successfully reduced the number of automobile-related accidents in the United States.

LEARNING OBJECTIVES

- Understand the scope and magnitude of morbidity and mortality stemming from gun violence.

- Grasp and appreciate the significance of lost quality of life that results from gunshot injuries (understand QALYs).

- Delineate and describe public health approaches to reducing gun violence.

- Understand that structural-level solutions to the crisis of gun violence have been largely untapped in the United States.

- Explain the trends in deaths and injuries from automobile collisions.

- Describe the structural-level approaches that have been applied to highway safety.

- Describe the structural-level approaches that have been applied to improving the safety of automobiles.

- Compare and contrast the public health approach to preventing gun violence with that for preventing deaths and injuries from automobile collisions.

A strictly structural-level approach is also appropriate to the public health challenge of ending the **epidemic of gun violence**. But due in part to the strength of the American industries that manufacture and sell guns and ammunition, this has yet to occur. Thus, this chapter draws a contrast between the success in controlling the public health problem of traffic fatalities/injuries and the failure to control the growing public health problem of gun violence. The primary case in point is the tight regulation of the auto industry and constantly evolving safety standards used to construct our nation's state and federal highways. Although averting traumatic injuries may lack the heroism inherent in saving lives through improved emergency medical services, it is vital for you to understand that the prevention-based approach greatly adds to what is known in public health practice as **quality-of-life years**. Indeed, this chapter provides you with an introduction to the concept of **quality-adjusted life years (QALYs)**.

As you read this chapter, be aware that the thread weaving the various prevention targets into a coherent whole is the eloquence of **structural-level interventions**. In fact, it is no longer considered competent public health practice to simply rely on information provision as a method to alter the risk factors leading to violence and traumatic injury. The toll of gun violence demands a far more active public health approach – and this is where your citizenship as an American comes into play. Gun violence is always a heated political issue and demands a fully educated electorate (i.e., your generation of new voters) with an in-depth understanding of the issues and how to prevent needless deaths and long-term disabilities caused by guns. The overwhelming racial disparities characterizing gun violence further exacerbate the urgency for this type of public health action. As you should well guess by this point in the book, people of color are most affected by the national epidemic of gun violence; thus, ignoring the issue of gun violence also ignores the glaring issue of racial injustice in the United States.

this chapter draws a contrast between the success in controlling the public health problem of traffic fatalities/injuries and the failure to control the growing public health problem of gun violence

ignoring the issue of gun violence also ignores the glaring issue of racial injustice in the United States.

Gun Violence Is a Pervasive Public Health Problem

Americans seem to love sensationalistic media coverage of events, both good and bad in nature. Tragic events such as mass shootings are a case in point. In 2016, for example, a lone gunman entered an Orlando, Florida nightclub and killed 49 people, wounding another 53. The shooting occurred in the early morning (around 2:00 am.). By daybreak, the story was being broadcast and published throughout the nation – a mournful President Obama expressed anger, outrage, and hope for a time when our nation would take far more active measures to control gun violence. Yet the 59 people who died that day represented only .014% of the annual average death toll (estimated at 40,600 per year) from gun violence in the United States (Everytown Research & Policy, 2020). So, the real news is that most acts of gun violence rarely make the news – they have become an unfortunate part of everyday life in America.

The annual number of homicides from gun violence in America is 26 times greater than in other high-income nations. This uniquely American problem is clearly amplified for Black Americans, who are 10 times more likely to be homicide victims of gun violence than their white counterparts. Sadly, the American problem of gun violence is the leading cause of death for children and teens; again, a pronounced disparity places Black children and teens at a 14 times greater risk of death by gun violence than their white counterparts.

You may be surprised to learn that of the estimated annual death toll from gun violence, nearly 6 of every 10 are victims of suicide. It has been estimated that simply having access to guns increases the odds of suicide via gun violence threefold (Everytown Research & Policy, 2020). In this regard, of course, the lack of public health attention to suicidality in America is a problem dramatically exacerbated by easy access to guns.

the lack of public health attention to suicidality in America is a problem dramatically exacerbated by easy access to guns

That America is constantly improving and evolving makes a lovely undertone for a political speech; however, statistics released by the CDC in May 2022 showed the nation (and the world) that U.S. gun violence resulting in homicide increased by 35% in just a single year (from 2019 to 2020). Because this 25-year U.S. high in homicides from guns coincided with the start of the COVID-19 pandemic, it is convenient to attribute it to mental health issues stemming from the pandemic. Such an attribution, however, would ignore competing theories, such as the rampant gun violence occurring in our nation's capital on January 6th, 2021.

Although gun violence resulting in homicide is an obvious metric of public health, for every homicide, at least three other incidents of gun violence will result in long-term injuries and/or disabilities. A case in point is a person named Jim Brady, who served as press secretary for President Ronald Regan. In 1981, an assassination attempt on the president left nearby Mr. Brady with a gunshot wound to the head – an injury resulting in permanent partial paralysis (Brady, 2022). Think about this two ways: from a purely human perspective, being physically incapacitated for a lifetime is clearly tragic; and from the larger public health perspective, consider the ongoing medical costs, lost years of being a fully productive member of the workforce, and countless losses in quality of life.

This larger perspective sheds light on the question of what the costs are, to our nation, of the gun violence epidemic. While medical costs and lost productivity are fairly straightforward to calculate and understand, the "costs" of loss in quality of life require the application of a commonly used public health tool. The next section introduces the public health concept of **quality-adjusted life years (QALYs)**.

What Is a Quality-Adjusted Life Year?

To begin, think of your own life in terms of one year of perfect health – no issues with injuries, disease, or long-term disabilities. Then, for a second year, imagine that you (like Jim Brady) sustained a traumatic gunshot wound that caused paralysis and thus greatly limited your movement and mobility. Your physical inabilities are most likely shared by thousands of other gunshot victims; thus it is likely that experts in QALYs have developed a multiplier for your condition. For example, let's say that multiplier is .66 (it is always a value of less than 1.0). So, that the value of that second year is reduced by one-third:

$$\text{Year 1 : One year at } 1.0 = 1.0$$
$$\text{Year 2 : One year at } .66 = .66$$
$$\text{Total for the two years} = 1.66 \,/\, 2.00$$

So, you experience a loss of quality of about one-sixth over the two-year period.

The concept of QALYs is vital to public health practice. In a nutshell, this concept robustly justifies advanced and even intensive prevention efforts. Although QALYs are used primarily as part of economic analyses of public health intervention programs and policies, it behooves all citizens of our nation to constantly be reminded – in very clear terms, such as QALYs – of the deeper extent to which issues such as gun violence impact our lives. Clearly, death by gun violence is the most tragic consequence; however, we should also be aware of the consequences for the victims who survive gun violence. Like death rates from gun violence, the number of injuries caused by gun violence has been steadily increasing. For instance, an organization known as Gun Violence Archive (2022) reported 22,779 gun violence injuries in 2014 and (with mostly steady yearly increases) 39,492 injuries in 2020. This represents a stunning and sobering increase of 73.4%!

Given what you have learned so far in this chapter, it should already be clear that the uniquely American problem of gun violence is very much at crisis proportions, with every indication that the epidemic may continue to worsen. For example, consider two highly

The concept of QALYs is vital to public health practice

we should also be aware of the consequences for the victims who survive gun violence

publicized mass shootings: one occurring in Sandy Hook, CT, in 2012 and the other in Buffalo, NY 10 years later, in 2022. Despite all efforts by the 2012 White House administration under President Obama, Congress failed to pass bills controlling even handguns that could be signed into law by the president. As a result – and in stark contrast to nations such as Australia – the number of mass shootings in the United States between the events of Sandy Hook and Buffalo exceeded 3,500 (Parker, Pager, & Itkowitz, 2022)! It is exceedingly clear that our failure to control guns designed for taking human life has caused millions of needless deaths (mostly of young Black males) and uncounted lifelong injuries is a product of a divided (and thus weak) U.S. Congress. A take-home point here is that your voting future should be devoted as much to the careful selection of congressional representatives and senators as it is to local races and the always-popular presidential races.

your voting future should be devoted as much to the careful selection of congressional representatives and senators as it is to local races and the always-popular presidential races

Of course, the public health response to the escalating gun violence crisis must involve the voting public. Sadly, however, states are passing laws that make America even more "awash in guns" (using the phrase quoted from President Obama). For instance, in March 2022, the state of Indiana passed a law allowing anyone 18 or older to openly carry handguns in public places. This new legislation is known as **constitutional carry**, and supporters claim that this right is granted to them as part of the Second Amendment to the U.S. Constitution (see **Photo 11.1**). The Indiana governor signed the bill into law despite vocal opposition from law enforcement agencies throughout the state, including the director of the state police force (Lange, 2022) To be clear, the Indiana law does not require even the commonsense approach of background checks (part of the **Brady Handgun Prevention Act**; see the next section), despite the success of this approach in controlling gun violence in America. If conceptualized as a contagious disease, the epidemic of gun violence in the United States has no cure in sight. Moreover, due to the divisive nature of gun laws, true political courage is severely lacking when elected officials could be acting to save lives and prevent lifelong injuries caused by gun violence.

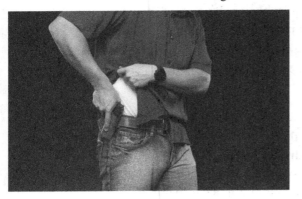

Photo 11.1   Indiana is only one of many states that freely allow any adult to openly carry guns in public places.
Source: Straight8Stock/Adobe stock.

BOX 11.1. A CLOSER LOOK AT THE SECOND AMENDMENT

Of value to you, as a public health professional, is the simple and obvious point that public health educators can easily fill this void. Perhaps it is time for health educators to begin debunking people's misconceptions about the value of gun ownership and the true wording of the Second Amendment. It reads as follows:

A well regulated Militia, being necessary to the security of a free State, the right of the people to keep and bear Arms, shall not be infringed.

It is not clear that private citizens (i.e., people not in the military) are the reference point of this rather outdated language. In fact, when this amendment to the Constitution was written, the phrase "bear Arms" referred only to the use of guns as part of military service. A person carrying a gun, hunting, or having a gun at home would not have been said to be "bearing Arms." Also, given the wording "being necessary to the security of a free State," you can easily see that this amendment was a constitutional method of ensuring that members of the military would always have the right to possess guns.

Despite the lack of any reference in the Second Amendment to non-military rights to gun use, millions of Americans have used this amendment as a type of false shield against what they perceive as an infringement on American life when they hear the term **gun control.** Gun control measures in the United States have always been tightly focused on handguns and assault weapons – which are a far cry from any type of weapon that a framer of the Constitution could have possibly imagined. Guns used for hunting and sport shooting have never been the subject of gun control measures. By falsely polarizing the issue as "taking our guns," those who use the Second Amendment as their argument are missing the larger point in the language about "being necessary to the security of a free State." Indeed, as you are learning in this chapter, America is far from a "free state" for those living in places where gun violence is an everyday occurrence. Its victims include children, shoppers in grocery stores, and people sitting in what should be the safety of their own homes.

This textbook's clear theme is that public health is a public responsibility. It is perhaps gun violence that most dramatically punctuates this principle. Although the next section of this chapter delineates a few best-known prevention-orientated approaches to gun violence, the root of this problem remains easy access to guns. Until "We the People" take control of our own safety and begin to vigorously remove handguns and assault weapons from the fabric of everyday American life, the public health crisis of gun violence will only continue to escalate.

Because this escalation is especially a crisis for people of color, gun violence highlights yet another glaring public health disparity. Consider the mass shooting in May 2022 at a supermarket in a predominately Black neighborhood. The shooter was an 18-year-old white male who believed that people of color would soon "replace" white people unless they were killed. His shooting spree was the topic of a commentary in the *Washington Post* that included these words: "The shooting Saturday afternoon at a Tops grocery store in a predominately Black neighborhood in Buffalo is the deadliest mass shooting in 2022 but is one of more than 200 so far. He [the alleged attacker/shooter] declared himself a white supremacist and anti-Semite; he laid out his plan to target a Black community" (Givhan, 2022). So, again, think of guns (especially automatic weapons designed for massive killing) as the pathogen in a disease of epidemic proportions. The hatred that fuels these mass shootings gives the pathogen a type of stage where it can thrive, but in the absence of access to guns designed as weapons, that same hatred would not result in the massive killings that rage across America.

Approaches to Reducing Gun Violence

As previously mentioned, through the joint efforts of Jim Brady and his wife, Sarah Brady, Congress passed an act in 1993 known as the Brady Handgun Prevention Act (Brady, 2022). The most enduring and important aspect of this legislation is the **Brady Background Check System**, which has blocked more than four million potential gun buyers from possessing a gun. Because handguns are small, they are typically used to commit gun violence. Unfortunately, handguns have taken on the properties of assault weapons with the capacity to repeatedly fire several large bullets in only a few seconds (see **Photo 11.2**).

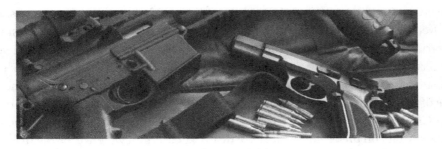

Photo 11.2   If gun violence was a contagious disease, the pathogen would be these types of weapons.
Source: Mariusz Blach / Adobe Stock.

Until our nation begins to act more like other high-income countries of the world by imposing commonsense restrictions on gun manufacturing and sales, the best few approaches to controlling gun violence are those described in this section of the chapter.

Buy-Back Programs

Although far stricter controls on U.S. gun sales have been proposed for decades, these bills never reach the stage of congressional approval. In other nations, however, great strides have been made. For example, in 1996, Australia mandated a national ban on all semi-automatic weapons, pump-action rifles, and shotguns. A key part of this ban was a **buy-back program**. As implied by the name, buy-back programs purchase (at retail price) banned guns already owned by private citizens. In the Australian example, the government purchased a total of 68,727 handguns from private citizens and then destroyed them. The program worked extremely well. For instance, one study showed that between 1979 and 1996 (again, 1996 is the year this ban took effect), Australia had 13 mass shootings. In contrast, no mass shootings occurred between 1997 and 2013. The same study showed that the average rate of deaths from gun violence between 1979 and 1996 was 3.6 for every 100,000 people; the rate dropped to 1.2 for every 100,000 people by 2013 (Chapman, Alpers, & Jones, 2016).

Making "Safer" Guns

One way to make guns a bit less dangerous, especially for children, involves the concept of manufacturing "smart guns." This idea is an extension of using technology for other public safety measures, such as the multitude of features mandated for cars and highways that help avoid injury and death from auto collisions. Smart gun technologies include

- Touch memory
- Voice recognition
- Fingerprint recognition
- Radio frequency identification

Of these technologies, radio frequency identification appears the most promising and popular so far. The gun owner wears a specialized watch, bracelet, or ring synced to the trigger. Without a signal from one of these wearable devices, the gun will not fire.

Of course, the idea of these methods is to limit the use of a gun to its owner. As you might guess, this does not provide as much control as a ban on guns, because gun owners are still free to fire at will! Although the technology can be very useful in keeping children and teens from using a gun stored in the home, the idea lacks the strength of a ban accompanied by a buy-back program. In America, we have more guns than people!

State Laws Regulating Gun Sales

As opposed to attempting to pass national regulations and bans on guns such as assault weapons, an alternate approach is to strengthen state laws that discourage gun ownership. A great deal of variation currently exists from state to state in terms of the number and strength of laws concerning gun sales. This variation naturally lends itself to a somewhat simple question: "Is the death rate from firearms lower in states that have more stringent laws concerning the purchase of guns?" That very question has been answered by a group of researchers who cleverly used CDC data for their study. As a type of clearinghouse for the nation, the CDC routinely collects data on preventable causes of death, such as gun violence. Using firearm-related fatalities as their outcome measure, a team of researchers categorized all 50 states relative to how many of five possible gun control measures were in effect. After ranking each state based on these five control measures, the researchers created quartiles (i.e., lower one-fourth through the upper one-fourth of the states) based on scores from zero (no gun control laws) to five (all five possible laws in effect). They found, as you might suspect, a strong linear relationship indicating that states with the most stringent laws had the lowest rates of firearm-related gun deaths and, by extension, states with the fewest laws had the highest rates of firearm-related gun deaths (Fleegler, Lee, & Monuteaux, 2013). Simply stated, the study provides compelling evidence that state-level laws regulating the sales and use of guns make a tremendous difference in terms of saving lives and averting the morbidity of gun-related injuries.

state-level laws regulating the sales and use of guns make a tremendous difference in terms of saving lives

A Public Health Approach

Think for a minute about what you have already learned about public health practice. You have learned, for example, that the social environment shapes and limits the health-protective behaviors of most people. You have also learned that a key superstructure of society (i.e., cultural beliefs) shapes behaviors and, in turn, is shaped by the collective behaviors of those who are part of a particular culture. Let's apply these concepts to the daunting task of at least stemming the rising tide of gun violence.

The Role of the Media

This textbook now turns attention to the **superstructure of the media** (a collective term for movies, television, music, music videos, and forms of news and print media). Here, the media is considered the root cause of much of the previously described U.S. gun violence. To illustrate this point, let's begin by considering a fascinating study published in the well-known medical journal *Pediatrics.* Using trained coders, the research team evaluated the presence of guns in violent segments of top-rated PG-13 movies released between 1985 and 2012. They found that the number of scenes with gun violence more than tripled during this period. This type of study by a journal devoted to raising healthy children and adolescents is crucial to understanding the root problem of children becoming adults who view gun violence as a somewhat acceptable and perhaps necessary part of life. A sentence from the conclusion of this highly cited article is noteworthy: "By including guns in violent scenes, film producers may be strengthening the weapons effect and providing youth with scripts for using guns" (Bushman, Jamieson, Weitz, & Romer, 2013).

Similarly, media and deeper structures of embedded American culture largely shape the concept of masculinity. The American version of masculinity is still somewhat patterned after cowboys, rugged fighting, and killing. Too often, masculinity becomes entwined with owning, carrying, and using guns. That 80% of all perpetrators and victims of gun violence are male is not spurious in any way. Indeed, a gender divide exists between males and females relative to gun ownership, with five males owning guns for every female owner.

Too often, masculinity becomes entwined with owning, carrying, and using guns

Traditional cultural norms define masculinity as being powerful. For millions of American men who cannot obtain power through wealth, prestige, or occupational status, a form of socially recognized and often socially sanctioned power is obtainable in the form of a firearm. When masculinity is also defined as being capable of committing violence – including gun violence – it becomes what is often referred to as **toxic masculinity** (see **Photo 11.3**). That toxic

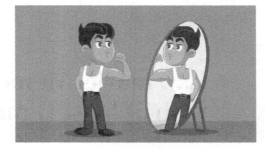

Photo 11.3   Toxic masculinity is a root cause of the American gun violence crisis.
Source: nicoletaionescu/Adobe stock.

When masculinity is also defined as being capable of committing violence – including gun violence – it becomes what is often referred to as **toxic masculinity**

masculinity is a root cause of the U.S. crisis in gun violence is well-researched by psychologists, sociologists, and criminologists. For instance, a notable report produced and published by the *Washington Post* in the spring of 2022 (just after the massive shooting in Buffalo, NY) included an exceptionally poignant section about masculinity being a root cause of gun violence (Parker, Pager, & Itkowitz, 2022).

The Role of Mental Illness

Although mental illness is not a main cause of gun violence, it does appear to play a somewhat prominent role in suicides and mass shootings (which typically conclude with the person doing the shooting committing suicide), so mental illness and delusions of hyper-masculinity may weigh heavily in the gun violence equation. To punctuate the rampant nature of mass shootings, an example of how mental illness sets the stage for gun violence occurred right after the Buffalo shooting described earlier. This shooting occurred on 24 May, 2022 in Uvalde, Texas. The gunman was only 18 years of age and began his killing spree by shooting his grandmother. In the days that followed, astute journalists made the general point that Texas has some of the least restrictive gun laws in the nation. They also questioned how a person as clearly psychopathic as the Uvalde shooter could so easily obtain assault weapons.

At the time, the Texas governor (Greg Abbott) had been making gun laws less restrictive (despite a highly publicized mass shooting in El Paso, TX, just two years before the Uvalde massacre of elementary children). For instance, under Governor Abbott, a Texas law was passed for permitless gun carrying (known as the **permitless carry bill**). The day following the Uvalde shooting, a prominent political figure, former Congressman, and candidate for Texas governor (Beto O'Rourke) publicly blamed the Uvalde massacre on Governor Abbott's lack of gun control. His remarks focused on two types of assault weapons: the AR-15 and the AK-47. He passionately made the following statement about gun control: "When we see that (assault weapons) being used against children . . . hell, yes, we're going to take your AR-15, your AK-47" (Svitek, 2022).

The larger point emphasized by many journalists at the time was how easily a psychopathic gunman could obtain these deadly assault weapons. Sadly, as Americans mourned the death of the school children massacred in Uvalde, the following Memorial Day weekend was a period when at least 11 other mass shootings occurred (see **Figure 11.1**).

The week following Memorial Day 2022, the nation's leading newspapers ran front-page stories predominately addressing gun violence and gun control. That week was marked by a televised presidential address to the nation on June 2. Among President Biden's most passionate statements that night was his plea that Congress pass more aggressive regulations. He stated, "For God's sake, how much more carnage are we willing to accept?" He then said, "The issue we face is one of conscience and common sense." He proposed several commonsense laws that Congress could easily enact, but congressional resistance to his pleading was obvious (Wagner & Scott, 2022).

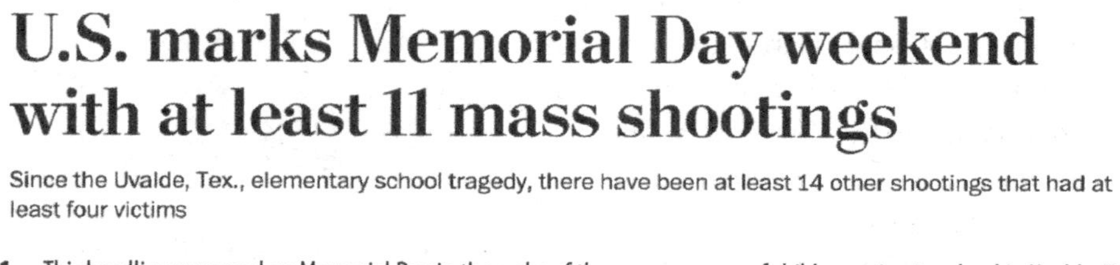

U.S. marks Memorial Day weekend with at least 11 mass shootings

Since the Uvalde, Tex., elementary school tragedy, there have been at least 14 other shootings that had at least four victims

Figure 11.1   This headline appeared on Memorial Day in the wake of the gun massacre of children going to school in Uvalde, Texas

The American Myth of "Self Defense"

Another root cause of the crisis lies in the great American myth that guns are needed for self-defense and thus gun ownership prevents crime. This American ethos is common but clearly misinformed.

The data debunking the myth regarding gun ownership making people safer is abundant in the research literature. For example, a comprehensive study of 27 countries correlated the per capita rate of gun ownership with the death rate from firearms (correlation is a common statistic for public health research – it yields a value ranging from zero to one that quantifies the strength of the association between any two factors). Across all 27 countries, a very strong correlation of .80 was found, indicating a substantial link between gun ownership and death from gun violence (Bangalore & Messerli, 2013). This same study observed an absence of a significant correlation between the per capita rate of gun ownership and the national firearm-related crime rate. Thus, nations with greater levels of per capita gun ownership did not experience the lower crime rates expected by the myth that gun ownership makes us safer.

The correlational study of 27 countries described in the previous paragraph also sheds light on the myth that gun violence is primarily caused by the crisis of mental illness in a nation such as the United States. In correlating the mental illness burden of the 27 nations with their death rate from firearms, the research team found a modest correlation of .52. Also, the study found an absence of a significant correlation between mental illness burden and national firearm-related crime rates. In a subsequent analysis relative to the firearm-related death rate, it was observed that the variable of gun ownership far outweighed the variable of mental illness burden in terms of predicting the national death rate from firearms (Bangalore & Messerli, 2013). Although hundreds of studies tell a similar story – that mental illness and gun violence are not strongly connected – one study arrived at a conclusion that is worth your consideration: even if the somewhat elevated risk of gun violence (which includes suicide) among persons with a diagnosed mental illness were reduced to the same level of risk as a person without mental illness, the overall population-level decline in gun-related violent death would be only about 4% (Swanson, McGinty, Fazel, & Mays, 2015).

> the variable of gun ownership far outweighed the variable of mental illness burden in terms of predicting the national death rate from firearms

In case you're wondering why so many **American narratives** (i.e., belief systems about a phenomenon) around gun violence focus on mental illness, consider that this explanation exonerates the gun industry and supports the millions of people who cling to an illusion that "guns don't kill; people kill." The logic of this illusion is akin to saying that opioids such as fentanyl are harmless – the user makes them dangerous. As for exonerating the gun industry, understand that, like the tobacco industry (see **Chapter 4**), the U.S. gun and ammunition industries produce nearly $30 billion per year in sales. It is in their best interest to promote misconceptions about the Second Amendment, support politicians who are against gun control, and shape the American belief system by constantly shifting the blame for events such as mass shootings to people suffering from mental illness. Thus, much like the Truth Campaign you learned about in **Chapter 4**, a reasonable approach to gun violence would be to expose the public to the deceptions promoted by the gun and ammunition industries.

> a reasonable approach to gun violence would be to expose the public to the deceptions promoted by the gun and ammunition industries.

The Social Aspect of Gun Violence

As a closing point to this part of the chapter, it is fair to consider gun violence as spreading much like an infectious disease. This idea involves understanding social networks, particularly social media-based social networks. Social networks tend to amplify small bits of misinformation into large amounts of distrust. They also promote alternative realities, such as those describing the need for all Americans to be "locked and loaded" with an adequate arsenal of guns and a long-lasting supply of ammunition. These networks can create norms that work against the majority's will to at least control assault weapons. These norms are relatively common – you may recognize them:

- Guns are an American freedom.

- Everybody has a gun – we should, too.

- Guns don't kill; people kill.

- Guns are safe in the right hands.

- You must have a gun to protect yourself from criminals and home invasion.

Because of the widespread proliferation of these norms, a basic public health challenge is to provide ongoing counter-narratives. The public health response must also involve engaging people in advocacy efforts to prompt safer behaviors and identify pro-gun lobbies that make huge profits from the sale of guns. With national surveys conducted in 2022 showing that most Americans favor gun control, advocacy efforts need to include supporting and electing politicians who can and will stand up for the public's safety by at least passing relatively straightforward legislation such as that banning the sale of assault weapons. This type of action from the public must occur to make a real difference in the gun crisis.

In contrast to a public health approach, gun control actions taken at the individual level are ineffective. For instance, The American College of Physicians recommends that physicians engage with their patients in conversations designed to elucidate the risks of having guns in the home. Data either supporting or refuting the value of these physician-patient discussions is lacking. This medical approach to the crisis is sadly misguided and predicated on assumptions about people at risk of committing gun violence even having a physician, let alone one who takes the time to engage patients in this type of conversation. Of interest, however, is that the state of Florida passed a law (which stood for several years before being repealed) restricting these recommended conversations between physicians and their patients (Hagen, Carew, Crandell, & Zaidi, 2019). The passage of this law illustrates the sheer power of gun lobbies such as the National Rifle Association.

Trends in U.S. Automobile Collisions and Injuries

Similar to the unique American experience of gun violence, American residents have a far greater rate of death and injury caused by automobile collisions than most high-income counties (Evans, 2014). However, unlike our gun violence crisis, fairly dramatic declines in automobile deaths and injuries have occurred since 1972 (Evans, 2014). These declines have been produced through decades of highly refined research studies and advanced research technologies designed specifically to understand car crashes, how they can be avoided, and how the damage to human bodies can be mitigated. The term **mitigation**, in this regard, is similar to the term **harm reduction** (see **Chapter 9**): the idea is that not all collisions can be prevented, but key regulations can greatly reduce the risk of death and the severity of injuries.

Perhaps the most valuable form of mitigation has been implementing required standards for automobile manufacturers regarding mandatory **driver-side airbags**. Developed and monitored by the National Highway Traffic Safety Administration (NHTSA), airbag technologies have continued to improve since 1 April 1989, when national regulations for automakers took effect that required the installation of driver's-side airbags on all newly built cars and small trucks. Airbags are known as a **passive restraint system**, meaning the user (in this case, the driver behind the wheel) is not given the option of using or not using the device – it is automatic and cannot be disabled.

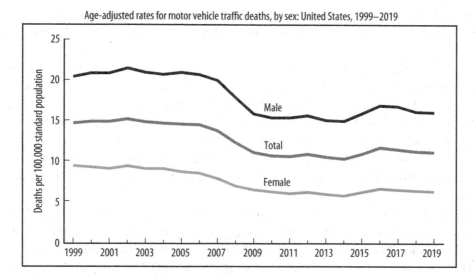

Age-adjusted rates for motor vehicle traffic deaths, by sex: United States, 1999–2019

Figure 11.2   Generally, the U.S. rate of death from automobile collisions has declined
Source: Spencer, M. R. et al., 2021 / CDC / Public domain.

So, right away, let's compare this national standard that protects the public's health to gun violence. People did not cling to images of freedom and independence, such as the prototype American cowboy. They did not claim a constitutional privilege to own and drive a car not equipped with an airbag. Further, people were generally not misled by falsehoods about airbags the way they are about gun ownership. Finally, any resistance from the auto industry was meager compared to the gun and ammunition industries' use of highly paid political action groups such as the National Rifle Association. As you read this section of the chapter, keep thinking about the stark contrasts between the two American problems.

Figure 11.2 illustrates the decline in death rates during just the 20-year period from 1999 through 2019. Most of the decline occurred in conjunction with improved safety standards for automobiles. From 2006 through 2010, the total rate declined by about 8% per year (Spencer, Hedegaard, & Garnett, 2021). The same 20-year period was also a time when a fairly dramatic decline occurred in terms of vehicle occupants (i.e., persons other than the driver), with that rate dropping by 37%.

Of course, the question you must have by now is, "What is the current rate, and how much of a public health problem is this compared with gun violence?" The answer is about 30,000 annual deaths, equating to about 90 per day (less than the 110 per day for gun violence). Although progress has been made in reducing deaths and injuries caused by automobile collisions, the 30,000 annual deaths still pose a substantial challenge to public health practice. The good news is that the downward trends signify that the structural-level approaches applied through numerous regulatory actions are working and can still be improved.

Regulatory Actions Applied to Highways

Have you ever noticed that raised reflectors are placed between lanes when you are driving on a four-lane highway (meaning two lanes of traffic in each highway direction)? Have you noticed that some sections of highways have grooved payment that slows down your car and even makes noise? Do you notice the heavy metal guardrails that line the right side of highway shoulders when that area of roadway is built on ground that goes downhill? How about the streetlights often used to brighten your vision when driving local roads at night? All these safety measures are the product of decades of research conducted by the National

Highway and Traffic Safety Administration (NHTSA). This administration was established as part of the federal National Highways Safety Act and is part of the U.S. Department of Transportation.

A critical function of the NHTSA involves an age-old public health action: **surveillance and monitoring**. Although public health surveillance systems count cases of nationally reportable diseases such as chlamydia and gonorrhea, the NHTSA version of this action collects data from all fatal car crashes. Known as the **Fatality Analysis Reporting System**, this extensive database enables a related monitoring function. Monitoring in this case involves using the database to make statistical projections relative to risk factors that appear to be most implicated in auto fatalities. Through this surveillance and monitoring system, data-driven improvements are made to America's roadways.

In stark contrast to the lack of congressional action against gun violence, the U.S. Congress has a stellar track record of creating and passing legislation that constantly improves the safety of highways and local roads. This type of legislation is constructed around data-driven conclusions. As always, an example is helpful. In June 2022, the NHTSA reported that data from the Fatality Analysis Reporting System indicated a 16-year high in traffic fatalities in 2021 (NHTSA, 2022) Compared to 2020, a 10.5% increase in auto fatalities was recorded in 2021 (creating a 16-year high of 42,915 deaths that year). Two points emerged from this data. First, the number of deaths most likely increased due to the COVID-19 pandemic (see **Chapter 1**). As lockdowns, restrictions, and general fear concerning COVID-19 abated in 2021, Americans traveled more miles than they had in 2020. Specifically, the NHTSA estimated that Americans traveled 325 billion more miles in 2021 compared to 2020. This equated to an increase of 11.2% in what is known as **vehicle miles traveled** (VMT). When looking at auto fatality rates in 2021 using VMT, it was reported that fatality rates were lower in 2021 compared to 2020 (a decline of 1.34 deaths per 100 million people). The second point was that the sheer number of auto fatalities prompted congressional and public support for implementing a federal program known as Safe Streets and Roads for All. This $6 billion program is now rebuilding and improving local roadways throughout the United States, thus serving as a complement to the high standards already applied to interstate highways. The required standards for local road improvement projects were, as you may have guessed, created through the monitoring function of the Fatality Analysis Reporting System. The take-home point here is that the public health functions of surveillance and monitoring have been applied with great fidelity to making America's roads safer.

The take-home point here is that the public health functions of surveillance and monitoring have been applied with great fidelity to making America's roads safer

Regulations Applied to Automobile Manufacturing

Perhaps even more impressive than creating safer highways and local roads, the NHTSA uses the Fatality Analysis Reporting System to make data-driven requirements for manufacturing autos sold in the United States. For example, data from this system was used to determine whether amber-colored rear turn signals are less implicated in rear-end fatal collisions than red-colored turn signals. This rather simple question was easily handled by the database: the finding was that amber was safer, but not by a wide enough margin to justify restricting auto manufactories from installing red rear turn signals if they choose to do so. On the other hand, using the database to address questions about the optimal safety of different types of front headlights in car design found evidence that one type outperforms another. This evidence was then used to place a manufacturing restriction on automakers relative to headlights. Everything used in making a car – from the headlights to the taillights – is regulated by the NHTSA.

Everything used in making a car – from the headlights to the taillights – is regulated by the NHTSA

One of the most remarkable and exemplary innovations that make cars and small trucks so much safer than in the past is the collapsible steering column. Rather than having a solid steel core, collapsible steering columns are constructed with an inner core of soft plastic that can bend in the event of a front-end collision. Whereas solid steel would be directed straight into a driver's head, the plastic core allows the column to bend upward and, therefore, above the driver's body. The NHTSA estimated that this innovation has the potential to avert 13,000 auto fatalities each year and an additional 23,000 non-fatal injuries (Riopelle, 2012). After decades of accumulating research and supporting data, the NHTSA made collapsible steering columns mandatory in new automobiles starting in 2022. Again, although this type of public health research is not disease-focused (see **Photo 11.4**), it exemplifies how research can and should be used to inform regulatory actions that ultimately avert morbidity and mortality.

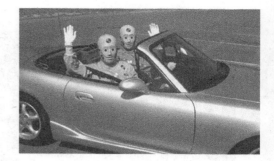

Photo 11.4   The National Highway and Traffic Safety Administration invests heavily is research that informs regulations.
Source: Nerdi~commonswiki / Wikimedia Commons / Public domain.

A final point relative to a car's safety is regulating its driver! Have you ever wondered, for example, why some areas of a roadway have posted speed limits of 25 miles per hour, other areas have speed limits of 35 miles per hour, and so on? The answer brings us back to decades of research conducted primarily by the NHTSA. For instance, using the Fatality Analysis Reporting System, the NHTSA was able to conclude that the odds of a pedestrian surviving being struck by a car declined substantially once the car's speed exceeded 30 miles per hour. Thus, on roadways likely to be populated with nearby pedestrians, you will typically see speed limits posted at 30 miles per hour, or less in the event of curved roads that create blind spots that prevent drivers from easily seeing pedestrians (see **Photo 11.5**).

Noteworthy relative to regulating drivers is that states and local municipalities must enforce laws such as posted speed limits. Sadly, it seems that too many drivers feel a need to constantly exceed the speed limits of highways and local roads. For 2019, the NHTSA estimated that 26% of all highway traffic fatalities resulted from speeding. This equates to the death of 9,478 people. The good news is that the 26% estimate is less than the estimates of closer to 33% for the years preceding 2019. The bad news is that our nation continues to somehow foster the idea that speeding is not dangerous (see **Box 11.2**).

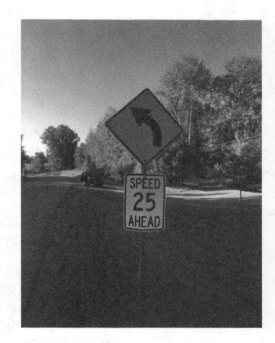

Photo 11.5   Intensive research is the basis for posted speed limits.

BOX 11.2. THE HUMAN SIDE: "IT WON'T HAPPEN TO ME"

Think for a minute about the daily lottery. Every day, millions of people lay down their money to purchase lottery tickets that have astronomically low odds of winning. Yet they play and continue to pay. State lotteries are important sources of added revenue because people are eager to take a chance. Players are aware of the astronomically low odds, so why do they continue? The answer to this question is known as **optimism bias** in the behavioral and social sciences and lies in a human tendency for individuals to assume that they are not ordinary – that they will somehow be the lucky one.

With the idea of optimism bias in mind, consider speeding on a highway. Chances are good that most students reading this box have been either the driver of or a passenger in a speeding car. If this applies to you as a driver, try to think about any reasoning that was part of your thought process at the time. Were your thoughts similar to any of these?

* I am a great driver, so this is OK.

* Traffic is not bad today – speeding is safe.

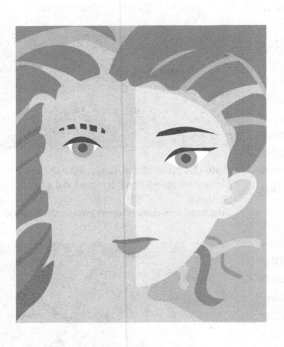

- I am in complete control of this car – nothing will happen to hurt me.

- My luck in avoiding bad things has always been really good.

- I am not the same as everybody else – I am destined to be OK at the end of each day.

The larger point here transcends speeding and applies broadly to health behaviors. Millions of Americans appear to have a protective way of thinking – something along the lines of "it won't happen to me." Although the protective side of this thinking can be good (i.e., it keeps us from a state of constant fear, anxiety, and worry), it also prompts people to push their luck regarding chances they knowingly take relative to becoming unintentionally pregnant (or causing an unintentional pregnancy), contracting COVID-19, exceeding dietary diabetes-related restrictions, missing daily medications such as those used to control hypertension, and (a classic) smoking tobacco despite being fully informed about the risks of eventually developing heart disease or cancer. Ultimately, it seems to be part of human nature for people to exempt themselves from the possibility of being a victim of tragic events – such as automobile collisions – that they know occur to "other people."

Similarities and Contrasts Between Controlling Gun Violence and Controlling Traffic Fatalities/Injuries

Before examining the contrasts, let's begin with the similarities between these two seemingly distinct forms of public health crisis. The most important observation is that both epidemics kill people of all ages, although victims are often young (especially regarding gun violence) and otherwise perfectly healthy. Thus, the total number of life years lost and QALYs are very high for both epidemics. Further, each crisis can be reduced in magnitude using structural-level approaches. Another important similarity involves the sudden nature of death and how this unexpected loss of loved ones impacts surviving family members and friends.

Turning now to the contrasts, the most glaring is that the U.S. federal government invests heavily in research and infrastructures needed to constantly improve the safety of driving a vehicle. Indeed, a principle of the NHTSA is that accidents don't just happen – they result from a set of predictable circumstances that can be altered to protect the public. By contrast, research and infrastructure investments in preventing gun violence are completely absent. Rather than viewing the problem as preventable, it is not unusual for state representatives or members of Congress to claim that some amount of death from gun violence is a price we pay to protect the rights given to people under the Second Amendment (again, see **Box 11.1**).

Next, because states receive federal funding to help build and maintain highways and roads, the federal government has a fair degree of control over the safety and design of America's roadways. This control simply does not exist regarding gun violence. Similarly, federal oversight of car manufacturing provides a strong intervention point, whereas a counterpart to this oversight does not exist relative to gun violence. Taken together with the first contrast, these two contrasts provide ample evidence as to why gun violence continues to escalate while the overall downward trend in fatalities from automobile collisions shows great promise in terms

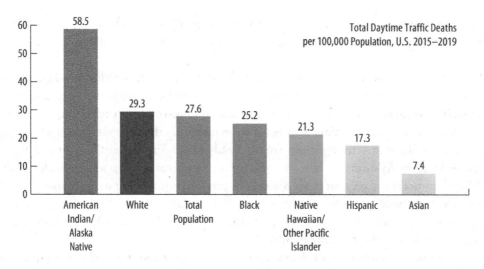

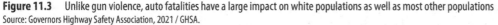

Figure 11.3   Unlike gun violence, auto fatalities have a large impact on white populations as well as most other populations
Source: Governors Highway Safety Association, 2021 / GHSA.

of ultimately ending this crisis. Clearly, investing in research and then applying the results through federal regulation is called for relative to the tragic loss of human lives, and countless long-term injuries, caused by gun violence.

A vital contrast involves the glaring racial disparity relative to gun violence, which places Black Americans at great risk, versus an absence of such as disparity for auto fatalities. White Americans are somewhat more likely than Black Americans to be killed in a daytime auto collision (Governors' Highway Safety Administration, 2021). As shown in **Figure 11.3**, except for American Indians/Alaskan Natives, significant racial disparities do not exist for auto fatalities.

Whether white Americans are a bit more likely than Black or Latinx Americans to be killed in an auto collision weighs into the more aggressive federal approach to reducing auto fatalities is a matter of speculation. It is, of course, possible that the largely white members of the U.S. Congress are less invested in averting a gun violence crisis that overly affects persons of color. Again, as a part of "We the People," your advocacy and personal voting record are perhaps the most vital public health actions that must occur to bring equity to future efforts directed at preventing gun violence.

Overall, the greatest contrast between the two common causes of death discussed in this chapter may be that we depend on automobiles, trucks, etc., for the tasks of daily living, whereas guns are not a necessity. Of course, some people will argue that we need guns to defend ourselves. This argument is predicated on the outdated idea that American citizens will need to fight in hand-to-hand combat with people from an invading nation. Although romanticized by movies, today's world of war between nations is marked by economic sanctions, nuclear build-ups, and sophisticated military operations involving air strikes and other tactics that go far beyond people on the ground shooting at each other. Given that guns are not a necessary part of life and automobiles are very much needed, the epidemic of gun violence is the one that could be quickly and efficiently ended.

Review and Key Terms

This chapter brought you into the sphere of federal regulation as a primary form of promoting the health of the public. The two forms of crisis (gun violence and automobile accidents) will not be solved by easy public health tools such as education, social marketing, local ordinances, or organized communities devoted to reducing death from guns and/or auto collisions. Saving

investing in research and then applying the results through federal regulation is called for relative to the tragic loss of human lives, and countless long-term injuries, caused by gun violence

as a part of "We the People," your advocacy and personal voting record are perhaps the most vital public health actions

Saving lives through prevention requires a unified (i.e., national) approach that is data-driven and always grounded in science and technology

lives through prevention requires a unified (i.e., national) approach that is data-driven and always grounded in science and technology; anything less is akin to allowing either crisis to continue.

This chapter introduced you to the point that America has an **epidemic of gun violence**. As you learned, this epidemic is escalating, and its toll on human life is counted in deaths as well as **quality-adjusted life years** (QALY) lost due to long-term injuries. Uniquely, this chapter focused on the emerging **structural-level interventions** that can and should be applied to controlling the epidemic. Among these are the Brady Handgun Prevention Act and the **Brady Background Check System**; it is vital for you (as an American citizen and member of the voting public) to understand each of these legislative acts. An equally important type of legislation involves **gun buy-back programs**, which have been used successfully in other nations: the government pays people a retail price for guns they own that become officially banned, as well as some types that are not officially banned.

As the chapter progressed, you learned about the **superstructure of the media** and how it has shaped a long-standing American culture that glamorizes guns in the hands of strong men. This culture around guns is the **root cause** of much of the gun violence epidemic. As part of this culture, most people have been widely exposed to **American narratives** related to guns, shooting, killing, perceptions of self-defense, and "justifiable homicide." These narratives escalate to much greater danger when combined with **toxic masculinity**. This concept has been broadly applied to multiple forms of violence perpetrated by men. Again, given the superstructure of the media and its portrayal of manly power so frequently linked to the image of men holding and using guns, it should be clear to you that toxic masculinity greatly exacerbates gun violence and is thus a root cause of the problem.

The chapter then discussed the epidemic of automobile collisions and the death/injuries that occur each year as a result. You learned about regulations put into effect by the NHTSA. Although many of these regulations are centered on preventing collisions, others focus on **mitigation**. This term represents the concept of minimizing harm to the driver, passengers, and others by regulating both the design of highways and the design of vehicles used on the highways. The driver's-side airbag is an excellent example of a well-research innovation that was codified into law for all new cars manufactured and sold in the United States

[The general downward trend in America's epidemic of automobile collisions is an exemplary model for public research and practice]. The NHTSA, for example, constantly and diligently engages in the two practices of **surveillance** and **monitoring**. Through the planned use of these two tools, our highways and vehicles are undergoing continuous improvements focused on protecting human life. A paramount example in this regard to the **Fatality Analysis Reporting System**. This organized method of surveillance creates an idea database that allows for monitoring the degrees of success with each passing year of safety improvements. In conjunction with this system, you also learned that death rates alone are not necessarily a reliable indicator of trends. This was illustrated in the example of a post-COVID increase in traffic fatalities that was actually not an increase at all when considering the huge added number of **vehicle miles traveled** in 2021.

America has successfully harnessed the political will to protect ourselves against the crisis of automobile collisions

The chapter concluded by providing several examples of the stark contrasts between the two epidemics. Ultimately, the essence of these contrasts is that America has successfully harnessed the political will to protect ourselves against the crisis of automobile collisions; however, we have barely scratched the surface of our expanding crisis of gun violence. Until "We the People" take ownership and demand that our elected representatives act in favor of public safety over the wishes of the gun and ammunition industries, the U.S. gun violence crisis will continue.

For Practice and Class Discussion

Practice Questions

1. Which of the following terms is least implicated as a root cause of homicide caused by gun violence?
    a. Toxic masculinity
    b. Superstructure of the media
    c. America's mental health crisis
    d. American narratives about guns

2. Which safety feature of a car is the best example of a mitigating device?
    a. Collapsible steering column
    b. GPS sensor that warns of an impending collision
    c. Raised reflectors on four-lane highways
    d. Grooved pavement that warns drivers of an impending road hazard

3. One common American narrative is that "the government wants to take away our guns." Which statement is false in this regard?
    a. Buy-back programs will pay people for guns.
    b. People who own assault weapons purchased under the background check system would be exempt from any ban.
    c. Federal and state proposals to ban weapons are not focused on guns designed to hunt game.
    d. These programs have been very successful in other high-income nations.

4. Although mass shootings garner a considerable amount of coverage by the media, they represent a very small portion of the total gun deaths that occur annually in the United States.
    a. True
    b. False

5. The dual actions of surveillance and monitoring are best exemplified in this chapter by the:
    a. Gun buy-back program
    b. Brady Handgun Prevention Act
    c. Fatality Analysis Reporting System
    d. Regulation of the auto industry

6. Which statement relative to passing federal laws banning assault weapons is true?
    a. As of 2022, Congress had yet to pass any legislation on to the executive branch (i.e., the White House).
    b. Presidential bills that ban assault weapons have been vetoed by Congress.
    c. Laws banning assault weapons constantly change with each new White House administration.
    d. Only the Brady Act has ever been used to successfully ban assault weapons.

7. Which issue is not characterized by a racial disparity that favors White Americans?
    a. Long-term injuries from gun violence
    b. Deaths from gun violence
    c. Daytime deaths from auto collisions
    d. Being the victim of gun violence

8. One solution that may contribute to reducing gun violence involves the use of manufacturing technology so that guns can be used only by their licensed owner. These are:
   a. Safe guns
   b. Smart guns
   c. Registered guns
   d. Non-repeating weapons

9. As you learned from reading this chapter, the general decline in auto fatalities is a product of engineering based on research, with federal mandates used to make innovations mandatory. The current trend is for this same pattern to be applied to controlling gun violence.
   a. True
   b. False

10. If guns, gun purchasing, and gun carrying were regulated along the same lines as currently regulations for cars and other vehicles, all of the following would be likely to occur except:
    a. Sales may be limited to non-felons
    b. The speed at which guns can fire multiple rounds of bullets could be regulated
    c. The Second Amendment would be revised by the U.S. Congress
    d. Assault weapons would only be sold to persons trained and certified (annually) in using these weapons.

Discussion Questions

11. The appeal of the Florida mandate relative to physicians counseling patients about the risks of gun ownership was unsuccessful. Why would Florida want to prevent these conversations? Also, what role did the NRA play in defending the 2011 decision during the 2014 appeal? Since the 2014 appeal, many opinions and controversies have been published in newspapers, blogs, magazine articles, etc. Locate at least two opinion articles: one defending the decision and another opposing it. Then, compose a two-page double-spaced paper summarizing each position, concluding with a paragraph providing your commentary on these two positions.

12. This chapter concluded by delineating a few key contrasts between the crises of gun violence and automobile fatalities. Other stark contrasts exist. Paired with one or two other people also taking this course, consider other stark contrasts and then come to a consensus as to which one of these is the most important and also lends itself to a structural-level intervention. Have one group member make and post an audio file describing your thinking.

13. Using any national newspaper or internet-based news site of your choice, go online to find a news story about a recent mass shooting. Using no more than two double-spaced pages, describe the story in terms that relate to what you learned in this chapter. If applicable to your class, post this to the discussion board of the learning management system and be ready to promptly engage with others students as they reply to your post.

References

Bangalore, S., & Messerli, F. H. (2013). Gun ownership and firearm deaths. *The American Journal of Medicine, 126*(10), 873–876.

Brady (2022). History of Brady. https://www.bradyunited.org/history

Bushman, B. J., Jamieson, P. E., Weitz, I., & Romer, D. (2013). Gun violence trends in movies. *Pediatrics, 132*(6), 1014–1018.

Chapman, S., Alpers, P., & Jones, M. (2016). Associations between gun law reform and international firearm deaths in Australia. *The Journal of the American Medical Association, 316*(3), 291–299.

Evans, L. (2014). Traffic fatality reduction: United States compared with 25 other countries. *The American Journal of Public Health, 104*(8), 1501–1507.

Everytown Research & Policy (2020). Gun violence in America. https://everytownresearch.org/report/gun-violence-in-america/

Fleegler, E. W., Lee, L. K., & Monuteaux, M.G. (2013). Firearm legislation and firearm-related fatalities in the United States. *Journal of the American Medical Association – Internal Medicine, 173*(9), 732–740.

Givhan, R. (2022, May 18). A week of violence punctuates generations of hate. *Washington Post.* https://www.washingtonpost.com/nation/2022/05/18/weekend-violence-punctuates-generations-hate/

Governors' Highway Safety Administration (2021). An analysis of traffic fatalities by race and ethnicity. https://www.ghsa.org/sites/default/files/2021-06/An%20Analysis%20of%20Traffic%20Fatalities%20by%20Race%20and%20Ethnicity.pdf

Gun Violence Archive (2022). www.gunviolencearchive.org

Hagen, G., Carew, B., Crandell, M., & Zaidi, Z. (2019) Patients and guns: physicians are not asking. *Southern Medical Journal, 112*(11), 581–585.

Hutto, E. (2022, May 26). Why are we blaming gun violence on mental illness? *Medpage Today.* https://www.medpagetoday.com/special-reports/exclusives/98933

Lange, K. (2022, March 21). Gov. Holcomb signs bill eliminating permit requirement to carry handguns in Indiana. *Indianapolis Star.* https://www.indystar.com/story/news/politics/2022/03/21/indiana-gov-holcomb-signs-constitutional-carry-handun-laws-bill/7088876001/

National Highway and Traffic Safety Administration (2022). Newly released estimates show traffic fatalities reached a 16-year high in 2021. https://www.nhtsa.gov/press-releases/early-estimate-2021-traffic-fatalities

Parker, A., Pager, T., & Itkowitz, C. (2022, May 22). From Sandy Hook to Buffalo: Ten years of failure on gun control. *Washington Post* https://www.washingtonpost.com/politics/2022/05/22/guns-biden-democrats-buffalo/

Riopelle, C. (2012). What are the benefits of an energy-absorbing steering column? http://www.ehow.com/facts_7580516_benefits-energy-absorbing-steering-column.html

Svitek, P. (2022, May 25). Beto O'Rourke confronts Texas Gov. Greg Abbott at Uvalde press conference: "this is on you." *The Texas Tribune.* https://www.texastribune.org/2022/05/25/beto-orourke-greg-abbott-uvalde-shooting/

Swanson, J. W. McGinty, E. J. Fazel, S., & Mays, V. M. (2015). Mental illness and reduction of gun violence and suicide: Bringing epidemiological research to policy. *The Annals of Epidemiology, 25*(5), 366–376.

Wagner, J., & Scott, E. (2022, June 2). Biden calls for Congress to ban assault weapons, high-capacity magazines. *Washington Post.* https://www.washingtonpost.com/politics/2022/06/02/house-judiciary-emergency-gun-legislation/

CHAPTER 12

CLIMATE CHANGE: THE IMPORTANCE OF WATER

You can't always get what you want, but if you try sometimes, you'll find you get what you need.

—*The Rolling Stones, "You Can't Always Get What You Want"*

Overview

For decades, the topics contained in introductory textbooks for public health have been relatively the same (see **Chapters 2–11**). Then came climate change, with a multitude of consequences ranging from overpopulation of insects (including those that transmit disease) to emerging diseases caused by warmer climates, famine, and drought. These and other consequences of climate change collectively present an entirely new and daunting set of public health challenges that were previously unknown to public health practice. Food (see **Chapter 13**) and water are the two most pressing public health consequences of climate change. This chapter will help you understand the global water crisis and introduce you to some emerging solutions to this life-threatening problem.

By way of context, you need to understand that water is the most essential part of anything we, as humans, can possibly consume. The millions of chemical reactions that occur daily in the human body do so within water. Water flushes waste from the body via the kidneys, dissolves essential minerals that we consume from foods, regulates body temperate, lubricates the joints in the body, and even provides a sense of fullness when we may otherwise be over-consuming foods. Given that the human body is composed of 60% water, a public health priority involves providing everybody with ample amounts of clean water from birth through death. Nothing else is as immediately vital to our survival.

As you study this chapter, notice that the emerging solutions to the global water crisis imply a need for humans to make several adaptations. Although many people fervently resist adaptation, the ability and willingness to adapt define the survival of any species – including humans. Because climate change has progressed past the point of being reversible, the necessary adaptions now become pressing goals for all of us. From a public health perspective, water cannot become a commodity for only those who can afford to pay a high price: it must be accessible to all people. Falling short of this objective will translate water into yet another ongoing health disparity.

LEARNING OBJECTIVES

- Understand the urgency and importance of addressing the global water crisis.

- Articulate the basic causes of the global water crisis as a direct result of climate change.

- Delineate and describe U.S. public health approaches to the water crisis that focus on **reducing** consumption.

- Delineate and describe U.S. public health approaches to the water crisis that focuses on **reusing** water.

- Apply the four pillars of public health practice to protect the U.S. water supply.

Because climate change has progressed past the point of being reversible, the necessary adaptions now become pressing goals for all of us

This chapter focuses on the necessary adaptations created by the already dwindling global supplies of the most basic chemical compound of human existence (i.e., water). The opening quote for this chapter comes from a rock group that was famous in your grandparents' generation. The words apply nicely to this chapter's theme: we have to give up many things we want (e.g., private swimming pools, car washes, flushing toilets after each use, long showers, and watering lawns). If our species can give up so many of the things we want when it comes to water, we may find that we will get what we need to sustain life, including a food supply. To be clear, these and other adaptations are mandatory for our survival as a species. It is not wise or even rational to ignore the crisis or hope for some scientific breakthrough that will instantly solve it.

the global water crisis represents perhaps the single most urgent public health problem in your lifetime

To optimally understand the global water crisis, you will need to gain at least a cursory understanding of climate change and how it has created massive water shortages even at this relatively early stage of its progression. You will learn that we exist in a delicate balance between nature and humanity's all-too-consuming needs and desires. One chapter in an introductory-level textbook cannot, of course, cover it all. Thus, this chapter is devoted only to those aspects of climate change and the water crisis that are amenable to solutions that are already ingrained in public practices, such as public education, promoting and incentivizing behavior change, regulating water use, and legislating the protection of water. Study this chapter carefully, because the global water crisis represents perhaps the single most urgent public health problem in your lifetime.

we must work together to avoid clean water becoming a commodity that is affordable to only segments of the human population

Keep in mind that the World Health Organization has emphatically stated that access to clean water is a fundamental human right. When this does not occur – as is true globally for nearly 6 of every 10 humans – people use and drink substandard water, a marvelous vector for the easy propagation of pathogens such as cholera. Thus, a lack of clean water equates with inflated rates of water-borne infectious diseases, many of which (especially infant diarrhea) lead to death. It is vital for you to understand that we must work together to avoid clean water becoming a commodity that is affordable to only segments of the human population.

The Meaning of a Global Public Health Problem

Too many Americans (including their elected officials) believe that public health issues can be defined and corrected only for our citizens. The controversy raised by the World Health Organization over the global disparities in access to vaccines against COVID-19 is a case in point. As much as people in the United States would like to believe that taking both initial doses and all recommended follow-up booster doses will protect us from COVID-19 until all humans are protected, the virus will always have free rein to mutate and spread in new and potentially more dangerous forms around the world (see **Chapter 1**). Climate change is global in origin, and its ramifications will not exempt any area of the planet. Thus, a first take-home point for you in reading this chapter is that the United States is already very much affected by the global water crisis (see **Figure 12.1**).

Climate change is global in origin, and its ramifications will not exempt any area of the planet

Again, just thinking about the United States, consider the Colorado Rocky Mountains. Famed in movies, music, and legend, these majestic mountain tops (see **Photo 12.1**) have for centuries served as a primary source of yearly water for much of the southwestern

In worsening drought, Southern California water restrictions take effect

Outdoor water use limited to one day per week in parts of the Los Angeles area

Figure 12.1   Americans are not exempt from the global water crisis

United States. The once nearly constant accumulation of snow during the long Colorado winters could culminate in snowpacks of 30 feet or more. Snowpack, in turn, serves as a way for the earth to store and slowly release water during the spring, summer, and fall of each year. Many streams and rivers in Colorado are close to full capacity in the early spring months as the snowpack begins an initial period of melting (see **Photo 12.2**). Streams and rivers that empty into the Colorado River take water to much of the Southwest, including southern California. They are also sources of irrigation water for farmers and are protected and regulated by local ordinances (see **Photo 12.3**).

Although snowpack is the lifeblood of many southwestern states, its annual depth is quickly diminishing, and the melt-off starts sooner with each passing year. Estimates suggest that the western states lost 20% of their annual snowpack between 1950 and 2020. However, we should not expect that pace (a 20% decline over 70 years) to continue. Future declines are projected to be more severe in a much shorter time period: for example, an additional 25% decline between 2020 and 2050 (Siirilla-Woodburn, Rhoades, Hatchett, et al., 2021). Over the entire United States, the 2021 snow cover was recorded at 6% – the lowest since record-keeping of snow cover began in 2003. As the earth warms and weather patterns change, the United States will see some years in the near future marked by a near absence of snow cover and dramatically low amounts of snowpack (Siirilla-Woodburn, Rhoades, Hatchett, et al., 2021). Thus, as you can easily imagine – or may have experienced firsthand – the western states, in particular, are already challenged by the global water crisis.

Now that you understand that this global problem truly means all nations, let's consider the question many people ask: "What can just one person do?" The answer is difficult to fully understand as it involves the concept of very small acts ultimately adding up to large-scale changes. The small acts of one person quickly magnify when all of his/her friends and family members also engage in these small acts. As the number of people engaging in seemingly small acts continues to expand, entire **social movements** can occur. Ultimately, these social movements will culminate in substantial change. For example, consider the social movement associated with the symbol shown in **Figure 12.2**.

You are probably familiar with the "Reduce, Reuse, Recycle" logo. However, this form of social movement takes on new meaning when we consider the high stakes involved in the global water crisis. As this chapter progresses, you will learn that **reuse** and **reduce** are the primary options available to Americans as a way to protect our immediate and long-term health and security.

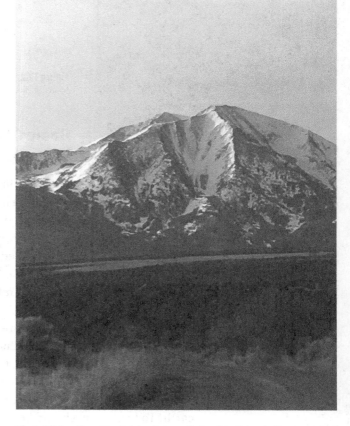

Photo 12.1   Mount Sopris is located near Carbondale, Colorado. Its snowpack is visible throughout much of the year.

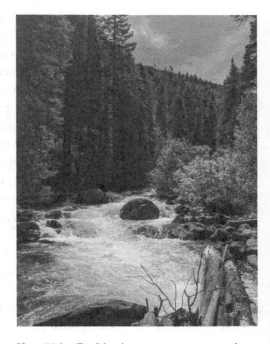

Photo 12.2   This Colorado stream transports snowmelt from the higher elevations of the Colorado Rockies to the Colorado River.

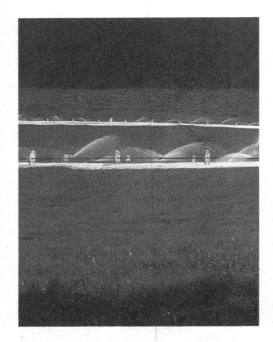

Photo 12.3   Because rain is sparse in many western states, farmers rely on snowmelt to grow even ordinary fields of hay. This field is being irrigated on a cold spring morning.

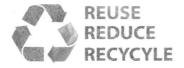

Figure 12.2   Small acts by millions of people always make a big difference
Source: suradeach seatang/Adobe stock.

Basic Causes of Climate Change and the Global Water Crisis

First, if you have been wondering whether climate change is legitimate (given the large numbers of politicians and industry executives who deny this reality), you should be aware that the level of international commitment to solving climate change issues has been extremely strong (and well-funded) for decades. Top-ranked scientists from all over the world hold conferences at least twice yearly. These meetings are a time to share findings and reach consensus on the substance of reports generated each year and published by what is known as the **Intergovernmental Panel on Climate Change** (IPCC) (IPCC, 2022). So, if you are skeptical about climate change, please read one or more of the reports generated by the IPCC.

The two most basic causes of climate change are the release of massive amounts of **carbon** and **methane** into the atmosphere that surrounds and protects the earth. To begin, you should be thinking about your own **carbon footprint**. This is a term used to denote the daily amount of carbon produced as a result of any given action. For instance, let's say you have a job located six miles from where you live. When you ride a bike to that job, the carbon expenditure is zero. However, when you drive an average size car six miles, you emit about 2,500 grams of carbon into the atmosphere. Almost any daily activities you take for granted are likely to add to this carbon footprint. The energy used to heat water for your shower adds to the daily footprint, as does the energy used to cool your home or apartment in the warm months or heat it in the cold months. The daily carbon footprint is further expanded by your shopping choices! For example, having a package delivered to your home leaves a carbon footprint in your name. Purchasing foods, wine, and so on from a grocery store or restaurant that are not from local sources also costs energy for shipping, thus adding to the daily footprint. Just considering fruit, strawberries, peaches, pears, pineapples, bananas, oranges, and apples are all typically consumed on a year-around basis in places like New York and New Jersey that do not grow these foods or grow them only during short periods in the summer. Thus, for example, it takes energy to bring fresh strawberries from a California valley to your door in any of the other 49 states.

The question becomes, "Why the focus on fossil fuels"? When we use fossil fuels for energy, carbon is released. Energy harnessed from wind or the sun does not have this same effect. To quickly understand why only fossil fuels release carbon, think back to high school when you learned about photosynthesis. You should recall that most green plants live by converting sunlight, water, and carbon dioxide into oxygen and organic chemical compounds (energy). Trees, for example, are tremendously important for using carbon dioxide to create oxygen and energy (see **Photo 12.4**).

The process of photosynthesis also **binds carbon**. This is why, for example, the purposeful destruction of the Amazon rainforest for short-term profits threatens the human species. Ironically, when a tree is destroyed, not only do we lose its ability to bind carbon, but if it is burned, that bound carbon is released into the atmosphere. Think of this release as a type of **reverse photosynthesis**. Burning centuries-old sources of bound carbon, such as coal, is infinitely worse in terms of releasing bound carbon.

Although not as massive in volume as carbon, methane gas has a more devastating impact on the earth's ozone layer and is much more efficient at trapping heat, thereby warming the planet. Thus, methane is widely considered the second main cause of climate change. Methane is a leading **greenhouse gas**, meaning it is part of a mixture with other gases (including carbon dioxide) that is responsible for progressively trapping warm air, leading to what is known as the **greenhouse effect** (warm air become trapped in the atmosphere, while a deteriorating ozone layer lets in more heat via the sun). Although methane gases dissipate more quickly than carbon dioxide gases, they are much more destructive than carbon dioxide. The good news about methane is that the human-made sources of this gas can be controlled (primarily by eliminating beef, dairy, and rice from the global diet).

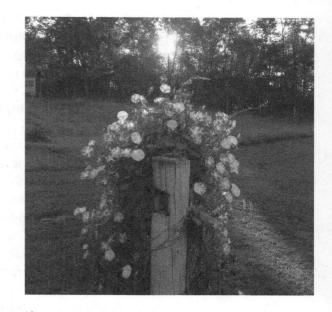

Photo 12.4   Trees, grass, and flowers all bind carbon, thus helping to slow global warming.

With the planet progressively warming, we can expect equally progressive changes in the following:

- Levels of evaporation of existing above-ground water supplies such as lakes, rivers, streams, and estuaries

- The speed at which glaciers melt and thus raise ocean levels (as ocean levels rise, saltwater seeps into estuaries and may render freshwater unfit for drinking)

- Overall annual snowfalls, translating into a loss of snowpack

- Periods of drought leading to substantially lower amounts of annual rainfall

Solutions Based on Reducing Consumption

For added emphasis on the importance of humans adapting to the realities of climate change, you must understand that our species has a very long history of adapting to the demands of harsh environments. However, these adaptations have been less demanding in the past 100 years. Climate change may force our species to once again make dramatic changes in our culture and our daily behaviors. A primary adaptation – one already occurring on a small scale – takes the form of simply using less water. The challenge here is to educate the public about what parts of our culture and daily habits consume the greatest amounts of otherwise **potable** water (meaning water that is safe to drink).

First, let's consider how much water it takes to produce different types of food. As you can easily imagine, meat is the most water-intensive, simply because an animal must be kept alive for months or years (years in the case of beef or pork) before it can be slaughtered and turned into supermarket packages of meat. So, for example, it is estimated that it takes more than 1,800 gallons of water to produce one pound of beef.

it takes more than 1,800 gallons of water to produce one pound of beef

You may be surprised that producing non-meat sources of food and drink also require substantial amounts of water. For example, the cultural tradition of drinking coffee consumes a large amount of water just to grow the beans (it takes more than 1,000 gallons of water to produce 1 gallon of coffee). Growing grapes for making wine is not much better, with nearly

900 gallons of water needed to make a single gallon of wine. Even seemingly simple and whole-some foods require massive amounts of water, such as the nearly 300 gallons it takes to grow what will become 1 gallon of rolled oats sold in a store or the 50 gallons of water needed to produce 1 gallon of cow's milk. It takes just over 50 gallons of water to produce a single egg for your breakfast!

Known as a **water footprint**, the amount of water necessary to produce various foods and drinks provides us with a guide as to how we might better conserve water. This is the critical starting point when it comes to reducing the amount of water we use. It is critical because estimates suggest that at least 80% of the available water in our nation is used for agriculture. Sadly, a great deal of the food produced is not even eaten; thus, a first step to improved water conservation is for people in high-income nations, such as the United States, to begin treating food more respectfully and never to let it go to waste (Water Footprint Calculator, 2022).

If you explore the Water Footprint Calculator just cited, you should be able to quickly arrive at the conclusion featured in the summary report of the website: that animal-based food products leave a much larger water footprint than plant-based food products. A top offender is beef! Beef cattle produce a large amount of the earth's total methane gases. Thus, being a consumer of beef not only exacerbates the methane problem but also leaves a very large water footprint (**Chapter 13** will examine this issue in greater detail).

At this point, you may be pessimistic that humans can make dramatic changes such as giv-ing up beef. If so, your pessimism is well founded. Nonetheless, given that the theme of this chapter is adaptation, it is vital to appreciate the power you have as a consumer. The foods and beverages you buy will shape demand for more of the same product, thereby perpetuating a cycle of what may be a large water footprint or perhaps, after reading this chapter, a cycle of a much smaller water footprint. To emphasize this point, let's consider the following model.

The Demand-Supply-Waste Model

As already noted in this chapter, the collective actions of people can make a difference in how well we adapt to the global water crisis. Ultimately, people are also consumers, and consumers are the market force that shapes industries – including those that expend massive amounts of water. As an example, consider **fracking**. This is a method of forcing either natural gas (i.e., gas for cooking and heating homes) or oil from its ground source of shale (a type of soft rock). Fracking uses water pressure to force either gas or oil to the surface, where it is harvested for consumer purchase. The average fracked well for natural gas consumes about 6 million gallons of water (water that cannot be recycled for human or agricultural use). By contrast, the average fracked well for natural gas consumes less than 2 million gallons of water. So, some quick math tells you that being a consumer of fracked natural gas gives you a water footprint that is approximately three times greater than would occur by being a consumer of fracked oil. And of course, not being a consumer of fracked oil would greatly reduce your water footprint. With this example in mind, let's consider how fracking could be greatly reduced even in the absence of legislative action or regulatory actions.

Figure 12.3 depicts the **demand-supply-waste model**. The gears in this model indicate that the primary driver of waste is consumer demand. Waste in this example, applied to frack-ing, is the huge volume of water that cannot be recycled. Let's think about demand regarding the larger offender: fracking for natural gas. Across America, professional chefs and even mom-and-pop dinners prefer the quality and speed of cooking with natural gas compared to electric stoves/ovens. This preference for quickly cooked food and gourmet dishes that are best made on a gas stovetop is a type of consumer demand that drives supply. Making the adaptation from foods cooked with gas to those cooked with electric heat may be going too far

animal-based food products leave a much larger water footprint than plant-based food products

being a consumer of fracked natural gas gives you a water footprint that is approximately three times greater than would occur by being a consumer of fracked oil

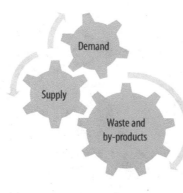

Figure 12.3   The demand-supply-waste model

for some restaurant owners and experienced home chefs; however, this relatively minor adaptation could be something consumers ask for – meaning they demand good foods cooked with clean electric energy rather than natural gas that may have been harvested through the water-intensive process of fracking. For example, as demand declines for new gas stoves for home use (replaced by demand for electric induction stoves), the manufacturing of gas stoves will slow at an equal pace, thereby also slowing the need for – and production of – natural gas. As the total yearly production of fracked natural gas declines, so will the massive waste of water used to make this product.

Current Approaches to Reducing Water Consumption

Although reining in the rampant use of water for agriculture will be the big-ticket item relative to reducing America's water use, several other options are already being implemented in some parts of our country. Three frontiers in this regard are particularly noteworthy.

The first requires a change in American culture. For decades, our culture has revered the idea of neatly groomed suburban lawns. The idea of lush green grass growing densely and cropped neatly seems to be nearly an obsession in the United States. Given their already massive water shortages, a few western cities now incentivize people not to grow grass in their suburban yards. For instance, the city of Los Vegas, NV, and the surrounding communities served by the Southern Nevada Water Authority offer residents and businesses what is known as the Water Smart Landscape Rebate. This program pays people $3 per square foot of grass sod permanently removed and replaced with desert landscape plants and materials (e.g., cacti, rocks, and bark). The water authority notes on its website that the average savings in water is about 825,000 gallons per 15,000 square feet of converted grass lawns. This rebate program began at a time in Nevada's history when the governor had recently signed a bill requiring the removal of decorative grass like that used on residential streets in communities that have a homeowners' association, businesses, highway and road medians, and traffic circles. Before the rebate program, the water authority noted that most water consumption in its service area was used for outdoor watering of greenery. Yes, most of us like to see green grass, trees, and shrubs as we walk, bike, or drive a car; however, this "want" is not helping us keep what we need: a sustainable supply of water for human use.

Second, although you may not have realized it, chances are good that you have visited a city or lived somewhere that restricts the amount of water available for everyday functions such as showering and flushing toilets. More broadly, the U.S. Environmental Protection Agency (EPA) promotes the residential installation of water-conserving innovations like the **WaterSense toilet**. Flushing toilets is the most water-intensive household expenditure of this

the U.S. Environmental Protection Agency (EPA) promotes the residential installation of water-conserving innovations

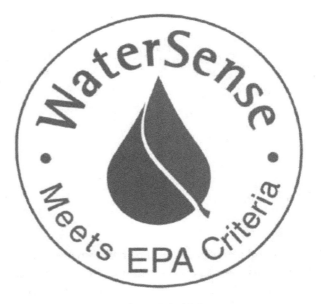

Figure 12.4   Be sure your home or place of residence has toilets with this label
Source: U.S. Environmental Protection Agency.

precious resource (30% of all water use), and WaterSense-labeled toilets (see **Figure 12.4**) are those engineered to greatly reduce the amount of water it takes for one flush. The older generation of toilets used an average of 6 gallons per flush. Conversely, WaterSense-labeled toilets use only 1.28 gallons per flush (even less than the current federal standard of 1.6 gallons per flush). The EPA estimates that these water-conserving toilets can save the average household about 13,000 gallons of water annually. Magnified across the entire United States, the possible savings is 520 billion gallons of water per year (EPA, 2022)!

As suggested by the simplicity of water-conserving toilets, an emerging and critically valuable solution to the global water crisis involves engineering. In a sense, think of this as **public health engineering**. To punctuate the importance of this approach, consider a study conducted by the Water Research Foundation. By randomly selecting 1,000 households and studying their annual water usage, water use behaviors, and use of water-saving devices (e.g., WaterSense-labeled toilets, showerheads that restrict water flow, high-efficiency dishwashers and sinks), the Water Research Foundation found a remarkable 22% decline in average household water use between 1999 and 2016. The most important finding was that this decline occurred because of water-saving devices as opposed to more conscientious use of water by consumers. So, again, you can see that public health is better served by structural changes (in this case, public health engineering) than by changing people's behaviors. One conclusion of the study was that any given household could save 35% of its annual water use by installing 100% of all recommended water-saving devices (DeOreo, Mayer, Dziegielewski, & Kiefer, 2019). Of course, this does not mean public health should give up on promoting human actions that conserve water. In fact, the critical action to promote is the installation of water-saving devices in homes that are not regulated by building codes or in older homes that are exempt from new building codes. Other behavioral-based solutions should not be ignored! For instance, look closely at **Box 12.1** to learn more about how much water can be conserved by not using dishwashing machines.

the critical action to promote is the installation of water-saving devices in homes that are not regulated by building codes

The Importance of Protecting Sources of Potable Water

Despite what average Americans increasingly do to conserve water, a constant counterforce is that some industries still dump waste (including heated water and waste with toxins) into

BOX 12.1. THE HUMAN SIDE: WE REALLY ARE WORLDS APART WHEN IT COMES TO WASTING WATER

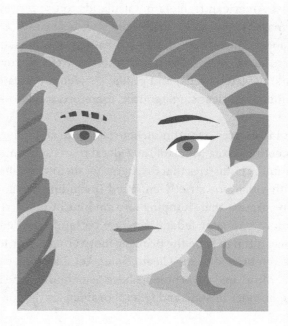

Let's begin with a fictional character: Juanita, a teen female living in an arid part of the world. She spends much of her time tending to family chores, most of which involve some form of cooking and meal preparation. To prepare even a modest meal of rice and beans, she must have at least one to two quarts of potable water. About 1.5 miles from her home is a community water supply. It is used by hundreds of others, and the water is not potable. Juanita uses two one-gallon containers to collect this precious water and carry it home. She strains it through cloth to remove any coarse debris and then lets it sit for most of the day, hoping most of the sediment will sink to the bottom of the containers. Late in the day, she cautiously pours the water from containers into cooking pots, being careful not to also pour any visible sediment. She then boils the collected water (now measuring much less than two gallons) over a hot fire for at least 20 minutes. The water is then suitable for cooking and possibly drinking. Much of her day was consumed by this task.

In another world, three people living in a typical U.S. household consume food and water all day long, leaving their dirty dishes in a sink full of water. In the evening, they wash these dishes in a fairly standard dishwashing machine. It is estimated that most dishwashers (other than a new generation of low-water machines) use between four and nine gallons of water per load. With only three people in the household, the dishwasher is never full, but the small family does not take the time to wash their dishes by hand (a process that may use less than two gallons of water).

What would a person like Juanita think about how a family of three so quickly consumes potable water to save a small amount of effort and time? This "worlds apart" story is important because only about 41% of the human population has reliable access to a supply of potable water. To treat water as a source of life is a stark contrast to areas in the world where water is taken entirely for granted. Ironically, taking water for granted is often not even a recognized part of the culture in a water-secure part of the world – the thought of 59% of all humans struggling for enough water to survive is foreign.

> only about 41% of the human population has reliable access to a supply of potable water

waterways that are used – or could be used – for potable water supplies. Thus, a key aspect of conserving water is to regulate **pollutants** that can be discharged into bodies of water.

Pollutants can take one of two forms when it comes to water contamination: **point sources** and **common sources**. To help you understand the difference, think of two scenarios. The first example is the state of Kentucky, which allows homes abutting some waterways to discharge wastewater (including feces) directly into important water sources, such as the

Kentucky River. When feces, urine (often containing remnants of medication and illicit drugs), and even blood (from menses) are flushed through a pipe directly into a river, that cause of water pollution is clearly identifiable. This is known as a point source. In the second scenario, it is common practice for countless American farmers in farmlands to use fertilizers, manures, herbicides, and pesticides in massive quantities. Especially after heavy rain, the runoff from fields treated with these substances finds its way into streams, rivers, and lakes. It is also common for these agricultural products to find their way into the wells of rural homes, thereby contaminating private drinking water (wells) and public (city/county) water supplies. This type of water pollution does not have a clear single source; therefore, it is known as common source water pollution.

Regardless of whether pollutants are point sources or common sources, state and federal governments have a large role to play in protecting water. Much of the federal role is subsumed by the **Clean Water Act.** This federal law requires industries that discharge waste into a waterway to report the amounts to the EPA, with violations strictly enforced (including possible closure of the business). Of course, it can be argued that dumping any amount of industrial waste into a waterway should be illegal (more stringent federal acts are certainly needed). Unlike fines, however, the fear of lawsuits may ultimately be the primary motivating factor for industries to comply with laws such as those embodied in the Clean Water Act. Lawsuits can also be brought against entire municipalities. Municipal governments have been found to be in violation of the Clean Water Act and a large number of state and federal ordinances that protect the safety of household drinking water.

A classic lawsuit that may favorably shape the future of public health regarding water occurred in the state of Michigan. In 2017, criminal charges were filed in Michigan against state officials involved in the delay and cover-up of a famous public health disaster referred to as the **Flint water crisis.** In 2014, the city of Flint decided to supply households with water drawn from the Flint River rather than continuing to rely on piping water from the Detroit City Water System. The failure of these officials to invest in the mandated treatment of the river water created the crisis, which primarily involved very high levels of lead (as much as 100 times the safe levels established by the EPA) that suddenly appeared in the water in peoples' homes. Lead is a toxin, and its ill effects are especially damaging to the developing brain tissue of young children. The corrosiveness of the untreated river water acted on the outdated lead pipes in these homes to release lead into the water used for cooking, drinking, bathing, brushing teeth, and so on. An estimated 9,000 children were exposed to these extreme levels of lead, and the toll on their mental development is perhaps the most tragic aspect of this highly preventable crisis (see **Figure 12.5**).

Now that you are thinking about pollutants, try to remember the last time you purchased a food or drink product to go. Was it served to you in a Styrofoam container? Also recall the last time you bought groceries or made a purchase at a drugstore. Were the things you bought put in a plastic bag? Most to-go containers are made from a type of plastic, just like plastic bags given out at stores. These and myriad other plastic products form massive amounts of daily trash. Sadly, much of it ends up in waterways. **Box 12.2** describes one of the most pressing public health issues of our time: how plastics in waterways become **microplastics**.

Blood Lead Levels Among Children Aged <6 Years — Flint, Michigan, 2013–2016

Weekly / July 1, 2016 / 65(25)

On June 24, 2016, this report was posted online as an MMWR Early Release.

Chinaro Kennedy, DrPH[1]; Ellen Yard, PhD[2]; Timothy Dignam, PhD[2]; Sharunda Buchanan, PhD[2]; Suzanne Condon, MS[3]; Mary Jean Brown, ScD[2]; Jaime Raymond, MPH[2]; Helen Schurz Rogers, PhD[2]; John Sarisky[2]; Rey de Castro, ScD[1]; Ileana Arias, PhD[1]; Patrick Breysse, PhD[1] (View author affiliations)

Figure 12.5   Each week, the CDC features leading public health news, such as this report about the Flint, Michigan water crisis

BOX 12.2. WHAT ARE MICROPLASTICS ALL ABOUT?

Plastics are a necessary part of our daily lives, but they also have a design flaw: they never decay! So, you can imagine that an issue exists as to what should be done with the massive amounts of plastic waste produced by humans every day. Landfills are, of course, the best answer. Unfortunately, a large percentage of this plastic ends up being discarded into waterways. Just considering the earth's oceans, estimates suggest that about eight million metric tons of plastic waste are dumped into oceans yearly, with 99% of floating ocean debris being some form of plastic. Again, this plastic will never decay. Instead, it breaks apart into progressively smaller and smaller pieces that are ultimately invisible to the eye but still very much present. Thus all plastic waste eventually becomes microplastics.

Measured in nanometers, microplastics are so tiny that fish, marine mammals, and even mollusks (such as mussels and clams) inevitably consume them. In turn, the fish, shellfish, and mollusks that humans harvest and eat equate with the human consumption (albeit indirect) of microplastics. So, why is this a problem? Because beyond the offensive sight of plastic debris floating in waterways and oceans, the eventual human consumption of microplastics has been linked to issues with reproductive health, oxidative stress (an overproduction of cells that can damage the body), toxicity to the human liver, and cellular mutations (Baldwin, Spanjer, Hayhurst, & Hamilton, 2020).

The levels of microplastics in our waterways are expected to greatly increase by 2050. You should be aware that single-use plastics (e.g., Styrofoam cups, candy bar wrappers, bags that hold vegetables together in a grocery store) are the primary culprit when it comes to blatant human lack of action. Ironically, the top offenders of all single-use plastics are water bottles! Because companies have convinced Americans that drinking bottled water is superior to drinking water from their own homes, the market for single-use plastic bottles of water provides approximately 50 billion servings of bottled water to American each year. The irony, of course, is that a large portion of this massive number ends up in waterways and oceans, thus creating microplastic pollution that adds up year after year. It is difficult to imagine even 1 billion of anything the size of a single-use water bottle; the concept of 50 billion yearly staggers and defies the human imagination. It is estimated that about 14 million tons of plastic water bottles are added to the world's oceans each year (Earthday.org, 2022). Keep in mind that the damage keeps accumulating (remember, plastic never fully disintegrates).

If reading this box has made you want to do something positive to prevent microplastic pollution of the foods we harvest from water, the best response you can have is to stop buying products that include single-use plastics.

Solutions Based on the Reuse of Water

Think about potable water as a finite resource. As such, we can either use less of the supply or somehow replace the supply. This section of the chapter addresses how it is increasingly possible to give back to the finite supply. In this section, you will learn that public health engineering is the backbone of this strategy. Three basic options exist:

- Making ocean water into drinking water
- Using greywater wisely, and constructing stormwater recapture systems
- Taxing industries that most affect the needs of water treatment plants

What Is Desalination?

Salt in water creates what is known as saline. Thus, **desalination** is the process of removing salt from water. The approach uses ocean water (which is highly salinated) to create potable water. If the technologies of desalination progress to the point that ocean water can be claimed and reused for potable water, the global water crisis will be somewhat reduced in magnitude.

Desalination can be achieved through distillation or reverse osmosis. Of these two methods, only distillation is used to provide potable water to people in areas of the world with the least rainfall. The concept is relatively simple: it involves heating ocean water and then letting the evaporated water contact cool air so that condensation occurs (this is why grass on a lawn quickly picks up a layer of dew at nightfall). The technology challenge is not so simple: distilling massive amounts of water in an energy-efficient way using an approach that is affordable for even the poorest nations. It is up to your generation to discover technologies that will achieve affordable and massive desalination.

Another method of reclaiming water is focused on conserving potable water by reusing **greywater** for purposes such as flushing toilets, watering vegetable gardens, washing cars, etc. This process is less reliant on technology than it is on plumbing! Yes, you are reading this correctly – the last sentence ended with the word *plumbing*. Greywater is nothing more than water used for showers, baths, dishwashing, washing clothes, food preparation, brushing teeth, etc. Greywater does **not** contain urine or feces.

Most of the current greywater reuse in the United States is designed to provide irrigation for vegetable gardens, lawns, and yard trees. The designs may be as simple as rerouting drains pipes from sinks, showers, and washing machines to empty into an outdoor catchment container that can use gravity (or a small pump) to use this recaptured water for the photosynthesis needed to grow outdoor plants (thus binding carbon). A more sophisticated (and therefore less affordable) design captures greywater inside the home and stores it as a source of fluid for flushing toilets. A drawback to this in-home reuse is that even greywater that looks clean may have contaminates that require a filter before the greywater enters the separate plumbing system used only for toilets. Thus, periodic maintenance and replacement of these filters is a behavioral adaptation that must be made by persons opting to reuse greywater for toilet flushing.

Another method of reusing water involves (once again) public health engineering. This method is based on the premise that rainwater falling in urban areas cannot soak into the ground as it does in rural areas. A negative result of urbanization is that most permeable ground is covered in pavement, concrete, or buildings. Rainwater is left without a purpose or a place to flow. If its flow eventually empties into a waterway, the problem is magnified because the rainwater picks up pollutants along roadways, sidewalks, and rooftops. These pollutants, complete with heavy metals such as lead, then contaminate the potable water in nearby lakes, rivers, and streams.

The solution to this largely urban problem involves both a passive and an active approach. The passive approach is easy enough to understand. This is best exemplified by the city of Seattle, WA and a program known as Green Stormwater Infrastructure (Environmental Protection Agency, 2017). Because city governments have the authority to issue or deny building permits, they can mandate that designated amounts of space be set aside for soil to grow greenery. The city makes and implements plans for the use of these spaces, including planting trees, grasses, and perennial flowers. Because the spaces remain permeable, they allow rainwater to enter the earth and provide the substrate for photosynthesis to grow greenery, thereby binding carbon. The Seattle plan also designates roads with permeable pavement, allowing water rainwater to flow through some roads and thus enter the ground.

The active approach involves engineering and concrete. Again, mandated by zoning regulations and building codes (two very important tools that protect and promote the health and safety of the public), the city requires newly constructed areas to include plans for building and maintaining stormwater drainage systems that ultimately capture even heavy rains and channel the water to treatment facilities. An important observation to make here is that Seattle is one of the most progressive U.S. cities regarding stormwater drainage systems, and thus it can serve as a model for other U.S. cities that will eventually understand and even embrace the need to reuse rainwater.

It is up to your generation to discover technologies that will achieve affordable and massive desalination

periodic maintenance and replacement of these filters is a behavioral adaptation that must be made

Water Treatment Facilities in the United States

Although far from new, a vital public health practice – one that is highly regulated and closely monitored – is reusing residential and industrial water by treating it to remove solids (including human feces), toxic chemicals, pathogens, human urine, and a host of other non-visible substances. Think about this process when you hear somebody say, "government should keep its nose out of our business." The funding of county and municipal water treatment facilities must always be maintained and even enhanced if people want to have adequate supplies of potable water. Again, recall the statement previously cited in this chapter that access to clean water is a fundamental human right. It makes little sense to spend billions on medical care unless we first ensure that sources of disease are removed that might harm people whom medical care would otherwise try to fix.

> The funding of county and municipal water treatment facilities must always be maintained and even enhanced if people want to have adequate supplies of potable water.

City sewage and water treatment is the very origin of public health practice. One of the first water treatment facilities in the United States was constructed in Lowell, MA. This occurred at a time (ca. 1890) when typhoid fever was epidemic and death from this bacterial infection was relatively common. This first attempt at water treatment used sand filters to eliminate typhoid bacteria from treated water.

At the dawn of the 20th century, chlorine was first used to kill water-borne bacteria in Jersey City, NJ. As chlorinating public water supplies became more common, a segment of the population objected because the safety of this chemical was unknown. Then, in 1916, a water treatment plant in Milwaukee, WI, experienced a very brief (seven hours) failure of its chlorination system. Soon afterward, as many as 100,000 consumers of this water experienced severe cases of diarrhea, and approximately 500 new cases of typhoid fever were diagnosed (60 people died as a result). A clear turning point in public support for water treatment facilities was marked by this tragic set of circumstances that nonetheless produced impeccable evidence demonstrating the value of water treatment.

At this time in history, water treatment has become an advanced science. The remaining issue involves the disposal of what is known as **sludge**. Think of sludge as the solid remains of treated water (see **Photo 12.5**). As sewage is filtered, more non-water substances are distilled from their original form. These include remnants of drugs, medications, or hormones that people excrete in their urine. These solids also comprise a host of chemicals used for cleaning, laundry, personal hygiene, hair coloring agents, and a large array of soaps and shampoos that produce microplastics. As an advanced science, the water treatment process now provides the public with a great deal of protection against the spread of infectious diseases by reusing public water. What is lacking is a method of safely disposing of the sludge. This is a public health issue

> At this time in history, water treatment has become an advanced science

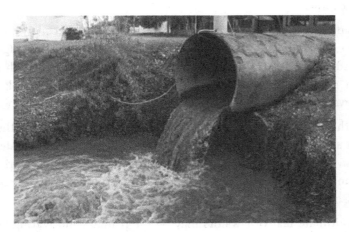

Photo 12.5   Raw sewage will become reclaimed water, with sludge as a by-product.
Source: Vastram / Adobe Stock.

of great importance because federal regulations allow for the use of sludge as fertilizer to grow food consumed by people. The legal use of sludge as an agricultural fertilizer relabels sludge as **biosolid compost**.

Because some of the compounds, chemicals, and substances (particularly hormones) in biosolid compost can easily travel up the food chain (meaning they move from plants to animals and from animals to people), its use in agriculture is a threat to the health of the public (Center for Food Safety, 2022). To punctuate this point, it is important for you to now learn about **persistent organic pollutants** (POPs). These are carbon-based compounds that contaminate the human food and water supply. The word "persistent" is important because POPs never dissolve, dissipate, or disappear! Biosolid compost is a primary source of POPs. At this juncture, it is well worth noting that most POPs enter the food and water supply as industrial waste. For example, regulating the industrial discharge of POPs into waterways remains an ongoing public health challenge, despite the EPA's efforts to enforce the 1974 Safe Drinking Water Act. Again, this is an example of how you, as an informed citizen or resident of the United States, must be aware and willing to participate in regulating the destruction of the food and water supply brought about through the discharge of POPs by industries.

Applying the Four Pillars of Public Health to Protecting Water

In your lifetime, water will become increasingly vital and more valuable. As such, it is likely to become the leading public health issue. Thus, this juncture in the course is an ideal place for you to learn about the four main pillars of public health action:

1. Educate

2. Regulate

3. Legislate

4. Litigate

Each pillar applies nicely to the challenges we face as result of a dwindling supply of potable water. Let's work through one example for each of these four pillars:

1. Before people begin to reuse greywater, public health efforts will have to design and implement massive **education** programs that teach the public about basic options (such as rerouting the drainpipe from a washing machine into an outdoor garden or installing a greywater system that is used for flushing toilets). To make a difference, these education-based efforts cannot be small or confined to selected communities; they must be large-scale and widespread.

2. California's Safe and Affordable Drinking Water Fund is an excellent example of how we (meaning "We the People") can conserve water via **regulation**. Taxing the water use of businesses and industries is similar in principle to other public health actions you have learned from reading this textbook, such as taxing tobacco, alcohol, and even sugar-sweetened beverages.

3. Passing laws that incur criminal and/or civil liability to those breaking them is a third vital public health action. Just two years before the passage of the 1974 Safe Drinking Water Act, the Clean Water Act was passed and mandated by law. Fifty years later, the United States has found that this legislation has made a tremendous difference relative to regulating what is discharged into public waterways.

4. Ultimately, legitimate fear of lawsuits may be the primary motivating factor for municipalities, businesses, and industry to comply with laws such as those embodied in the Clean

Water Act. For instance (and as previously noted in this chapter), in 2017, criminal charges were filed in Michigan against the state officials involved in the delay and cover-up of the Flint water crisis (via lead).

Although these four pillars have served public health quite well in the past, a key challenge regarding the global water crisis is to recognize that the root of the problem (i.e., climate change) will constantly exacerbate it. Thus, a race will occur between humans and the ever-dwindling water supplies on earth – a race that must be won by humans dedicated to making the necessary adaptations to survive. These adaptations will require change and personal sacrifice. But change can be a good thing, right? Each new generation makes changes from the previous generation – for example, it would be odd if the Rolling Stones (cited for the quote that opened this chapter) remained a favorite rock group of your generation. In much the same way that music cultures change, our culture must change relative to how we conserve and reuse water.

Key Terms and Review

In many respects, this chapter represents a set of urgent priorities for each of us who inhabit the planet. A theme in the chapter is that humans must be willing to adapt to a series of harsh realities brought about by climate change. The necessary adaptation regarding water may be the most formidable. Think about your **water footprint** as a case in point. Much like a **carbon** or **methane** footprint (i.e., how much **carbon** and **methane** you indirectly produce in one day), the question to always ask yourself is, "How much water does it take to support one day of my life?" With water being such a central part of daily life, especially in the United States, it will be important that public health education, regulation, legislation, and even litigation become the common **four-pillar** approach to water conservation and reuse.

The cautionary note at the end of this chapter is critical for you to understand and embrace. We cannot ignore the reality that climate change is moving ahead without apparent slowing. To help keep pace with the expanding water crisis, people must reduce their **carbon (and methane) footprint**. From reading this chapter, you now know that plants (especially trees) bind carbon. Carbon is released through burning; this is a type of **reverse photosynthesis**. The release of carbon and methane gases is causing the planet to warm – this is known as the **greenhouse effect**. This warming is directly responsible for the steady decline in annual rainfall and snowfall (with **snowpack** measurements dropping each passing year).

Despite the clear loss of water from the planet, humans continue to waste this resource. **Fracking**, for instance, uses tremendous amounts of water to pump natural gas from the ground (gas that is then a primary source of methane release). As long as people continue to prefer natural gas to clean energy (or even green energy), that demand drives the need for increasing the supply, and the increase in supply adds more and more to the greenhouse effect. Thus, you should fully appreciate how the **demand-supply-waste model** applies to the water crisis in particular and to public health more broadly.

The chapter provided you with a considerable focus on methods of conserving water. For example, you learned that **WaterSense**-labeled toilets use only 1.28 gallons per flush. The innovation of high-efficiency toilets is just one example of how **public health engineering** can be used to conserve even more water. Another case in point is redesigning household fixtures such as showerheads, dishwashers, and washing machines for laundry.

Reusing water is increasingly an efficient public health engineering response to the water crisis. Paramount among these methods is the reuse of **greywater**. Unlike **desalination**, the systems for affordable water reuse are already created relative to greywater. The next step is to create widespread adoption of these systems via social movements that endorse this form of water protection. Ultimately, however, regulations, legislation, and even litigation will help us build and maintain progressively more effective water treatment systems. Despite their technological advances, water treatment plants cannot remove microplastics from water, and they cannot remove a host of other pollutants that must also be regulated. **Point source** pollutants are highly identifiable (such as lead during the **Flint water crisis**). Conversely, **common source** pollutants are hard to trace back to a specific cause. With either type of pollutant, legislation such as the **Clean Water Act** must be kept in place, updated, and constantly enforced. This is especially applicable to industries that deposit **persistent organic pollutants** into our public waterways.

A central challenge for the future (and this one is owned by your generation) will be how to safely dispose of **sludge**. Clearly, the current solution to call sludge **biosolid compost** and allow its use for producing animal and plant products that become part of the human food chain is not a responsible action. Controlling this problem will require more intense regulation and legislation from our federal government. As a high-income nation, we also have a high price to pay for the privilege of being part of the 41% of the human species with adequate supplies of **potable** water. Part of that price is a willingness to impose regulations and enforce laws on our American industries.

For Practice and Class Discussion

Practice Questions

1. A natural form of annual water storage takes the form of:
   a. Snowpack
   b. Greywater reuse systems
   c. Desalination systems
   d. Potable greenhouse effects

2. Which human action leaves the largest water footprint?
   a. Eating a serving of oatmeal
   b. Eating beef
   c. Consuming organic vegetables as an entire meal
   d. Drinking a glass of wine

3. Which human adaptation would most reduce the amount of methane gas entering the atmosphere and also conserve water?
   a. Less use of gasoline-powered cars
   b. Using electric heat and ovens rather than heating and cooking with natural gas
   c. Reusing greywater for vegetable gardens
   d. Enforcing the Clean Water Act such that all industries must fully comply

4. Which term represents the **least** advanced technology for adapting to the water crisis at this time in history?
   a. Fracking
   b. Public health engineering
   c. Desalination
   d. Reverse photosynthesis

5. The Flint water crisis was mostly a problem caused by a heavy metal: lead. The contamination of water with excess heavy metals also comes from:
   a. Stormwater that enters treatment plants
   b. Acid rain

    c.   Greywater recapture and use

    d.   Microplastics

6. A large industry located on the banks of the Ohio River produces soaps and other products that all contain POPs. The company was fined for dumping some of its industrial run-off into the river. The POPs will:

    a.   Ultimately dissolve and thus become harmless to humans

    b.   Be completely removed from any water used for humans when it is processed at water treatment plants

    c.   Enter the food chain via the use of this water for agriculture

7. The industry described in Question 6 is an example of:

    a.   Point source pollution

    b.   Common source pollution

    c.   Microplastic poisoning

    d.   The need for improved public health engineering

8. Building codes are used to conserve water! The best example listed here is:

    a.   Mandating the use of WaterSense-labeled toilets

    b.   Offering incentives for people to install greywater recapture systems

    c.   Using green space to reduce the amount of stormwater running into streets

    d.   Calculating the average water footprint of a newly constructed home

9. The Johnson family has owned and operated a 2,000-acre cattle ranch in Utah for more than 100 years. None of the family members ski or care about snow-related recreation activities. However, every year they measure the snowpack depth in the Colorado Rockies. Why?

    a.   Snowpack in the Colorado Rockies supplies the Colorado River with most of its water. The river, in turn, supplies water to much of the southwestern United States, including parts of Utah.

    b.   Snowpack is an organic pollutant that may carry heavy metals into waterways that eventually are used to provide water to the family's cattle. This creates beef that will not pass standards setting limits on heavy metals in human food.

10. Sludge is a solid substance that the Clean Water Act mandates must be safely disposed of in state-operated landfills.

    a.   True

    b.   False

Discussion Questions

11. One of the cited sources for this chapter is a fact sheet posted by Earthday.org. Read this fact sheet carefully. As you do, think about how you would explain the statements expressed in millions and billions to a young child who does not comprehend how massive 1 million plastic bottles are (let alone 1 billion). Try to come up with your own version of this fact sheet – one that could be used to teach elementary school students about the need to stop the habit of buying single-use plastics. Be sure that your fact sheet emphasizes (in a very simple way) the point that microplastics are entering the food chain in progressively greater quantities.

12. As part of this chapter, you learned about the IPCC. Since the time of writing and publishing this textbook (2022), it is quite likely that climate change has progressed as predicted, or even faster than predicted, in 2022. The task is to go to the IPCC website and

read a summary of the most recent synthesis report. Then, write a one- to two-page paper that captures your reactions to the report. Post this for class discussion.

13.   Now that you understand what is meant by a water footprint, try estimating your own water footprint for just the water coming into your home for your needs (this does not count the water needed to grow the food you eat that day or frack the natural gas used to keep you warm, for example). Do this for one typical day in your life. So, from the time you wake up until the time you go to bed, keep track of all water use: for example, how many times did you flush a toilet, and how many gallons does the toilet use for each flush? Did you run a dishwasher, and if so, how much water does it use for one cycle? Did you shower, and if so, how many gallons per minute are used by your showerhead? Keep a diary of this water use throughout the day, and post it (with your estimated total usage) to an online source that other people taking this course can also view. After most students have made their postings, take a look at the totals and react by posting your thoughts for others to read.

References

Baldwin, A.K., Spanjer, A.R., Hayhurst, B., & Hamilton, D. (2020). Microplastics in the Delaware River, 2018: U.S. Geological Survey data release. https://doi.org/10.5066/P9QVIVX3

Center for Food Safety (2022). What is sewage sludge? https://www.centerforfoodsafety.org/issues/1050/sewage-sludge/regulation

DeOreo, W. B., Mayer, P., Dziegielewski, B., & Kiefer, J. (2019). Residential end users of water, Version 2, Executive report. Water Research Foundation. https://perma.cc/33LV-VC7M

Earthday.org (n.d.). Fact sheet: Single use plastics. https://www.earthday.org/fact-sheet-single-use-plastics/

Environmental Protection Agency (2017). Expanding the benefits of Seattle's green stormwater infrastructure. EPA 832-R-16-011. https://www.epa.gov/sites/default/files/2017-03/documents/seattle_technical_assistance_010517_combined_508.pdf

Environmental Protection Agency (2022). Fact sheet: WaterSense labeled toilets. https://www.epa.gov/sites/default/files/2017-01/documents/ws-products-factsheet-toilets_0.pdf

Intergovernmental Panel on Climate Change (2022). Synthesis report: Climate change 2022. https://www.ipcc.ch/report/sixth-assessment-report-cycle/

Siirilla-Woodburn, E. R., Rhoades, A. M., Hatchett, B. J., et al. (2021). A low-to-no snow future and its impacts on water resources in the Western United States. *Nature Reviews Earth and Environment, 2*, 800–819.

Water Footprint Calculator (2022). Food's big water footprint. https://www.watercalculator.org/footprint/foods-big-water-footprint/

CHAPTER 13

CLIMATE CHANGE: IMPLICATIONS REGARDING FOOD

There are people in the world so hungry, that God cannot appear to them except in the form of bread.

—*Mahatma Gandhi*

Overview

As you learned in **Chapter 12**, water is quickly becoming a scarce commodity around the world and in many parts of the United States. That same lesson also applies to the topic of this chapter: food. Even before the economic upheaval caused by COVID-19, agencies such as **Feeding America** generated estimates suggesting that about 12% of all Americans experience hunger on a daily basis (Feeding America, 2021). This is, of course, an average; that percentage ranges up to one-quarter of the population in states such as Mississippi.

It is unlikely that the true experience of hunger has ever occurred for most people reading this book. Fasting and the experience of hunger are not equivalent. If you have ever fasted, you may have felt a physical need to eat, but psychologically you were not left with no idea how – or when – you would eat again. When a person does not have enough food to keep up with the basic caloric demands of everyday living, their weight begins to drop daily. Once the body has burned all available fatty tissue for its basic energy requirements (i.e., energy to keep the heart beating, the lungs working, and the kidneys, liver, and other vital organs functional), it begins to burn protein for its basic fuel. Protein is available to the body in the form of tissues such as those forming skeletal muscle, blood, and lymphocytes (these are a basic part of the immune system), as well as vital organs – including cardiac muscle. Before the body sacrifices its ability to keep the heart beating, the immune system will be so dramatically compromised that most people who starve to death actually die of common forms of infectious disease. An organization known as **The World Counts** has created a stark summary for you to think about as you study this chapter: "Around 9 million people die every year of hunger and hunger-related diseases. This is more than from AIDS, malaria, and tuberculosis combined" (The World Counts, 2022).

Broadly known as **food insecurity**, this is perhaps the second most fundamental aspect of public health (with water being the first). The need for food takes

LEARNING OBJECTIVES

- Understand the urgency of solving the ever-expanding problem of food insecurity in America.

- Define the macro-level influences that must be addressed to reduce climate change.

- Understand and explain the point that climate change–induced food shortages are a threat to health equity in the United States.

- Explain how the global food crisis is both a cause and a consequence of climate change.

- Delineate and describe the change model known as diffusion of innovations, and apply it to American farming practices.

- Fully embrace the concept that small daily changes can have a profound impact on reducing climate change and increasing health equity in the United States.

- Understand that a plant-based diet provides ample protein and is part of controlling climate change.

Understanding the Science and Practice of Public Health, First Edition. Richard Crosby.
© 2023 John Wiley & Sons, Inc. Published 2023 by John Wiley & Sons, Inc.

precedence over most other human needs, including almost all desire a person may have to prevent disease or protect themselves from harm that may occur in the future. Among children, food insecurity has been clearly linked to learning disabilities. Moreover, as a nation becomes increasingly food insecure, so does its political stability. Thus, in many ways, the issue of food insecurity transcends public health to extend to the general welfare of society.

To provide a bit of symmetry with **Chapter 12**, this chapter will also give you more background on climate change and the somewhat faltering response of the U.S. government to its causes. This background is vital to understand, given that nearly all of the consequences of climate change will vastly increase the already high levels of health disparities in the nation. Climate change may become the most substantial driver of health disparities (with food insecurity being the top form of disparity).

As part of the larger mosaic of a public approach to food insecurity, this chapter also provides more information about the causes of climate change. Unlike water, food is an indirect cause of climate change. When it comes to animal-based foods, much of what we choose to consume adversely affects our climate via carbon and methane release. The level of adaptation needed to overcome the deeply ingrained cultural habits of constantly consuming animal-based foods is a focal point of this chapter. From a much broader perspective, it is also incumbent on America's farmers to make adaptations to move toward plant-based food systems. Therefore, this chapter will also introduce you to a model of change that can be applied nicely to the challenge of helping farmers make the needed adaptations.

This chapter will ultimately lead you back to a similar point made in **Chapter 12**. That key point applies broadly to public health; however, it fits this chapter perfectly: it is the small changes we make on a daily basis that matter the most. Ironically, when humans shift to plant-based diets, we will see not only a drop in carbon and methane release but also a greater abundance of food. A concluding point of this chapter is that all of us must work tirelessly to increase the food supply. By doing so, the growing chasm between the wealthy and poor in the United States will no longer be exacerbated by egregious differences in access to enough food to live, think, work, and stay healthy.

Food Insecurity in America

Although estimates vary based on the source, it is fair to say that about 41 million people go to bed hungry each night in this nation. As a so-called "super power," we are clearly neglecting the most basic public health need of these people. This astonishing and appalling figure includes one of every six children living in the United States. Given the rapid development of the brain in the first several years of life, malnutrition during early childhood has long-term repercussions for the mental capacity of millions as they grow into adulthood. Given that the average cost of a meal in the United States has been estimated at just over $3.00 (Feeding America, 2021), this is a public health problem that is within reach of economic solutions.

According to the landmark federal publication *Healthy People 2030*, poverty is the most common cause of food insecurity (CDC, 2022). As income levels across a population decline, so does the level of nutrition. Thus, food insecurity exists at various levels. The least severe is known simply as **food insecurity**, meaning ongoing and reliable access to nutritious food is absent. The key word in this definition is **nutritious**. Foods such as noodles, rice, bread, and corn products are plentiful in the United States and therefore very affordable, even for people living at income levels classified far below poverty. However, a steady diet of these grain-based, highly processed foods has been linked to a long list of chronic diseases and associated with decreased immune functions that consequently predispose people to infectious diseases.

The next and more severe level is **very low food security**. At this level, access to nutritious food is sporadic at best. The most severe level is often termed **food insecurity with hunger**.

Among children, food insecurity has been clearly linked to learning disabilities

it is the small changes we make on a daily basis that matter the most

about 41 million people go to bed hungry each night in this nation

At this level, poverty is typically extreme, and people are not consuming enough calories (regardless of the nutritional value of those calories) to maintain body weight. It is this level that is a rectifiable economic problem. For instance, one estimate suggests that the state of Mississippi (which has the largest hunger problem in America) could resolve this crisis with an influx of approximately $300 million per year (Nguyen, Cafer, & Deleveaux, 2021). Although this amount of money may seem large to you, consider that it is actually very small in comparison to the huge sums the federal government spends annually for non-crisis issues such as the exploration of space, expanding the U.S. Department of Defense, and repairing highways. As this chapter proceeds, however, you will see that the emerging public health solutions to food insecurity in America do not simply rely on hope for federal spending.

Macro-Level Influences Leading to Climate Change

A key theme of this chapter is that our food choices may be both a cause of climate change (when meats and other animal-based food products dominate the market) and an adaptation to help slow climate change (when plants are consumed directly by humans rather than first being fed to animals). The social and economic structures that drive our food choices can best be thought about as **macro-level influences** on behavior. As opposed to a term such as **micro level** (which applies to personal influences), **macro level** represents societal structures far beyond personal control. For example, you have probably seen advertising from the beef industry, such as "Beef – It's What's for Dinner." In addition to the way advertising shapes American food habits, the economic structure of price has a tremendous macro-level influence on our food choices. For instance, it is cheaper to buy a fast-food hamburger than a salad (and the hamburger provides a far greater number of calories and protein). Eventually, our food habits become part of American culture, and people go with the flow and select foods from a limited list of options – most of which are animal-based products.

As the earth continues to warm and water becomes increasingly scarce, the ability of farmers to easily grow a diverse set of crops is diminished. Unlike people, plants cannot make adaptations, so their one-time abundance can quickly disappear. To be clear, all food consumed by humans begins as various species of plants. Historically, people lived solely on a plant-based diet, with meat used as a method of subsistence only during winter months. As the Industrial Age reached full capacity, Americans (as well as citizens of other high-income nations) began to eat meat and other animal-based foods regularly, all year. As **omnivores**, humans can survive on either plants, which provide nutrients on a direct basis, or animal-based foods, which provide plant-based nutrients on an indirect basis (i.e., the plants are converted to animal tissue and animal milk, which is then consumed by humans). Keeping in mind that plants are increasingly less abundant, the issue of climate change now forces humans to conserve the food supply as much as possible. So, the question you must ask yourself becomes, "Is the process of consuming plants that have been converted to animal products efficient?" To answer this question, it is important to understand **feed conversion ratios**.

all food consumed by humans begins as various species of plants.

Feed Conversion Ratios

Consider this quote from a well-known author and activist regarding food security and climate change:

> Assume we have one acre of fertile land. We can use this acre to grow a high-protein plant food, like peas or beans. If we do this, we will get between 300 and 500 lbs of protein from our acre. Alternatively, we can use our acre to grow a crop that we feed to animals, and then kill and eat the animals. Then we will end up with between 40 and

Table 13.1   Feed conversion ratios (based on the edible weight of the animal)

Animal	% return in calories	% return in protein
Chickens	11	20
Pigs	10	15
Beef cattle	1	4

55 lbs of protein from our one acre. Most estimates conclude that plant foods yield about ten times as much protein per acre as meat does. (Singer, 1990)

eating plants directly yields 10 times more protein than eating animal tissues and milk.

The quote gives you an easy-to-remember rule of thumb: eating plants directly yields 10 times more protein than eating animal tissues and milk. Because protein is typically the limiting factor in ensuring adequate human nutrition, this rule of thumb is well worth remembering as climate change exacerbates the limitations of the food supply. Of course, the 10-to-1 rule is an average. Thus, the task for you is to understand which foods are least and most inefficiently converted into usable protein by the human body. This level of efficiency is known as a **feed conversion ratio**; however, it has also been suggested that the term **conversion inefficacy ratio** is more descriptive because no type of meat comes close to a reasonably efficient conversion of either total calories (i.e., the total fat, carbohydrate, and protein calories in a meat product) or protein-derived calories). **Table 13.1** provides a basic set of ratios for the most commonly consumed meats.

As you can quickly see from this table, eating beef or beef products is by far the most inefficient use of plants. For example, if the unit of measure is pounds, it takes 100 pounds of grain and/or grass to put 1 pound of edible beef on your dining room table. Had that same amount of grain been used as bread, pasta, or other foods directly consumed by humans, the earth would not have lost 99% of the usable energy gained from direct consumption versus the indirect consumption of beef. Another way to think about it is that humans use cattle to convert products like wheat and corn into a culturally cherished food such as a hamburger. The cattle become what is best described as a highly inefficient system of feeding people. **Table 13.1** also shows that chicken and pork products end up on your dinner table at a huge expense to the earth compared to consuming plant-based foods directly.

What feed conversion ratios do **not** provide is a metric for the cost to the earth relative to the carbon/methane footprint of these foods. Because cattle emit copious amounts of methane and take longer to mature to slaughter, the human love for beef creates a major portion of the atmospheric gases causing climate change to continually escalate. A take-home point here is that if humans insist on eating meat, they should choose chicken or pork and sacrifice beef in service of adapting to climate change and responding optimally to the global food crisis. Yet it is estimated that about 55 pounds of beef are consumed annually, on a per capita basis, in the United States. The term **per capita** means "per person"; thus this average of 55 pounds is an underestimate if, instead, the rate is calculated on a "per beef consumer" basis. Clearly (and despite the demands of climate change and the global food crisis), the beef industry continues to thrive in America (see **Photo 13.1**). Ironically, one key reason why this industry continues to thrive is based on the concept of **subsidies** (see **Chapter 6** for a review of this term).

Under the Trump administration – in just the two years of 2019 and 2020 – American farmers producing livestock (primarily cattle and dairy cows) received more than $14 billion in federal subsidies, as administered by the U.S. Department of Agriculture (Faber & Schechinger, 2022). Although the amounts have been reduced, these subsidies continue to be paid to farmers. This places the U.S. government in a position of directly supporting an industry consistently ranked as a top offender relative to the release of carbon and methane as greenhouse

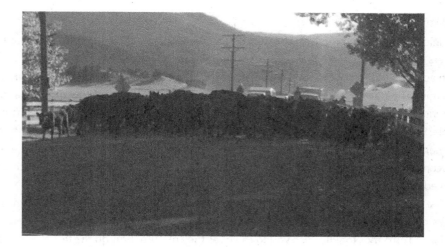

Photo 13.1   Cattle ranches of 1,000 acres or more are common in the United States.

gases accelerating the pace of climate change. (As you read this chapter, you will learn more about methane and its release from dairy cows; see **Box 13.1**.) These funds could be used for proactive approaches to slowing climate change, and their use for supporting American cattle and dairy farmers has been widely criticized by organizations determined to slow climate change (Faber & Schechinger, 2022).

BOX 13.1. GOT MILK?

Unfortunately, most people base their food choices on culture rather than science. Think about your own food choices: were they learned, or are they the result of reading summaries of science-based studies regarding food and human nutrition? Or ask yourself, "Why do I eat what I eat?" Is it because it was the food you were raised on as a child? Is it because it's easy to find in almost any store or corner restaurant? Is it because everyone else eats the same thing? As climate change escalates and food supplies – by necessity – shift from animal-based to plant-based, it will be vital for you to reimagine your food choices.

   Milk is a great example (**Photo 13.2**)! Today, you can buy milk made from nuts, hemp, and even oats. Yet most people continue to follow cultural habits and consume milk that comes from cows. But do you think most people truly understand the poor **protein conversion ratio** of milk? Similar to the feed conversion ratio, this is the ratio of converted protein relative to the amount of protein consumed by the animal in question. For cow's milk, every 1 gram of plant protein fed to a dairy

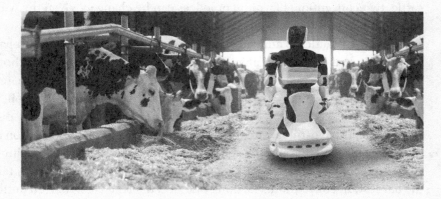

Photo 13.2   Dairy cows are the source of milk, cheese, butter, yogurt, and ice cream – is it worth the cost to our planet?
Source: scharfsinn86 / Adobe Stock.

cow yields .24 grams of protein in the milk that is then consumed by humans. So, about three-quarters of the protein is lost in the process of converting plant protein to milk protein.

In addition to the poor protein conversion ratio, it is important to understand the nature of cow's milk. The dairy industry is very guarded about the reputation of this product and produces videos that provide a somewhat less-than-accurate version of how milk goes from farm to table. Similarly, people in the vegan movement and those involved with People for the Ethical Treatment of Animals (PETA) produce less-than-accurate videos that give the public a worst-case scenario regarding how milk goes from farm to table. So, this box provides you with a more balanced description.

First, you need to know that cow's milk is the ideal nutrition for a calf! The milks comes from a series of mammary glands in the mother cow and contains a mixture of hormones, blood plasma, and enzymes that nourish young calves as they mature through the first few months of life. These substances are, of course, not meant for humans, so issues arise as to the risks of consuming cow's milk. For instance, a substance known as C-reactive protein is relatively abundant in milk, but human consumption of it has been linked to inflammation and an increased risk of metabolic syndrome (see **Chapter 5**) (Haug, Hustmark, & Harstad, 2007).

Milk and its numerous products are tightly linked to a great deal of American culture. For instance, it is likely that many of you reading this consumed milk as your only source of food after you were born. Nearly one-half of all U.S. infants are bottle-fed cow's milk (as opposed to milk from human mammary glands) for at least the first six months of life. America's dairy industry has cultivated a stellar reputation for milk as being wholesome. Given its backing by this industry, it would seem almost un-American to be critical of milk and its products. But the average dairy cow emits about 220 pounds of methane per year, and that gas is 28 times more potent than carbon dioxide relative to its destructive effect on our planet (Quinton, 2019).

Conventional Farming Practices

Although plant-based foods are much more earth-friendly, it is important to understand a second macro-level influence on climate change: conventional farming. **Conventional farming practices** have led to over-use of the land that is exacerbated by a lack of rainfall. Unless these practices change – particularly the use of land for grazing cattle– our ability to grow plant-based foods consumed directly by humans will continue to dwindle. Beyond the issue of cattle, two conventional farming practices can be changed, given the willingness of American farmers to do so: plowing and cover crops.

The first practice is annually **plowing** (i.e., tilling) farmland to prepare it for spring planting. Plowing releases huge amounts of carbon from the soil (see **Photo 13.3**): carbon that otherwise would remain in the soil to help retain water. One estimate suggests that no-till farming practices could greatly increase the water capacity of the soil, with an approximate gain of 40,000 gallons for every 1% increase in carbon that is not distributed by plowing (Cosiers, 2019). No-till farming practices also equate with the retention of microorganisms in the soil, leading to more fertile soil with a greater ability to grow nutritious foods.

The second practice involves an economic shortcut that farmers take each fall following the harvest. In conventional farming practice, the land is left barren until spring. An emerging alternative that protects the world's precious and limited supply of topsoil is planting **cover crops** following the fall harvest. Cover crops are generally hearty grains that can withstand late fall frosts and thus germinate (i.e., grow) before winter brings daily freezing temperatures.

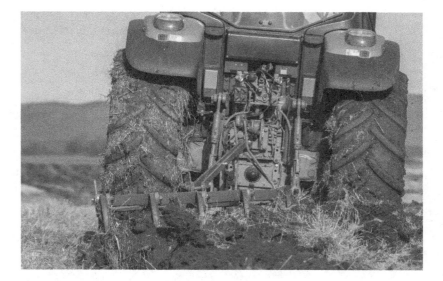

Photo 13.3   Farmers plow millions of acres annually, releasing large volumes of carbon.
Source: Kalina Georgieva / Adobe Stock.

Crops such as buckwheat, rye, and winter wheat are popular options for ground cover until spring planting occurs. The cover crops physically protect the topsoil from erosion (caused by heavy rainfalls and high winds) and also serve as a source of added **nitrogen** in the soil. Nitrogen is vital because it is the one ingredient of soil that produces protein in the foods humans consume. Plants such as peas (see **Photo 13.4**) take nitrogen from the soil and convert it into edible protein for humans. Given that at least one estimate suggests our world could be nearly depleted of topsoil and its precious nitrogen by 2080 (Cosiers, 2019), it is important that farmers in America and worldwide adopt no-till practices and plant annual winter cover crops.

> Nitrogen is vital because it is the one ingredient of soil that produces protein in the foods humans consume

Pollination of Plants

One last macro-level influence that warrants attention is the growing problem of insufficient insects (especially bees) to pollinate plants so those plants can produce the fruits and vegetables that sustain our health. Known as **pollinators**, the insects (again, mostly bees) that carry pollen between the male and female parts of plants are critical to the global food supply. Bees, for instance, pollinate approximately one-quarter of the global supply of directly consumed plant-based foods (see **Photo 13.5**). Recent dramatic declines in pollinators, especially bees, can be attributed to extreme temperatures caused by climate change, the sadly quickening pace of deforestation (discussed later in the chapter), and the common use of agricultural pesticides. The one type of pesticide ingredient that has been primarily implicated in the declining bee population is a class of chemical compounds known as **neonicotinoids**. Despite copious evidence of neonicotinoids destroying the U.S. bee population, this class of chemicals has yet to be regulated by the **Environmental Protection Agency** (EPA). So, once again, as part of "We the People," one of your civic obligations is to at least question why the EPA has failed in its responsibility to help protect the food supply by allowing the use of neonicotinoids.

> one of your civic obligations is to at least question why the EPA has failed in its responsibility to help protect the food supply by allowing the use of neonicotinoids

Noteworthy at this point in the chapter is that on the last day of June 2022, the U.S. Supreme Court ruled that the EPA does not have the authority to regulate carbon emissions and other damaging emissions that stem from industries (see **Figure 13.1**) This ruling figuratively took the teeth out of the EPA and opened the way for industries to have extremely large carbon footprints, as opposed to the once widely held goal of becoming carbon neutral. As you have probably also surmised, this ruling also will be applied to other regulatory actions of the EPA,

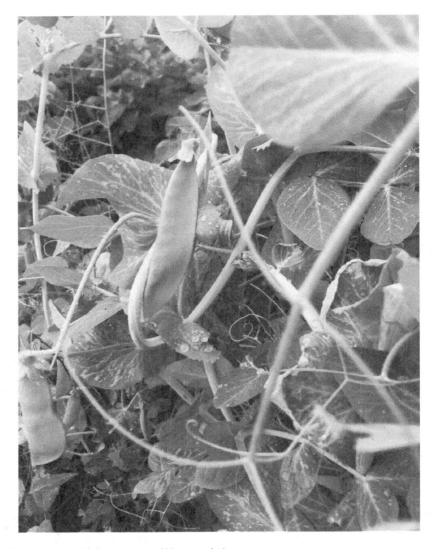

Photo 13.4   Plants such as peas "fix" nitrogen into edible protein for humans.

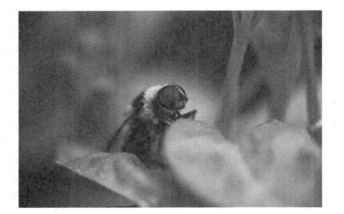

Photo 13.5   Bees give us food!

including any future efforts to eliminate the use of neonicotinoids. An informed electorate (i.e., members of the voting population in the United States) is perhaps the single most important counterforce to the numerous issues that collectively will lead to the continued depletion of our food supply. Stated differently, one of your obligations is to be proactive at the voting polls,

E.P.A. Ruling Is Milestone in Long Pushback to Regulation of Business

The decision created greater opportunities for business interests to challenge regulations, reflecting conservative legal theories developed to rein in administrative agencies.

Figure 13.1   In 2022, America's progress toward slowing climate change was altered by the U.S. Supreme Court
Source: Savage (2022).

thereby creating a backlash effect to Supreme Court decisions such as the one featured in **Figure 13.1**.

Climate Change–Induced Food Shortages Create Health Disparities

The simple economic principle of supply and demand means that as food becomes scarce, its price increases. This does not translate broadly into a lack of food for economically marginalized people. But it does translate into a divide in the quality of food consumed. Think back for a moment to **Chapters 5 and 6** – chapters that taught you several reasons why eating largely unprocessed foods (e.g., fresh produce) is necessary to avoid heart disease and cancer. The food industry will always manufacture highly processed foods (e.g., pasta, canned vegetables, and foods primarily constructed around sugar) that remain affordable to most people and thus relieve hunger and resolve food insecurity. As you know, however, the difference in quality between fresh foods and highly processed foods equates with a difference in the risk of chronic health issues such as metabolic syndrome, diabetes, hypertension, and obesity. Thus, in many ways, America is experiencing a food divide driven by income. As always, an example is helpful.

Let's assume that the basic public health agenda of consuming fresh foods rather than processed foods becomes a panacea in the United States (meaning it is embraced by everyone as the road to health). Now, keeping in mind that many highly processed foods can be purchased cheaply in America (e.g., canned beans, white rice, cookies, noodles, and hamburgers at fast food chains), consider a study conducted between 2019 and 2021 that derived average price increases for selected fresh foods (see **Table 13.2**).

As you might already know from experience, or as you can garner by studying **Table 13.2**, America's food divide is more than an academic theory. This divide is consistent with an unfortunate theme you have seen in nearly every chapter of this textbook: our health inequities

Table 13.2   Average percent price increase of selected foods, 2019–2021

Food product	Percent increase in price
Broccoli	141.3
Granny Smith apples	42.3
One gallon of milk	34.7
Skinless chicken breast	43.8
Cottage cheese	32.9
Red onions	10.5
Sweet onions	11.9
Russet potatoes	14.1

Source: Adapted from McNair, 2021.

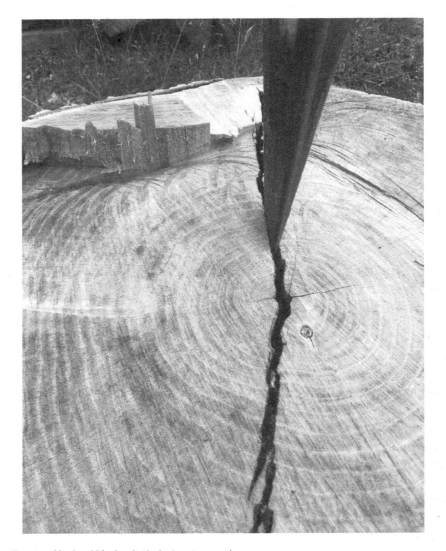

Photo 13.6   The price of food could further divide the American people.

our health inequities continue to expand, leaving millions of people at-risk – mostly those of Black race and/or Latinx ethnicity

continue to expand, leaving millions of people at-risk – mostly those of Black race and/or Latinx ethnicity. Of all the public health issues that appear to be driving a wedge (see **Photo 13.6**) deeper and deeper into the health of Americans, the forces of climate change will most likely make food the one issue that may someday become the primary factor that makes or breaks any one person's health. People who can afford a consistent diet of fresh foods will prosper in comparison to those forced to consume their calories in the form of highly processed foods. This will further expand the already severe health disparities relative to the most common chronic diseases in the United States. Just in case you may be reading this as "then people who have higher incomes will not be impacted," let's take a few minutes to consider the high costs of treating disease as compared to preventing disease.

For every person who goes through much of life consuming highly processed foods, the entire U.S. healthcare system becomes a fallback position to avert death and disability. Given the excessive outlay of money for both the Medicaid and Medicare systems in the United States, absorbing some of the costs of fresh food by providing vouchers to those with low incomes would be a wise investment by the federal government. This is already occurring to a small degree through the federal **Supplemental Nutrition Assistance Program** (SNAP). But as forward-thinking as SNAP is, it is heavily focused on providing low-income families with

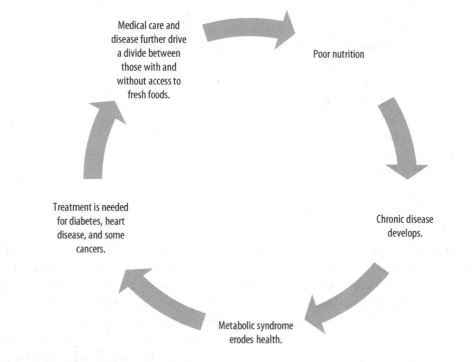

Figure 13.2   A cycle of dependence on costly medical care

adequate calories as opposed to a diet that is less focused on highly processed foods. This, of course, could be easily altered in the future because SNAP is tied to a debit card that can also be linked to bar codes on food products, thereby allowing and disallowing purchases based on nutrition science in the context of disease prevention. Barring this level of innovation, the current wedge that is separating the income classes in the United States into those who can and cannot avail themselves of a steady diet of health-protective foods will continue to feed a cycle of chronic diseases costing the U.S. economy an ever-increasing amount of the gross domestic product. Climate change will accelerate the cycle that continually misses the chance to save billions of dollars by averting chronic diseases. **Figure 13.2** provides a visual illustration of this cycle.

Climate change will accelerate the cycle that continually misses the chance to save billions of dollars by averting chronic diseases

Climate Change Is Both a Cause and a Consequence of the Global Food Crisis

From reading **Chapter 12**, you already know that the dwindling global water supply is a direct cause of climate change and the growing problem of food insecurity. Thus, it is quite clear that climate change has the consequence of causing the global food crisis via an ever-expanding scarcity of water and fertile soil. However, it is also the case that what we eat is a primary contributing factor to climate change. For instance, earlier in this chapter, you learned about feed conversion ratios; therefore, you understand that humans greatly contribute to the earth's warming via an overreliance on the inefficient conversion of plants to meat that is then consumed as beef, pork, or chicken. The next point to consider is that the human demand for beef has created very large financial incentives for what has become an incredibly devastating cause of climate change: deforestation.

what we eat is a primary contributing factor to climate change

Deforestation simply means that massive stands of woodland, timber, and smaller trees (all of which bind carbon) are torn from the ground. The process releases huge amounts of carbon into the atmosphere. The trees and their roots are then burned, releasing even more

Table 13.3   Land required (in square meters) to produce one kilogram of food

Food product	Land required
Average vegetables	.3
Potatoes	.2
Fruits (including citrus)	.5
Beef	20.9
Pork	8.9
Poultry	7.3
Butter	13.8
Cheese	10.2

Source: Adapted from Fairlie S. 2010.

carbon. The long-term effects are the most consequential because the absence of vast forests that once bound carbon means the warming of the planet occurs even faster. As if this human-caused catalyzing of climate change is not enough, the reason for the deforestation is typically to create pastureland and cropland to support cattle, which (as you already know) release methane that is even more powerful than carbon in terms of greenhouse gases.

the reason for the deforestation is typically to create pastureland and cropland to support cattle

As always, an example is helpful. Known as the "lungs of the world," Brazil's Amazon rainforest binds an extremely large percentage of the global carbon that would otherwise be quickly destroying the planet. Evidence indicates that the main reason for deforestation in the Amazon involves Brazilian farmers being paid large sums of money to produce beef for companies like McDonald's (Brice, 2022). Although such corporations deny a role in deforestation, it is extremely difficult for the Brazilian government to monitor and thus regulate cattle herds sold to global meat companies without records of origin. Moreover, the Amazon rainforest has a long history of exploitation by businesses and industry, despite laws and regulations designed to protect it.

Pause for a moment and think about what you can do! Multinational meat companies are very powerful and difficult to regulate, but an alternative approach can be much more effective. If the people of your generation and all who follow simply stopped eating beef, much of the global demand would fall dramatically, and all of this could end. But look at the line in any McDonald's drive-through during the lunch hour. You now understand that this high level of consumer demand is one of the primary causes of global warming.

Estimates suggest that since 1978, about 1 million square kilometers of Amazon rainforest have been destroyed, with about three-quarters of this land used to support cattle (Butler, 2021). Deforestation was stalled from about 2005 through 2014 due to intensified government regulation and law enforcement. However, after 2015, deforestation of the Amazon increased rapidly and continues to do so at the time this chapter was written.

after 2015, deforestation of the Amazon increased rapidly and continues to do so

Beyond beef, it is important to understand that the human affinity for eating any animal-based product is a primary – and preventable – cause of climate change. Using the international metric of kilograms, **Table 13.3** provides detailed information relative to how much of the earth's fertile land is needed to raise plant-based versus animal-based products. The table shows how much land it takes to produce a kilogram of average vegetable crops versus a kilogram of typical animal-based foods.

Again, with the global food crisis being very much a reality, this table provides stark evidence that an important small change is to adopt a plant-based diet. In addition to being a responsible steward of the planet and the earth's future, you may remember learning (in **Chapters 5, 6, and 7**) about the tremendous health-protective benefits of eating a plant-based diet.

Will Farming Practices Change in Response to a Warming Planet?

Farming in America is both a business and part of an inherited culture. Most farmland in the United States is owned and managed by large-scale companies known as **agribusiness**. You may, for instance, be surprised to learn that 90% of all farm animals never see the outside of the "factory" where they are raised for slaughter or for products such as eggs and milk (Reese, 2018). Iconic American images of farmers herding cattle, cows grazing in fields, or chickens happily pecking bugs in a lush green field are rapidly becoming the exception rather than the reality. The meat and dairy industries are heavily supported by the U.S. government, and they are following the industry model to create more and more products at costs that are within reach of most Americans. Agribusiness and its cost-cutting philosophy also control most of our plant-based food supplies, particularly wheat, corn, oats, soybeans, and sugar.

But even in agribusiness, farming practices are as much a result of past practices (given that the machinery is already in place at a huge price) as of what makes sense economically. Culturally, agribusiness thinks of animals as the primary source of human protein rather than plants. Culture also dictates that milk products should be based on dairy milk instead of plant-based milk. Agribusiness fills this demand as well. Whether driven by culture, farming practices, or economic benefit, America's farming methods are not being adapted to the needs of land that is slowly becoming less productive based on climate change. Unless farming practices change, it is unlikely that American consumers alone will be able to make a substantial difference in how quickly our food supplies dwindle with each passing year. Ironically, one of the first theories of change used widely in public health practice was initially used to promote the practice of planting hybrid crops among American farmers. Known as **diffusion of innovations** (Rogers, 1995), this theory of change can be applied to entire industries, including agribusiness. Let's use the example of no-till farming to understand how this theory works (and how it can be applied to other large-scale adaptations that will serve the public's health).

> America's farming methods are not being adapted to the needs of land that is slowly becoming less productive based on climate change

Diffusion of innovations (DOI) theory dates back to 1943, when it was applied to promoting the use of hybrid corn seeds among Iowa farmers. The best way to think about DOI is to consider a basic tenet of human behavior: people tend to follow the lead of others. In somewhat simplistic terms, people are more likely to adopt a given innovation (e.g., no-till farming practices) if they observe that others they respect have adopted the innovation. This spread of adoption is especially likely when it is easy to observe others experiencing a positive outcome. DOI suggests that the highly visible influence of **peer modeling** starts a chain reaction of adoption. This chain reaction can lead to geometric growth (even exponential growth) in the number of people who adopt a given practice or behavior. That some innovations spread very rapidly while others languish is likely a product of how openly the **social network** enables peer modeling of the adoption process and its results.

> DOI suggests that the highly visible influence of **peer modeling** starts a chain reaction of adoption

With these basic principles of DOI in mind, let's work through the example of no-till farming as an innovation to reduce carbon release from the soil and enhance agricultural productivity. The entire process relies on several key opinion leaders being willing to talk about and potentially try this innovative practice. In this example, key opinion leaders are farmers who are open to change and well-respected among their peers. It is important to remember an earlier point about farming being partly rooted in culture. Culture can and does evolve over time (e.g., the use of landlines is now limited to a small percentage of the U.S. population – a cultural shift to cell phones was successful). Creating a culture shift via key opinion leaders is analogous to using one spark to start a fire.

Key opinion leaders are heavily connected within their respective social networks. They tend to have elevated social status and frequent contact with others in the network. Further, they are well connected to people outside their immediate social networks (this is important for diffusing the adoption beyond just social networks). The key opinion leaders who first adopt the practice of no-till farming are only a small percentage of the overall population that will eventually decide to change their practice to no-till farming. These key opinion leaders are known as **innovators** once they adopt the practice.

DOI theory suggests that about 2.5% of any given population (e.g., farmers) will be innovators. In turn, innovators will influence many other farmers who become **early adopters** of the innovation. Early adopters are less bold than innovators but nonetheless willing to be among the first few to make the change to no-till farming. The theory posits that about 13.5% of any given population are early adopters.

Let's imagine now that about 16% of the farmers in a given area have made the switch and are planting at least some crops using no-till farming methods. With nearly one in six farmers adopting the innovation, you might imagine that social networks begin to include discussions among farmers about why people chose to make the switch. When no-till farming becomes part of daily social interactions among farmers, DOI theory considers this the true starting point. Up to this point, the speed of adoption may have been sluggish; however, the theory suggests that it will quickly increase as early adopters influence the **early majority** of farmers (about 34% of any given population). Once this early majority begins trying no-till practices, it will become a new norm among farmers, triggering most of the remainder (another 34%) to conform to this new norm. Known as the **late majority**, these farmers will be slow to change until they notice that everyone is doing it. DOI theory is realistic about the remaining 16%: **known as laggards**, these farmers are unlikely to ever follow the lead of others or conform to a new norm – they are therefore unlikely to convert to no-till farming practices.

As you may suspect, DOI theory is much more involved than this brief presentation. In the example, farmers would need a source of reliable information about the benefits of no-till farming as well as access and financial support or incentives to change their farming practices without high costs. Farmers making the switch would also need ongoing help and advice from an expert such as a county extension agent (these positions exist throughout the United States, and thus agents can play a key role in helping to align farming practices with the need to reduce carbon emissions).

A final note about DOI theory is useful here. Having been applied to public health issues as diverse as contraceptive use, HIV prevention, highway and automobile safety, and cancer screenings, this theory has been a staple of public health practice for several decades. It can and should be applied to meeting the challenges of climate change to food security in the United States and elsewhere. However, it is simply a tool to employ rather than a grand, sweeping answer to the problems of public health. For instance, whether the theory would be useful in helping cattle and dairy farmers convert to more earth-friendly products is unknown but unlikely. The change from beef and dairy cows to other food sources will most likely be driven by consumer demand. So, once again, overcoming climate change – in whole or in part – is in the hands of "We the People."

Small Changes Add Up

Before reading about the changes that any person one can make, it is important to acknowledge that millions of people in the United States do not accept the idea that our earth is rapidly warming and thus causing a shift in weather patterns that threatens human existence. **Box 13.2** describes the psychology of denying climate change and is therefore well worth reading at this time.

At this point in the chapter, it is time for you to think about your own carbon footprint as it relates specifically to obtaining the food you eat. For instance, if you live in the Midwest,

BOX 13.2. THE HUMAN SIDE: THE PSYCHOLOGY BEHIND DENYING CLIMATE CHANGE

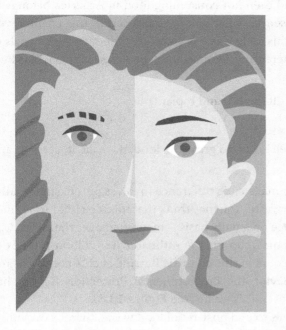

You may have traveled outside the United States by this time in your life. Many of you reading this book may be citizens of other countries. However, it is a safe bet that very few (if any) of the students reading this have been to either *Arctica* (i.e., the North Pole) or *Antarctica* (the South Pole). Global warming (which is the cause of climate change) occurs two to three times faster at the earth's poles compared to its midsection. Rapidly rising ocean levels worldwide result from the steady melting of glaciers and sublayers of **permafrost**. The evidence of climate change in these extreme parts of the world is iniquitous and undeniable. Yet without being there in person to see this firsthand, people elsewhere on the planet can easily slip into a mindset of **defensive denial**. This form of denial is a coping strategy – it lets us remain in a state of being OK with the status quo. For instance, if a person's income is based on the automobile industry, the oil or gas industry, or a manufacturing plant that is far from carbon neutral, then one way to still feel good about that job and income in the age of climate change is to dismiss climate change as a potential exaggeration or a scientific conspiracy.

Sadly, many of our elected members of the U.S. Congress fall into the all-too-human trap that promotes doubt about the urgency and scientific realities of climate change. Despite widely available photos from satellites showing how hot the earth has become, a fair number of congressional representatives and senators have become emblematic of the larger population in terms of what has been termed the **climate-change countermovement**. Consisting of millions of people, this movement is widely amplified by social media. As noted in one journal article that thoroughly addressed this counter-movement, it is characterized by "well organized efforts to undermine public understanding of human-caused climate change by promoting uncertainty" (Dunlap & Brulie, 2020). As you might guess, the movement may have hidden corporate sponsors (e.g., companies involved in the oil/gas industry and cattle associations in various countries). Moreover, part of the "well organized efforts" is often the use of poor science or deliberately falsified science to sow the seeds of doubt in the public mind and therefore create a counter-narrative. The counter-narrative then becomes an easy way for those already engaging in defensive denial to justify their apathy and/or inaction toward climate change.

East, South, or Pacific Northwest, think about your reaction to finding fresh strawberries for sale at the grocery store during winter. They may be a bit pricy, but chances are good that you have bought these (or other types of berries or fruit that are not in season where you live). Now, let's consider the distance those berries had to travel to reach you, carried by large semi trucks that burn copious amounts of diesel fuel. The distance is quantified as **food miles**. Food miles add to your carbon footprint in a modest way (because of massive shipments that reduce the number of food miles per product shipped). So, while not as substantial as giving up the consumption of beef, for example, eating locally grown foods is a daily habit that – while seemingly small – can add up to a large difference when magnified over a lifetime and multiplied by the number of people willing to make these adaptations.

Moving now to a potentially far more food- and earth-friendly practice that may seem small at first, consider that about 40% of the food grown in the United States is never consumed (U.S. Department of Agriculture, 2022). Although some of this 40% is waste at the level of the producer or wholesaler, most of it (about three-quarters of the 40%) occurs at the

about 40% of the food grown in the United States is never consumed

post-retail level. This is hard to imagine, given the nation's high rates of food insecurity; however, it becomes more plausible when you consider the vast inequities previously described in this chapter. The practice of purchasing and then not consuming food in America belongs to the middle- and upper-income classes. Based on what you have learned in this chapter, you should be able to quickly understand how this daily waste is counterproductive to the goals of reducing greenhouse gas emissions and increasing food security in America. Consider how this daily waste impacts:

* Land use (creating an artificial need to till the soil and replant)

* Water use (see **Chapter 12**)

* Human labor and energy (e.g., fossil fuels) used to grow the food, package it, store it, and transport it

Accordingly, one little changes that can make a big difference involves purchasing smaller amounts of food to ensure that none goes to waste. You may think that this idea is far too minor in scale to matter; however, that small change on a daily basis – magnified over the entire U.S. middle- and upper-class population – can make up for the estimated 133 billion pounds of post-retail level food waste that annually occurs in this country. Barring such a collective and dramatic change in overall consumer behavior, the Environmental Protection Agency has developed a model that prioritizes other uses of this waste (see **Figure 13.3**).

the top priority is to end post-retail food waste

As shown in this figure, the top priority is to end post-retail food waste, thereby providing less overall burden on U.S. farmland, conserving bound carbon, averting methane release from cows, and even reducing fossil fuel consumption. The next-most-preferred priority is to reclaim this food to help resolve America's hunger issues (reclaiming food has become common in many U.S. states). Moving further down the pyramid, you can see that the next priority

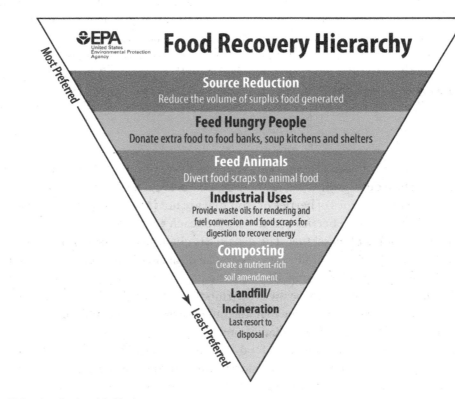

Figure 13.3   A national model of food recovery

is using food waste for animal feed. As a source of protein and calories for farm animals, this practice has the potential to reduce the demand for growing plant-based products that are converted by these animals into either meat or dairy products. Next, at the level of industrial use, notice that the model includes using food waste for biofuels. Close to the bottom of the model, composting food waste adds those nutrients back into the soil and thus helps to conserve a need to add nitrogen and other products that (as always) ultimately add to the carbon footprint of the food we eat.

Taking the idea of small changes to the level of communities, there is a growing trend to practice what is typically known as **food rescue** (also known as **food reclamation** or **food salvage**). The concept behind food rescue is to link sources of excess food to people in need of food. Given that as much as 8% of the total greenhouse gases emitted in the United States stem from food waste, this concept serves two purposes: (1) it avoids food waste, and (2) it distributes food to those who are otherwise food insecure. Using an app-based software program, a community can "harvest" reclaimed food from restaurants, dining halls, large and small grocery stores, and local farms that overproduce. This excess food may have been close to (or past) the expiration date, it may be left over from meals or restaurant hours that had fewer people than anticipated, or it may have been purchased in a quantity too large to sell within a reasonable time frame. Typically, food rescue relies on volunteers to pick up (harvest) this food and then distribute it to people who are food insecure. To learn more about the software and how this approach works, a case study of the program located in Boulder, Colorado, is well worth reading (Sewald, Kuo, & Dansky, 2018).

The current volunteer-based concept of food rescue could be applied to a public health model. Throughout the United States, state and local governments support approximately 3,500 **local health departments** (LHDs). The mission of LHDs is – as you might guess – to engage the community in health-promotion and disease-prevention actions. Thus, providing food to those without adequate amounts is entirely within the scope of their mission. Using the existing food-rescue software, it is entirely feasible for LHDs to transform food rescue from a volunteer-based program to one based on employees of LHDs.

A final small change that can have earth-saving implications takes you back to a previous section of this chapter where you learned about deforestation being driven by global meat companies, many highly reliant on you and others to buy beef products on a weekly, if not daily, basis. To dismiss the idea that greatly lowered consumer demand can bring down even giant corporations like McDonald's would be a mistake in basic logic and an apathetic response to what you now know is causing much of the global warming that will impact your generation and those who follow. In terms of DOI theory, think of yourself as a potential innovator relative to banning beef from your diet. You may be surprised how quickly your adoption of this innovation may spread through your social network. Perhaps our current beef culture (see **Photo 13.7**) will soon be replaced by foods that are earth friendly.

Throughout the United States, state and local governments support approximately 3,500 **local health departments**

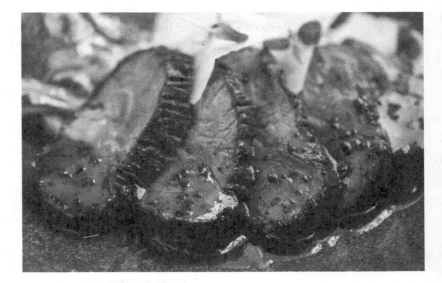

Photo 13.7   Summer fairs, carnivals, concerts, and farmer's markets typically feature grilled beef ribs and other meat cooked outdoors.
Source: Andrey / Adobe Stock.

To dismiss the idea that greatly lowered consumer demand can bring down even giant corporations like McDonald's would be a mistake in basic logic

A Plant-Based Diet Provides Ample Protein

By this point in the chapter, you certainly understand that consuming beef and other animal-based foods contributes to the massive problem of climate change. Further, consuming an animal-based diet drives the health equity wedge deeper into U.S. society by making less food available overall (recall what you learned about feed conversion ratios) when hunger in America is a crisis. What you may not know, however, is that a type of myth has been passed along from one generation to the next relative to needing meat to obtain adequate protein. This final section of the chapter provides a basis for understanding the fallacy of the idea that humans need meat for protein.

First, the mythology that typically surrounds protein involves how much we need to consume. As a result, Americans tend to greatly overconsume protein (by 50% or more). Approximately 40 grams of protein per day is ample for maintaining excellent health of the human body. The sources of these 40 grams are not relevant to the body because a varied diet of plant-based foods provides the same **essential building blocks** (known as **amino acids**) as the few types of meat we consume. Think of essential building blocks as being like colors of paint that can be used to make a portrait. Just as the portrait may require red, blue, and yellow colors (the primary colors you learned about in elementary school), the human body meets its basic tissue-building needs (including blood) through a strategic combination of what are chemically known as essential amino acids. Unlike the metaphor of using the three primary colors to create an entire portrait, the human body requires nine varieties of amino acids. Although no single plant-based food contains all nine, a steady and varied diet of plants easily provides the full complement of building blocks for maintaining health.

You should be aware that the term **plant-based diet** implies eating foods in their unrefined state. Plants include trees; therefore, nuts such as almonds are a rich source of protein. The edible seeds produced by plants (e.g., sunflowers, pumpkins, hemp, chia) are also rich in protein. The absolute best sources of protein, however, are foods classed in the legume family (these plants are adept at absorbing nitrogen and incorporating it into the food part of the plant). Rather than learning the term **legume**, just think about various types of beans (including chickpeas and lentils) as being the supreme source of plant-based protein. **Table 13.4** provides a hint of how quickly you can consume 40 grams of plant-based protein in one day.

a varied diet of plant-based foods provides the same **essential building blocks** (known as **amino acids**) as the few types of meat we consume

a steady and varied diet of plants easily provides the full complement of building blocks for maintaining health

Table 13.4   Sample of available proteins in common plant-based foods.

One-cup serving of . . .	Available protein
Soybeans	22
Lentils	18
Chickpeas	15
Beans (black, kidney, red, etc.)	15
Oats	7
Whole wheat pasta	6
Cooked spinach	5
Tofu	22
4 tablespoon serving of . . .	**Available protein**
Peanuts	9
Sesame or pumpkin seeds	7
Flax or sunflower seeds	8
Chia seeds	12
Walnuts or cashews	5

Source: Adapted from Davis, H 2022.

Review and Key Terms

In many ways, the most important term in this entire chapter is **food insecurity**. Although you learned about gradients of it (i.e., **very low food security, food insecurity with hunger**), the fundamental lesson of this chapter is that climate change has already magnified the global food shortage, and it will continue to do so during your lifetime. Accordingly, it is vital for humans to make a series of adaptations, all of which can add up to improved public health. Many needed adaptations depend on **macro-level changes**; therefore, reducing the scope of America's food crisis must involve government and industry support and cooperation.

climate change has already magnified the global food shortage, and it will continue to do so during your lifetime

An important take-home lesson in this chapter is that as **omnivores**, humans (especially those living in high-income nations such as the United States) all too frequently make the ecologically unsustainable choice of eating animal products rather than consuming a plant-based diet. The science behind this involves **feed conversion ratios** and a similar concept known as **conversion inefficiency ratios**. That the U.S. government continues to subsidize foods with highly unfavorable feed conversion ratios is a cause for concern among an informed electorate (i.e., people like you!).

You may have been surprised that much of this chapter focuses on **conventional farming practices**, such as failing to invest in the annual fall planting of effective **cover crops**. Unlike most forms of industry, farming in the era of climate change should be the business of the American people, given that so many current practices hasten climate change and increase a cycle of problems culminating in making the food crisis worse. Cover crops, for example, add precious **nitrogen** back into the soil. Also, we all have an obligation to be more vigilant about regulating pesticide use in **agribusiness** – especially a class of compounds known as **neonicotinoids** that are implicated in the declining bee population. Without **pollinators**, such as bees, our food supply will rapidly diminish. This vigilance must also be practiced at the federal level, especially by the **Environmental Protection Agency (EPA)**.

farming in the era of climate change should be the business of the American people

Components of the federal government other than the EPA are also critical to resolving the food crisis and slowing its cause (i.e., climate change). You learned, for instance, that the federal program known as the **Supplemental Nutrition Assistance Program** (SNAP) could be greatly improved by prohibiting the purchase of environmentally destructive foods, such as beef. You also learned that the United States and other nations worldwide are engaged in intense debates about how to best curtail or eliminate **deforestation** and the often illegal use of newly stripped land for grazing cattle to produce beef.

Regulating agribusiness is important, but the people of our nation will also need to make adaptations as soon as possible. Farming practices, for example, can become more responsible if public health practice applies **diffusion of innovations** (DOI) theory to the difficult task of adaptation among America's farmers. This theory posits that a small percent of the target population (2.5%) who are **key opinion leaders** will become **innovators**, and a larger portion (13.5%) will follow as **early adopters**. After this initial 16%, DOI theory is very much based on the concept of peer modeling within social networks as a trigger for the **early majority** and **late majority** of adopters. The theory acknowledges that about one-sixth of any given population (**laggards**) will not adopt the innovation in its current form (recall that the example applied to DOI was no-till farming).

Under the idea that small changes add up, this chapter may have prompted you to at least think about how your food choices contribute to your personal carbon footprint. The idea that your grocery purchases involve various food miles is one to think about over your lifetime of making food-buying decisions. Perhaps to your surprise in this regard, you also learned that about 40% of post-retail food is not consumed. In the age of a food crisis being fueled by climate change, this is nothing less than a blatant insult to the environment and to the millions of people who are food insecure. You then learned about **food rescue** and the public health opportunity to make this a part of standard practice among the 3,500 local health departments in the United States. Finally, related to making your own daily food choices (and conveying them to others to create a diffusion effect), you learned that **amino acids** are the **essential building blocks** of human tissue. More importantly, you learned that plant-based foods are a more than adequate source of these building blocks.

For Practice and Class Discussion

Practice Questions (answers are located in the appendix to this textbook)

1. A key point in this chapter was that small changes can add up to make large differences. Of course, this depends on a sufficiently large number of people making these small changes. Which bolded term in the chapter is **most** applicable in this regard?
   a. Diffusion of innovation theory
   b. Subsidies
   c. Pollinators
   d. Agribusiness

2. Which food has the most efficient feed conversion ratio?
   a. Farm-raised trout
   b. Lamb
   c. Walnuts
   d. Organically raised chicken

3. Clearly, the U.S. government can up its game to increase the food supply and reduce climate change caused by agribusiness. Which regulatory target is **not** within the realm of the federal government?
   a. The SNAP
   b. Deforestation of the Amazon rainforest
   c. Neonicotinoids
   d. Beef subsidies

4. Cover crops add nitrogen to the soil. This is important to humans because:
   a. It is the source of amino acids.
   b. It averts erosion.
   c. Nitrogen is vital to the lives of pollinators.
   d. It gives improved feed conversion ratios

5. Which food has the **least** efficient feed conversion ratio?
   a. Lean white pork
   b. Chicken breasts
   c. Roast beef
   d. Legumes

6. A young farmer in Nebraska makes this post on social media: "I will be changing 30% of my operation next year to no-till farming." Imagine that most other nearby farmers reading this post react by saying something like, "What is he talking about?" Applying DOI theory to this scenario, the young farmer making the post is **best** described as:
   a. An innovator
   b. Part of the early majority

   c.   A laggard
   d.   A spokesperson for agribusiness

7.   An entire community is devoted to redistributing excess farm produce. This is a practice known by the general name of:
   a.   Early adoption
   b.   Peer modeling
   c.   Food miles
   d.   Food rescue

8.   Sometimes, small things can be the reason for big problems. With that in mind, which term is actually no small thing relative to addressing the food crisis?
   a.   Conventional farming
   b.   Pollinators
   c.   Soil contamination
   d.   Omnivores

9.   Although meat is a superior source of dietary protein, plant-based sources rank a very close but clear second place.
   a.   True
   b.   False

10.   Imagine you have the power to suddenly change only one federal regulatory policy regarding food. Which action would produce the greatest return in terms of food causing climate change?
   a.   End the practice of subsidizing beef production.
   b.   Make more people eligible for SNAP.
   c.   Educate American farmers about no-till practices.
   d.   Genetically modify beans to produce greater levels of amino acids.

Discussion Questions

11.   One of the references cited in this chapter is a commentary from an organization known as EWG (Faber & Schechinger, 2022). Because this reference has a link to that commentary, this exercise asks you to begin by accessing it and reading it thoroughly. As you read, think about your reactions to these three questions:
   a.   Why are these subsidies provided, despite overwhelming evidence that cattle and dairy cows are top offenders relative to climate change?
   b.   What did you learn from reading this that was not covered in this chapter?
   c.   Are these climate un-friendly subsidies likely to end soon?

   Then, in less than two pages of double-spaced font, summarize your answers to these three questions and post them on a class-shared website for review and comment by other students taking this course.

12.   Two popular books broadly apply to this chapter: *Wheat Belly* by William Davis and *The Omnivore's Dilemma* by Michael Pollan. With the help of your course instructor, work with one or two other students taking this course to read and summarize either of these two books. Then, in a group meeting, present an oral summary to a few other students who chose to read the book you did not select (they will then present their oral summary to your group).

13.   Find a restaurant you like, and introduce yourself to a manager. Go there late in the day (or toward the time they close), and ask if you would be allowed to take a quick picture of

the waste container in the kitchen – the container where food is discarded (food from customers, food spoiled in the kitchen, etc.). Using any web-based learning management system that applies to the course you are taking in conjunction with this textbook, post the photo and a caption describing your thoughts about the amount of food being thrown away each day at that restaurant.

References

A Well-Fed World (2022). *Conversion inefficiency ratios.* https://awellfedworld.org/feed-ratios/

Brice, J. (2022, March 30). *McDonald's linked to Amazon deforestation in new report.* https://pulitzercenter.org/stories/mcdonalds-linked-amazon-deforestation-new-report

Butler, R. A. (2021, November 23). *Amazon destruction.* https://rainforests.mongabay.com/amazon/amazon_destruction.html

CDC (2022). *Healthy people 2030.* https://health.gov/healthypeople

Cosiers, S. (2019, May 30). The world needs topsoil to grow 95% of its food – but it's rapidly disappearing. *The Guardian.* https://www.theguardian.com/us-news/2019/may/30/topsoil-farming-agriculture-food-toxic-america

Davis, H. (2022). *Your guide to muscle building: plant-based proteins.* San Francisco, CA: Stone Pier Press.

Dunlap, R. E., & Brulie, R. J. (2020). Sources and amplification of climate change denial. In D. C. Holmes & L. M. Richardson (Eds.), *Research handbook on communicating climate change.* Cheltenham, UK: Edward Elgar Publishing Limited.

Faber, S., & Schechinger, A. (2022). *Climate change isn't high priority for the 1.2 billion USDA farm stewardship program.* https://www.ewg.org/news-insights/news/2022/04/climate-change-isnt-high-priority-12-billion-usda-farm-stewardship

Fairlie, S. (2010). *Meat: A benign extravagance.* Permanent Publications.

Feeding America (2021). *Hunger in America 2014: Executive summary.* https://www.feedingamerica.org/sites/default/files/research/hunger-in-america/hia-2014-executive-summary.pdf

Haug, A., Hustmark, A. T., & Harstad, O. M. (2007). Bovine milk in human nutrition: A review. *Lipids in Health and Disease, 6*: 25.

McNair, K. (2021, October 18). *Organic food is more expensive, but conventional food prices are catching up.* https://www.magnifymoney.com/news/organic-vs-conventional-food-study/

Nguyen, J., Cafer, A. J., & Deleveaux, J. (2021). *Mississippi health and hunger atlas 2021.* https://cps.olemiss.edu/wp-content/uploads/sites/183/2021/11/Mississippi-Health-and-Hunger-Atlas-2021.pdf

Quinton, A. (2019). *Cows and climate change: Making cattle more sustainable.* https://www.ucdavis.edu/food/news/making-cattle-more-sustainable.

Reese, J. (2018). *The end of animal farming.* Boston: Beacon Press.

Rogers, E. M. (1995). *Diffusion of innovations* (4th ed.). New York: Free Press.

Savage, C. (2022, June 30). E.P.A. ruling is milestone in long pushback to regulation of business. New York Times.

Sewald, C. A., Kuo, E. S., & Dansky, T. L. (2018). Boulder food rescue: An innovative approach to reducing food waste and increasing food security. *The American Journal of Preventive Medicine, 54*(5), S130–S132.

Singer, P. (1990). *Animal liberation* (2nd ed.). Pimlico.

The World Counts (2022). *Global challenges.* https://www.theworldcounts.com/challenges/people-and-poverty/hunger-and-obesity/how-many-people-die-from-hunger-each-year

United States Department of Agriculture (2022). *Food waste FAQs.* https://www.usda.gov/foodwaste/faqs

CHAPTER 14

OVERPOPULATION AND THE PREVENTION OF UNINTENDED PREGNANCY

Everything you see exists together in a delicate balance. As king, you need to understand that balance and respect all the creatures, from the crawling ant to the leaping antelope . . . we are all connected in the great circle of life.

—*Mufasa (*The Lion King, *1994)*

Overview

Much like Chapters 12 and 13, this chapter has a global focus. This is because **overpopulation** in Africa and Asia (the two continents primarily affected) will have severe ramifications for all humans, regardless of where they live. The chapter also addresses the very real (but difficult to imagine) possibility that human extinction – as a consequence of overpopulation – is a possibility. The concept underlying this possibility comes down to what is known as a **J-curve**, in which a species (in this case, humans) "crashes" because they have depleted the pool of resources needed to sustain life.

This chapter may be a bit challenging for you! It describe three basic public health actions that may avert human extinction. The first is to control the birth rate through policies and programs accelerating the use of highly reliable contraceptives. The second pertains to one of the most important global public health strategies: educating school girls and advancing their education as women. The third is about the overuse of the medical systems in developed nations (such as the United States) to extend life beyond a point desired by many people who are terminally ill (so, this deals with the death rate).

Understanding the Malthus Hypothesis

Just prior to the year 1800, a scholar named Robert Malthus published his predictions regarding any species (including the human species) "crashing" if its rate of growth exceeded the amount of available resources needed to sustain life. Although we seem readily capable of grasping and accepting this concept when it comes to the hundreds of species now being counted as extinct every month, too many people have ignored this possibility for the human species. Malthus suggested that as populations outpaced their resources, people would fight for survival; thus, wars

LEARNING OBJECTIVES

- Understand the Malthus hypothesis.

- Describe the differences between the S-curve and the J-curve.

- Understand how some countries have reduced population growth.

- Describe public health policies and opportunities relative to controlling the birth rate, including providing greater levels of education for school-age girls.

- Articulate possible public health solutions to the lack of equal education for females of all ages.

- Explain why death rates in many developed nations may be unnecessarily low.

would result. Further, he suggested that famine would be a second leading cause of human death. His hypothesis also included the point that great waves of disease (plagues) would follow, thereby leading to more death. Far from being mere speculation, the predictions of Malthus have already played out in parts of the world where populations have exceeded the **carrying capacity** of the environment.

The concept of carrying capacity is based on the availability of food, water, and oxygen. An example that is easy to think about is a fish tank. As long as the size of the tank can oxygenate the number of fish living inside, and there is ample food for the fish, everything is fine! But once other organisms growing in the tank begin to consume oxygen, the weaker fish will die. The same applies to a lack of food. This die-off will continue until the number of fish left alive is small enough that the diminished life-sustaining capacity of the tank can handle the life needs of those remaining. The fish tank is an example of a closed environment – its resources are limited. Now, think of the earth as a closed environment with limited food, water, and oxygen. In places on the planet where these three essential ingredients of life are lacking, the carrying capacity will be exceeded. A key point is that the phrase "where these three essential ingredients of life are lacking" implies that vast global disparities will exist in terms of death (because carrying capacity is not uniform).

The **Malthus hypothesis** is generic – it is not specific to any one species. So, let's take a few minutes to explore how well the predictions made by Malthus have held up over the past 200+ years. According to the International Union for Conservation of Nature, nearly 130,000 species are in danger of extinction, with about 35,000 in imminent danger. Further, the World Wildlife Fund has noted that the number of animal species declared extinct represents a 70% decline in the number of these species in the past 50 years (Jones, 2020). To help you personalize these sobering statistics a bit, **Box 14.1** provides a case study of the gray wolf. This box also gives you a bit more context as to how the extinction of any one species poses issues for all species.

*the predictions of Malthus have already played out in parts of the world where populations have exceeded the **carrying capacity** of the environment*

*The **Malthus hypothesis** is generic – it is not specific to any one species*

BOX 14.1. DIMINISHING BIODIVERSITY

Biodiversity is a term denoting a richness of species on earth that creates a functional ecology of plants, insects, birds, mammals, etc. As this biodiversity erodes, so does our fragile ecology that supports and protects the human species, thousands of other species, the climate, water supplies, the soil, and even the air we breathe!

As an example of how quickly this biodiversity is shrinking, consider the gray wolf. By 1930, this species was nearly destroyed (via hunting) in the Yellowstone Park area of the United States. Wolves prey on elk and deer, and thus, in the absence of wolves, these two species thrived. As the elk and deer population sizes expanded, their food supply began to include willow trees (which grow along streams and control erosion) and Aspen saplings (aspen trees house a variety of bird species). The result was massive soil erosion and, in the absence of birds, an overpopulation of mosquitoes. As you can easily imagine, the erosion led to issues with water management, and mosquitos have a significant potential to carry diseases such as malaria. Fortunately, by 1995, the wolves were reintroduced to Yellowstone Park. It has since been documented that the ecology there is returning to normal relative to the disrupted state caused by overhunting wolves. Of course, Yellowstone Park is a highly controlled environment: what about the rest of the nation?

Although the gray wolf made a stunning comeback after it was placed on the list of endangered species in the United States, this success was reversed during the Trump administration. The reversal occurred because animals removed from that list are no longer protected by federal law. Thus, the gray wolf became fair game for hunting by humans. Added to the existing lack of food (most gray wolfs die of starvation after about four years of life), the hunting drove the species back to a dangerously low number. However, this allowed a federal judge to reinstate the endangered status of the gray wolf, thereby giving them at least some protection against being hunted by humans.

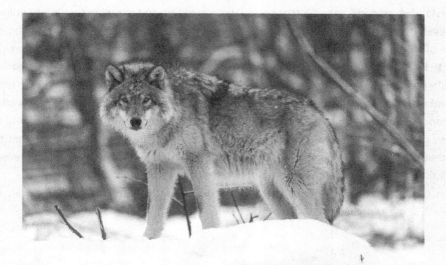

Source: Joe / Adobe Stock.

The S-curve and the J-curve

Understanding the issue of overpopulation involves learning about what are known as the S-curve and the J-curve. **The S-shaped curve** (see **Figure 14.1**) shows a point of diminished growth once the population nears the limits of carrying capacity. In human terms, this is when the birth rate and death rate are equivalent. The common term for this is **zero population growth**. So, you can think about this as one surviving birth for every one adult who dies.

The terms can be a bit confusing, so it helps to discuss just two for now. First, the **birth rate** is the number of live births per 1,000 people in any given population. For instance, birth rates in many economically challenged African nations are as high as 40 per 1,000 (a rate often deemed necessary by governments to keep a population from rapid decline). Second, the **fertility rate** is the number of live births divided by the number of females aged 15–50 in a given population. Hong Kong is an example of a city with an extremely low fertility rate: 1.9. The global average is 2.5 (see **Box 14.2**).

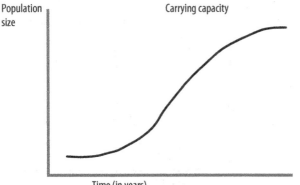

Figure 14.1   The S-shaped curve of population growth, plotted against carrying capacity

BOX 14.2. THE SUCCESS OF HONG KONG, CHINA

Why does Hong Kong – a city of considerable wealth – have such a low fertility rate? The answer is complex but nonetheless important to understand. A primary reason is that young women are having great success in obtaining higher education and, thus, greater levels of career placement early in life. This leads to deliberate actions designed to postpone pregnancy (i.e., the vigilant use of contraceptive practices). Further, the mean age of marriage for young women in this city is steadily rising. This appears to be based on the success enjoyed by young women in their careers, making marriage a far less attractive option (especially given China's gender-based expectations about the role of a wife in tending to household duties and being a primary caretaker of the very young and the very old). Also, as a thriving city, Hong Kong is an expensive place to raise a child. This economic reality leads to further deliberate action designed to postpone childbearing or even end fertility (via tubal ligation) so that children are never born to many women. Interestingly, despite government-based financial and other incentives to have children, an escalating number of young women in this city express a preference for having only one child in their lifetime, and growing numbers opt not to have children at all.

Ultimately, then, the success and independence of women explains the extremely low fertility rate in this major global city. Do you envision this occurring in any U.S. city at this time?

both the birth rate and fertility rate are based on the numerator of live births

Look again at the definitions of the birth rate and fertility rate. Notice that both the birth rate and fertility rate are based on the numerator of live births. Thus, neither statistic takes into account infant mortality. This is accurate because these rates are intended to help nations monitor population growth, meaning infants not surviving to the age of 5 years cannot reasonably be counted. Thus, to keep a population at zero growth, nations with high infant mortality rates are somewhat dependent on fertility rates also being high.

In terms of climate change and diminished carrying capacities (see **Chapters 12 and 13**), the S-shaped curve is an optimistic scenario. However, bear in mind that zero population growth has two sides to the equation: the death rate is equally important. As nations become progressively more adaptive relative to public health and more progressive with respect to healthcare, people will live longer lives, thereby decreasing the death rate. Often – and optimistically – this decrease in the death rate is offset by a corresponding decrease in the birth rate (or fertility rate). When this optimistic scenario occurs, it is known as a **demographic transition**. As you might imagine, the transition is from a population with a younger average age to one with a much older average age. Such transitions – occurring on a nation-by-nation basis – are reliant on **family planning**. One downside of this kind of transition in high-income nations is that healthcare costs for people later in life are typically several times greater than for young adults.

Moving now to the **J-shaped curve** (see **Figure 14.2**), the concept is simply that the rapid growth of a population will soon reach and exceed the carrying capacity, thereby triggering a

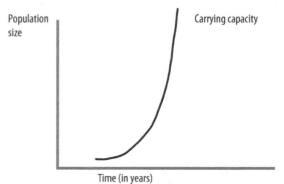

Figure 14.2   The J-shaped curve of population growth, showing the rapid escalation of population size and how it exceeds carrying capacity

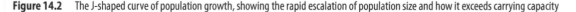

Malthus effect. After a population peaks at a birth/fertility rate that greatly outpaces the death rate (the top of the J-curve), the use of finite resources (soil for food, water, fish, etc.) leads to a depletion that has a cascading effect on the ecology and then triggers a die-off of the species. Again, remember that this occurs frequently with a large percentage of living species.

Negative Health Effects of Urbanization and Overpopulation

Let's go back to COVID-19 (see **Chapter 1**). As people crowd together, the odds of airborne infections propagating rapidly increase. In highly urbanized areas, this is true even in outdoor spaces. Consider, for example, most streets in New York City (see **Photo 14.1**) during much of the day. Although the air exchange rate in outdoor settings does not favor the transmission of infections such as COVID-19, expired droplets from coughing or sneezing in crowded outdoor settings can be highly transmissible vectors of airborne pathogens.

expired droplets from coughing or sneezing in crowded outdoor settings can be highly transmissible vectors of airborne pathogens

Ironically, an old public health theory known as a **miasma** appears applicable in the era of COVID-19 and other emerging airborne diseases. A miasma is an unpleasant smell or order; however, it was the focus of a predominant theory in the global era of the plague (Black Death). Originated by Hippocrates, the theory held that "bad air" was the cause of many common infectious diseases. This theory continued to be popular until the middle of the nineteenth century! It certainly was off the mark relative to diseases such as chlamydia, cholera, and hemorrhagic diseases. But as modern times arrived, it became apparent that some diseases were readily spread through the air among people residing in close contact with one another (including outdoor spaces). An example was the 1918 influenza pandemic (see **Chapter 1**) that claimed the lives of more than 50 million

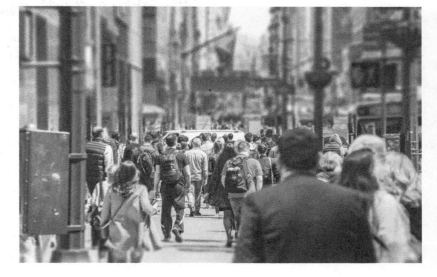

Photo 14.1   In heavily urbanized areas, even outdoor spaces can pose a risk of spreading airborne pathogens.
Source: Rawf8 / Adobe Stock.

people worldwide. Urban centers were especially hard hit, given that the virus could spread easily on crowded subway trains, buses, and even sidewalks. Thus, the seemingly primitive idea of "bad air" played out during this time, as Hippocrates had once suggested. With COVID-19, the same crowded conditions also served as an efficient means for the virus to propagate and claim lives.

Moving from airborne disease to waterborne disease, consider the Hudson River in New York. As more people came to reside near this river, it was increasingly used by boats and jet skis that discharge gas and oil into the water. It also became an increasingly attractive river for industries looking to construct new plants and factories. From the viewpoint of some industries, the Hudson offered a convenient waterway for dumping heated water (a common waste product) or any factory-produced chemicals that could not be stored or otherwise discarded. As urbanization continued near this historic river, the water was also filled with waste and garbage generated by people (bottles, cans, and debris). Moreover, the river was polluted as the result of agricultural practices in the area scaling up production by using more fertilizer – much of which ran off the fields and entered streams and smaller rivers that eventually spilled into the Hudson (see **Photo 14.2**).

A final point about urbanization involves the loss of trees, grass, and other plants that bind carbon into the soil. If you have lived (or live now) in a fast-growing city, you have doubtlessly

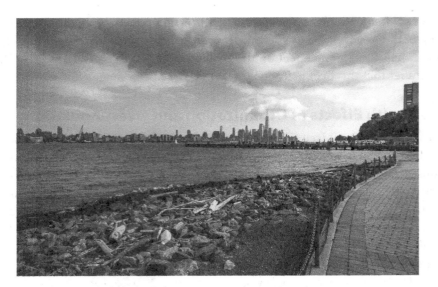

Photo 14.2 Many urban waterways, such as the Hudson River, are far from the standard of "fishable and swimmable" specified in the Clean Water Act.
Source: Ezume Images / Adobe Stock.

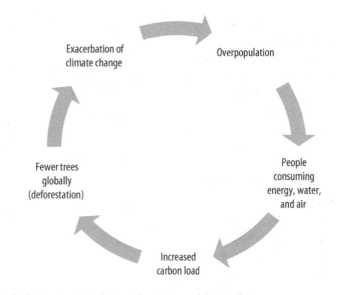

Figure 14.3 The relationship between overpopulation, deforestation, and climate change

witnessed how quickly trees and green space disappear as housing developments spring up. To this point, think about the effects of urbanization in terms of augmenting the pace of climate change. Of course, it is a bit unfair to attribute the destruction of trees only to urbanization. Instead, think of urbanization as a logical and necessary outgrowth of population growth. With this larger point in mind, study **Figure 14.3** to learn how overpopulation indirectly poses negative health effects for people due to deforestation leading to climate change.

think about the effects of urbanization in terms of augmenting the pace of climate change

Reduced Population Growth Is Possible

A key aspect of controlling climate change (which is seldom recognized in major global initiatives, including the Paris Climate Agreement) is controlling birth rates. The realities of overpopulation necessitate the question of how public health can play a role in at least preventing **unintentional pregnancy**. In the United States, nearly half (about 46%) of all births result from an unintentional pregnancy. To be clear, *unintentional* does not always imply *unwanted*; it simply means that one or both people involved in conceiving the pregnancy did not desire the pregnancy to occur at that time or at any time in the future.

As you can easily guess, a key population-level factor in any given nation's rate of unintended pregnancy is the use of **contraception** (methods that prevent pregnancy from occurring). More specifically, a public health guideline known as the **Four A's** applies nicely here. The Four A's are typically applied to products (e.g., medicines, vaccines, screening tests, vitamins, nutritional supplements, and – of course – contraceptive methods and devices). These four terms, which are used widely in global health (but are also applicable in high-income countries such as the United States), are as follows for any given product:

- **Availability:** An ample supply is available for public use.

- **Affordability:** The cost is within the financial reach of those who need the product most.

- **Accessibility:** The product is relatively easy to obtain (long traveling distances are not required).

- **Acceptability:** People desire to use the product.

Applied specifically to contraceptive options, the Four A's are described by these basic questions:

- Availability: Is the method/device widely found throughout the population?

- Affordability: Is the method/device fully or mostly covered by health insurance?

- Accessibility: Is the method/device easy to obtain close to where people who need it the most reside and work?

- Acceptability: Does the method/device carry a social stigma or have a negative moral overtone? Is the method/device trusted as safe and reliable by the users?

As you can garner from thinking about the Four A's applied to contraception, multiple public health strategies can be employed to promote its use. For instance, government subsidies can greatly reduce the costs associated with obtaining highly reliable contraception on an ongoing basis. An example is the birth control pill. From a global perspective, the United States is in the middle of a divide over government subsidies for contraception. All the former Soviet nations, Asia, India, and an impressive number of African nations are advanced in this regard because they provide the pill completely without charge to any female citizen who wants to avoid pregnancy. These nations are ultimately protecting women's rights, particularly among four populations of women most likely to experience one or more unintended pregnancies: (1) women of color, (2) low-income women, (3) women 18–24 years of age, and (4) unmarried women living with a cohabitating male partner. The concept of women's rights applies here because of the stunning change in the course of life that often occurs because of unintended pregnancy.

Unintended pregnancy followed by giving birth greatly decreases the chances of obtaining higher education and achieving career goals that provide adequate income. From a national perspective, a study of just one year (2010) found that public insurance programs throughout the United States paid for 68% of all unintended births, compared to just 38% of all intentional births. This same study estimated that the U.S. expenditure in that year for unintended births (as well as the costs of miscarriages and abortions for unintentional pregnancies) was $21 billion (Sonfield & Kost, 2015).

> Unintended pregnancy followed by giving birth greatly decreases the chances of obtaining higher education and achieving career goals that provide adequate income

Throughout the world, many nations have successfully controlled population growth via a reduction in the rates of unintended pregnancy. One of most advantageous ways to achieve this goal is the widespread use of **long-acting reversible contraception** (LARC). The long-acting aspect of LARC is based on the use of implants (either under the skin or in the uterus). LARC comes in two forms, which are commonly accepted as gold standards in highly reliable contraception: Mirena (an **intrauterine device**, meaning it is placed in the uterus) and Implanon (a hormonal contraceptive that works by slow release and is implanted under the skin of the upper arm). Because user error is not possible with either method, Mirena and Implanon are mistake-proof as long as the provider performs their role correctly when placing the implant. The reversible aspect of LARC is in comparison to tubal ligation (cutting of the fallopian tubes to render the female infertile), which is considered permanent. LARC implants function 3 to 10 years, with the option to have the provider remove the implant at any time.

Given the advanced biotechnology of LARC, the public health challenge lies in promoting the widespread use of these options. This is typically best achieved through the diffusion of innovation (DOI) theory you learned about in **Chapter 13**. Some of the key factors in applying LARC to DOI involve making both Mirena and Implanon

- Easy to *access* (every local village, town, or city neighborhood should have at least one provider of these services)
- Easy to *afford* (or completely free)
- *Acceptable* (meaning education programs dispel myths about side effects)

Fortunately for low-income women living in the United States, one national organization specializes in all three of these goals: **Planned Parenthood**. This non-profit, voluntary health organization provides a wealth of reproductive health care services – especially services relevant to contraception – in all 50 U.S. states.

Finally, it is well worth knowing that a longstanding federal policy/act (passed under the Nixon administration and known as **Title X**) provides free (or nearly free) contraceptive services to people with limited economic resources (these services include LARC).

The goal of widespread dissemination of LARC in the United States and elsewhere is further enhanced by lay health workers (defined as non-medical volunteers or people earning very low wages for their work) who assist women with family planning and birth. For example, a recent study in Ethiopia found that training lay health workers (known there as Community-Based Reproductive Health Care Workers) in promoting and inserting LARC significantly impacted the population-level use of LARC (Zerfu, Ayele, & Bogale, 2018). Simply stated, the lay health workers served as catalysts for aiding women to change from short-term contraception to LARC. The success in making this population-level change was stunning: 45% of women opted to have a LARC implant. This single study represents a world of possibilities for the widespread use of LARC in any nation where women do not have to pay for this method of contraception (including, of course, the United States).

Why Is the Widespread Education of Girls Important to Population Control?

For many students, the idea that educating girls is perhaps the single most important public health intervention may seem like a stretch. But when it comes to global issues such as climate change, this approach consistently emerges as the best possible investment in the future of the human species. The case for this high-level form of public health intervention was wonderfully articulated by Kristof and WuDunn (2010) in their book *Half the Sky: Turning Oppression into Opportunity for Women Worldwide*. They are reporters who work with boots on the ground, and their book describes not only the global atrocities experienced by young girls but also the tremendous success stories in parts of the world that have begun to embrace the idea that providing elementary and secondary education to girls (at a level on par with that provided to boys) ultimately leads to stronger economies, less violence against women, and a much later age of marriage; in addition, educated women have far fewer children than their counterparts who complete only a rudimentary education.

Although delving into the politics and sexism that have led to a widespread lack of education (and thus opportunity) for girls and young women is beyond the scope of this chapter, it is nonetheless valuable to have at least a basic understanding of the public health importance of expanding educational opportunities for females. First, many nations are largely **paternalistic** (meaning male-centered and male-dominated). This includes many parts of the United States; however, the degree of paternalism in many other nations translates into a blatant lack of opportunity for girls to attend school compared to boys. This gender-based disparity plays out into adulthood, leaving uneducated young women with extremely limited job opportunities (if any). These young women enter motherhood as a career; thus, conceiving children provides status, value in the community, and a form of employment. What has been gleaned by demographers is that any intervention that changes this equation will lower the nation's fertility rate. So, the question becomes, what interventions tend to work the best? Three of the most promising intervention approaches are worth your time and study at this point in the chapter.

any intervention that changes this equation will lower the nation's fertility rate

School Support

In reviews of randomized trials, Baird, Ahner-McHaffie, & Özler (2019) provided copious details about intervention approaches designed to keep girls in school and advance their education to post-secondary education. The concept of school support was a common thread in this review. This concept revolves around providing girls with a few basic needs that otherwise would preclude them from attending school. The most basic of these is the required school uniform (in many poorer nations, a household will only spend money on uniforms for its sons). Thus, providing funding for required school uniforms for girls is a very simple form of public health intervention (see **Photo 14.3**).

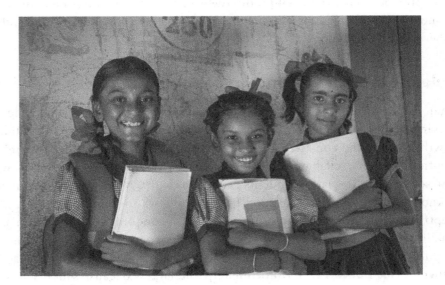

Photo 14.3   An inexpensive but worthwhile form of public health intervention is as simple as providing funds that pay for required uniforms for schoolgirls.
Source: paltu / Adobe Stock.

The second aspect of this support is paying all required school fees – including those that seem small, as even scant sums may be beyond the financial reach (or financial will) of the family/household. A final part of school support is assigning an adult mentor to help school-girls complete and excel in their homework and in-school assignments.

Cash Transfers

This intervention approach is either conditional (e.g., on having good grades) or unconditional. As opposed to school fees, these cash transfers happen regularly and are made to the household rather than the schoolgirls. Although nominal, this cash compensates households for any perceived loss of income/productivity that may result from girls attending school rather than performing other work at home or in the community.

Microcredit

Also known as microloans, **microcredit** is a form of financial assistance and an outstanding example of how very small investments can greatly benefit the future health and well-being of a nation. Applicable mostly to post-secondary education, microcredit is a method of lending money to young women. The money is used for advanced schooling or for starting home-based businesses that generate income to pay for advanced schooling. This intervention approach has been particularly effective for keeping girls in school (possibly into post-secondary education). In turn, this advanced education fosters their independence, creates greater equity with men, delays the age of marriage, and substantially reduces the number of pregnancies and births.

Of note, this type of public health intervention is extremely **distal** (meaning distant from the more ordinary approach of teaching about – and providing – contraception) compared to past approaches. Think of distal as meaning that the outermost layers of an ecological model (see **Chapters 2 and 3**) are the target of change.

the end results of educating girls and young women represent the most promising approach to ultimately reducing the global rate of population growth

Like most structural-level interventions, the end results of educating girls and young women represent the most promising approach to ultimately reducing the global rate of population growth. These approaches are also respectful and mindful of the point that women have a right to pursue lives independent of being a wife or mother. Even more vital is that the various approaches provide women with **economic freedom**, thereby reducing or ending dependence on men who may be careless about conceiving pregnancies or want to have more children than the number desired by women.

The Role of Males in Controlling Population Growth

Other than having a vasectomy (a simple surgical procedure that leaves the male incapable of conceiving a child), the one role that males can play in the service of controlling population growth involves the consistent use of condoms. Using condoms as the only form of contraception is a fairly reliable method. Data-derived estimates suggest that – when used correctly (see **Box 14.3**) – latex condoms can be up to 90% effective. This estimate implies what is known as **perfect use** (meaning the user follows the instructions exactly) of the contraceptive (in this case, condoms). The dual use of condoms combined with almost any other medically informed method used by a female sex partner is an ambitious yet highly valuable public health goal in a world that is quickly exceeding its carrying capacity for the human species (see **Photo 14.4**). Unfortunately, and largely because schools lack adequate sex education programs, far too many Americans do not know how to use condoms (see **Box 14.3**).

BOX 14.3. THE HUMAN SIDE: "OH, THE THINGS WE THINK!"

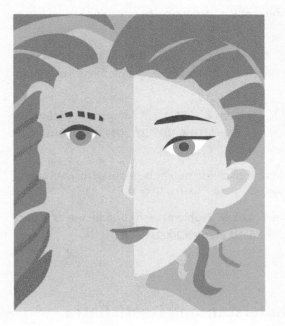

A somewhat odd aspect of human nature is the belief that we inherently know how to perform skill-based actions. For example, if you wear contact lenses, did anyone take a fair amount of time and effort to carefully teach you how to put them in? Or, if you run as an aerobic exercise, did anyone teach you the basics of this sport? Similarly, millions of people (both males and females) assume that they naturally know how to use condoms. It is amazing to ponder why humans so often think they know something when, in reality, they do not!

Even in a high-income nation like the United States, schools often neglect teaching teenagers (many of whom will never have other educational opportunities) about the intricacies of the correct and consistent use of condoms for the prevention of pregnancy and/or sexually transmitted infections (STIs). The result of this neglect is a lack of understanding and essential skills needed by the people choosing this method of contraception and/or disease prevention. Further, the ethic of "I just know" may preclude many people from bothering to learn through the use of credible internet sites or publications. Ultimately, people who thought they were being safe end up being surprised when conception occurs.

Starting at the turn of this century, a relatively small group of researchers began collecting survey data about to the types and frequency of condom-use errors reported by various populations at risk of unintended pregnancy and/or STIs (a short list of selected publications from the research is shown at the end of this box). The researchers typically found that seven condom-use errors (i.e., mistakes people make in the correct use of condoms) were common, meaning they occurred as frequently as one-third of the time for 10–30% of the subpopulations studied.

Based on the collective findings from these studies, an intervention program was designed and tested (Crosby et al., 2014). The program was simple. On a one-to-one basis, it provided people with the knowledge and skills to use condoms correctly (and thus more enjoyably). As an example of how a public health education program can easily teach people knowledge and skills, **Table 14.1** shows part of the manual used to train the educators who conducted the program.

Table 14.1   Common mistakes people experience when using condoms

Mistake	Solution	Comment
Condom slips off	Need a smaller size	Size is based on a fully erect penis. Another reason condoms may slip off is that the erection is not complete.
Condom breaks	This happens for two reasons: (1) the condom has come into contact with an oil-based lubricant or (2) it has been damaged by sharp fingernails, teeth, or jewelry.	Contrary to popular belief, condoms do not break because the penis is too big or there is too much ejaculate.
Condom is put on too late	Men need to learn about pre-cum and that they cannot penetrate a partner at all until the condom is on.	Pre-cum is not visible or something that can be felt easily – it is part of arousal.
Condom is taken off too soon	Men need to know that they cannot just take the condom off after they ejaculate and then have more sex.	Semen will remain on the penis, and this can introduce STIs to the partner or cause a pregnancy.
Condom is not put on correctly	Men need to be taught to pinch air from the receptacle tip with one hand while gently unrolling the condom with the other hand.	Also teach men that their partners should be encouraged to participate in condom application.
Condom becomes dry	Men need to be taught to pause sex every 5 minutes or so to add generous amounts of lubricant.	Lubricants must be water-based, silicone-based, or a combination of the two.
Condom slips off during withdrawal of the penis	Men need to be taught to hold the rim of the condom when withdrawing the penis.	This usually happens because the erection is lost soon after ejaculation.

The following are examples of studies about condom-use errors:

- Crosby, R. A., Charnigo, R., & Shrier, L. A. (2012). Condom use errors and problems among teens attending clinics: Better or worse than young adults? *Journal of Contraception, 3,* 17–22.

- Crosby, R. A., Milhausen, R. R., Marks, K. P., Yarber, W. L., Sanders, S. A., & Graham, C. A. (2013). Understanding problems with condom fit and feel: An important opportunity for improving clinic-based safer sex programs. *Journal of Primary Prevention, 34,* 109–115.

- Topping, A. A., Milhausen, R. R., Graham, C., Sanders, S. A., Yarber, W. L., & Crosby, R. A. (2011). A comparison of condom use errors for heterosexual anal and vaginal intercourse. *International Journal of STDs & AIDS, 22,* 204–208. doi:10.1258/ijsa.2011.010259

- Crosby, R. A., Graham, C. A., Yarber, W. L., & Sanders, S. A. (2010). Problems with condoms may be reduced for men taking ample time to apply them. *Sexual Health, 7,* 66–70. doi:10.1071/SH09020

- Crosby, R. A., Yarber, W. L., Graham, C. A., & Sanders, S. A. (2010). Does it fit okay? Problems with condom use as a function of self-reported poor fit. *Sexually Transmitted Infections, 86,* 36–38. doi:10.1136/sti.2009.036665

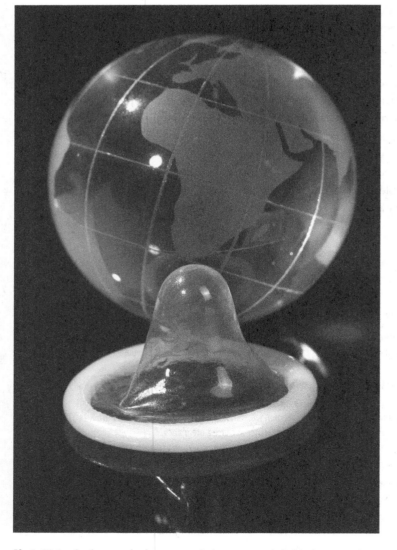

Photo 14.4 Condoms may be the answer to the long-term survival of the human species.
Source: Guy Shapira / Adobe Stock.

Understanding Death Rates

In many of the same nations experiencing a high birth rate, the **right to die** is often less of a right than a product of the surrounding medical culture. The medicalization of death often translates into people living longer than they wish to. This extended life is far too often of very low quality. The cost of extending life for a person with a terminal illness is far greater in the United States than other nations (between $30,000 and $45,000 per added year of life). In addition to this high cost, it is vital to consider several related points:

- In nations with healthcare systems that are government-based, resources are finite. Thus, using an unaffordable medication or surgery to extend life implies that healthcare services for much younger people must be sacrificed.

- Physicians and other medical professionals are trained to preserve life regardless of the cost. However, this ethic may not align with the will of a dying patient.

- Justifying out-of-range costs for dying patients based on private-payer health plans and fee-for-service healthcare creates a two-tiered society in which those with more money are prioritized.

Although end-of-life medical decisions are difficult and highly personal, many people who want the right to die may not be allowed to do so. As part of the medical ethic to preserve life at all costs, this right is commonly abridged in many U.S. states. Thus, just as overpopulation stems from a massive number of unintentional annual pregnancies, it also results from a medical industry designed to maintain life irrespective of its quality.

What About the Future?

Returning now to Malthus, it is worth noting that more recent scholars have moved beyond the concept of carrying capacity to describe overpopulation as a cause of emerging global pandemics such as Ebola, avian flu, severe acute respiratory syndrome (SARS), and COVID-19 (the most recent version of SARS) (Spernovasilis et al., 2021). As noted by these scholars, a common thread of emerging diseases that become national epidemics or global pandemics is that they are **zoonotic**, meaning the pathogen originates in a species other than humans. This consistent trend toward the emergence of zoonotic diseases is a likely consequence of overpopulation and its manifestations: particularly the rapid extinction of plant and animal species, creating a lack of **biodiversity**. Spernovasilis et al. (2021) described overpopulation as resulting in the global need for what have become known as **concentrated animal feeding operations** (CAFOs). In turn, the widespread proliferation of CAFOs provides an ecological advantage to zoonotic pathogens. The solution proposed by Spernovasilis and colleagues (2021) nicely summarizes this entire chapter by noting the tremendous public health opportunity relative to reducing unintended pregnancies, including a poignant direction for the future: "new methods of contraception that are more easily accessible and effective ought to be sought out."

Whether or not history shows that COVID-19 originated as a zoonotic disease, it is appropriate to end this chapter with the point that this disease created an upward trend in death rates, thereby slightly decreasing the otherwise rapid expansion of the human population (estimates suggest that the current 7.7 billion people inhabiting the earth will expand to 9.7 billion by the year 2050). From March 2020 through October 2021, COVID-19 was the third leading cause of death in the United States (Shiels, Hague, & de Gonzales, 2022). Whether other pandemics, or even the COVID-19 pandemic (see **Chapter 1**), may serve as a type of natural check and balance against the imminent dangers of overpopulation is a legitimate question for your future.

estimates suggest that the current 7.7 billion people inhabiting the earth will expand to 9.7 billion by the year 2050

Review and Key Terms

Building on the previous two chapters, this chapter has introduced the public health problems and challenges posed by global **overpopulation**. A species, including *homo sapiens*, is considered at risk of rapid decline when the population exceeds the **environment's carrying capacity**. Tragically, thousands of species become extinct with each passing year; this creates a loss in **biodiversity**. Extinction was famously explained by a scholar named Robert Malthus. Known as the **Malthus hypothesis**, this explanation currently applies to humans in parts of the world that have greatly exceeded the carrying capacity for humans, thus limiting the survival of those populations. The hypothesis posits that an **S-shaped curve** is a far more gentle response to the sharp decline in a population that occurs under the assumptions of the **J-shaped curve**.

One key to understanding the threat of overpopulation is considering the effects of urbanization (a necessary response to overpopulation) on public health. The fact that overcrowding of people creates an ecological advantage for airborne pathogens dates back several hundred years to the idea of a **miasma** (bad air). A second key is to understand that overpopulation leads to competition for a limited food and water supply, with this competition typically favoring those people with higher incomes over those with lower incomes and thereby creating further health disparities.

Given the emerging realities of the Malthus hypothesis, the goal of **zero population growth** has been embraced by many nations. Although this chapter differentiated between the **birth rate** and the **fertility rate,** it also emphasized the value and importance of approaching the problem of overpopulation by focusing on reducing the rate of **unintended pregnancies**. This can be achieved globally through increased public health efforts regarding access, availability, affordability, and acceptability (the **Four A's**) of **long-acting reversible contraception** (LARC). An example of LARC is the use of an intrauterine device. Regardless of the **contraceptive** choices women make, the rapid onset of climate change and its consequences relative to supplies of food and potable water necessitate increased public health attention to **family planning** efforts via organizations such as **Planned Parenthood**. In the United States, a particularly important piece of legislation (**Title X**) also helps provide equity relative to preventing unintended pregnancies.

This chapter may have surprised you by stating that one of the most **distal** yet powerful public health intervention approaches is focused on increasing the number of schoolgirls who complete elementary and secondary school programs. The enhanced education of girls and young women provides them with **economic freedoms** that are likely to result in fewer unintended pregnancies. Given that so many of the nations on earth are highly **paternalistic**, the public health goal of creating equitable educational opportunities for girls and young women has been largely pursued through approaches that involve cash transfers, providing uniforms, and **microcredit**.

Beyond unintended pregnancies, the overpopulation problem is exacerbated in many high-income nations (such as the United States) by a medical ethic to preserve human life regardless of cost, quality of life, or the desire of people living with a terminal disease or condition. The **right to die** is therefore a topic that also concerns public health. As more and more nations undergo a **demographic transition**, the issue of the right to die will become increasingly important in places with limited carrying capacity.

The chapter also focused on males as part of addressing the global problem of overpopulation. This focus took the form of enhancing public health efforts to greatly expand the use of condoms by males who may be at risk of causing an unintended pregnancy. A key aspect is that the **perfect-use** rating of condoms against conception is very high.

Despite the grim nature of the Malthus hypothesis, this chapter also made reference to the point that overpopulation may lead to rapid declines in the human population via **zoonotic** diseases. For example, you learned about **concentrated animal feeding operations** that provide emerging pathogens with large ecological advantages relative to propagating, thus affecting the human population on a large scale. This final point of emerging pathogens is a forerunner to the next (and last) chapter of this textbook.

For Practice and Class Discussion

Practice Questions (answers are located in the appendix to this textbook)

1. As part of a public health intervention program, social media marketing is used to promote the use of LARC as a responsibility to the earth. Which one of the four A's is the target of this program?
   a. Affordability
   b. Accessibility

c. Acceptability

d. Availability

2. The fertility rate will always be greater than the birth rate.

   a. True

   b. False

3. Which of the following is least associated with increased urbanization?

   a. Increased pollution of waterways

   b. Increased risk of airborne disease transmission

   c. Newborn deaths

   d. Fewer trees to bind carbon

4. Which one of the following best describes the concept of a demographic transition?

   a. Carbon dioxide levels accelerate global warming.

   b. The mean age of a population shifts to a much younger average.

   c. The birth rate exceeds the death rate by a 2:1 ratio.

   d. The fertility rate declines.

5. The Malthus hypothesis implies all of the following except:

   a. Zoonotic diseases will decimate a large number of people.

   b. Carrying capacity limits population expansion.

   c. A J-shaped curve involves a rapid die-off of the affected species.

   d. An S-shaped curve is a more optimistic outcome than a J-shaped curve.

6. Which one of the following public health actions is the least critical to reducing the rate of unintended pregnancy in the United States?

   a. Title X

   b. Microcredit programs

   c. LARC

   d. Programs that promote correct condom use

7. Thinking about all you have learned in this chapter, which form of public health intervention to reduce global overpopulation is the most distal in its goals?

   a. Widespread dissemination of LARC

   b. Teaching young males how to use condoms

   c. Enhancing the provision of low-cost (or free) contraception services for women

   d. Providing equal education opportunities for girls and young women

8. Which term represents "bad air" and is thus applicable to explaining the increased risk of respiratory diseases among urban populations?

   a. Right-to-die

   b. IUD

   c. Miasma

   d. Zoonotic

9. Educating girls and young women is vital to controlling overpopulation because this education focuses on teaching knowledge and skills regarding condoms and contraceptive options.

   a. True

   b. False

10. Carrying capacity is exceeded when:

    a. The population birth rate is above 2.0

    b. Finite resources supporting a population become insufficient

c. The S-shaped distribution reaches its peak

d. The fertility rate exceeds the birth rate

Discussion Questions

11. As part of this chapter, you learned about a 45% increase in LARC use that was achieved at a population level through the use of lay health workers. As you may recall, this occurred in rural Ethiopia, and the study citation is Zerfu, Ayele, & Bogale, 2018. Your task is to retrieve this article and read it entirely. Then, jot down at least three talking points you feel are worthy of posting on a class-based discussion board. Make your points very clear when you post!

12. This chapter briefly described the rapid extinction of species on the planet (creating a loss of biodiversity). Working with one or two other students, go online and locate a journal article that describes the recent (in the past five years) extinction of a species. Summarize what you learned into everyday words and share your summary with people not taking the same class via your preferred form of social media. How did your friends react to your posting?

13. As a rather ambitious yet valuable exercise that extends what you have learned in this chapter, consider reading the book *Under a White Sky: The Nature of the Future* (Kolbert, E. (2021). Crown: New York, NY). This book provides a vivid and gripping description of what your future could be like without immediately escalating the global response to overpopulation. After you finish reading the book, inspire others in the class by posting a one- to two-page summary of how it changed your thinking about overpopulation.

References

Baird, S., Ahner-McHaffie, T., & Özler, B. (2019) Can interventions to increase schooling and income reduce HIV incidence among young women in Sub-Saharan Africa? In R. A. Crosby and R. J. DiClemente (Eds). *Structural Interventions for HIV Prevention*. New York: Oxford University Press.

Crosby, R. A., Charnigo, R. J., Salazar, L. F., Pasternak, R., Terrell, I., Ricks. J., & Taylor, S. (2014). Enhancing condom use among young black males: A randomized controlled trial. *The American Journal of Public Health, 104*, 2219–2225.

Jones, H. (2020, December 31). Animals that went extinct in 2020 and ones that could disappear after 2021. https://metro.co.uk/2020/12/31/animals-that-went-extinct-in-2020-and-the-ones-that-could-disappear-after-2021-13780929/

Kristof, N. D., & WuDunn, S. (2010). *Half the sky: turning oppression into opportunity for women worldwide*. New York: Knopf Doubleday Publishing Group.

Shiels, M. S., Hague, A. T., & de Gonzales, A. B. (2022). Leading causes of death in the United States during the COVID-19 pandemic, March 2020 to October 2012. *The Journal of the American Medical Association, 182*(8), 883–886.

Sonfield, A., & Kost, K. (2015) *Public costs from unintended pregnancies and the role of public insurance programs in paying for pregnancy-related care: national and state estimates for 2010*. New York: Guttmacher Institute.

Spernovasilis, N., Markaki, I., Papadakis, M., Tsioutis, C., & Markaki, L. (2021). Epidemics and pandemics: Is human population the elephant in the room? *Ethics in Medical Public Health, 19*, 100728.

Zerfu, T. A., Ayele, H. D., & Bogale, T. X. (2018). Effect of deploying trained Community-Based Reproductive Nurses (CORN) on LARC use in rural Ethiopia: A cluster randomized trial. *Studies in Family Planning, 49*, 115–126.

CHAPTER 15

EMERGING DISEASES AND THE NEED FOR VACCINE RESEARCH

"Winter is coming."

—*Ned Stark; season 1*, Game of Thrones

Overview

After reading 14 chapters of this textbook, you may think the entire scope of public health practice is now within your understanding. In an ideal world, that would be true! But one defining characteristic of the 21st century is that it has been characterized by more emerging diseases than ever before. Therefore, the future of public health practice must include a response system for the inevitable outbreaks, epidemics, and pandemics of infectious diseases. This last chapter brings you back to where the textbook began: that the COVID-19 pandemic is simply one of many emerging threats to the health of the public. Consider, for instance, the 2022 outbreak of monkeypox (see **Photo 15.1**).

This chapter begins by providing you with a bit of history regarding the survival of the human race – which would not have been possible without vaccines for diseases such as smallpox and polio. Following the history lesson, you will learn how current medical and CDC recommendations greatly advance public health through routine schedules of vaccinations. Once you have a very clear image of how integral vaccines are to public health, the chapter then takes you into the realm of the most significant role of public health practice: preparedness for the emergence (or re-emergence) of highly infectious pathogens that have the capacity to end life. The cornerstone of this preparedness is a global system of vaccine development, manufacturing, distribution, and acceptance by entire populations.

This chapter is not for the faint of heart! Indeed, the grim realities of emerging diseases provide a somewhat dismal portrait of uneasy times for the health and livelihood of humans. Rather than shed light on tried-and-true intervention approaches, the chapter offers somewhat anxiety-provoking conclusions about the need to urgently intensify public health efforts focused on disease outbreaks and responses. However, just as the character Ned Stark in the *Game of Thrones* series used to warn ("Winter is coming"), we have time to prepare for worst-case scenarios. Whether this time is used wisely or squandered will be a product of global levels of financial and political commitment. Given the point (see **Chapters 12**

LEARNING OBJECTIVES

- Understand the history of vaccinating humans against smallpox.

- Appreciate that numerous diseases have been successfully controlled through childhood and adult vaccination efforts.

- Describe several types of emerging diseases that threaten humans.

- Understand that key organizations are already in place to respond effectively to emerging diseases.

- Understand the delicate balance between the ability to create vaccines and the mutation of emerging diseases.

CDC

Monkeypox Outbreak — Nine States, May 2022

Weekly / June 10, 2022 / 71(23);764–769

On June 3, 2022, this report was posted online as an MMWR Early Release.

Please note: This report has been corrected.

Faisal S. Minhaj, PharmD[1,2]; Yasmin P. Ogale, PhD[1,3]; Florence Whitehill, DVM[1,2]; Jordan Schultz, MPH[4]; Mary Foote, MD[5]; Whitni Davidson, MPH[2]; Christine M. Hughes, MPH[2]; Kimberly Wilkins[2]; Laura Bachmann, MD[3]; Ryan Chatelain, MPH[6]; Marisa A.P. Donnelly, PhD[1]; Rafael Mendoza, MPH[7]; Barbara L. Downes, MS[8]; Mellisa Roskosky, PhD[1,9]; Meghan Barnes, MSPH[10]; Glen R. Gallagher, PhD[4]; Nesli Basgoz, MD[11]; Victoria Ruiz, PhD[5]; Nang Thu Thu Kyaw, PhD[1,5]; Amanda Feldpausch, DVM[12]; Amy Valderrama, PhD[13]; Francisco Alvarado-Ramy, MD[14]; Chad H. Dowell, MS[15]; Catherine C. Chow, MD[16]; Yu Li, PhD[2]; Laura Quilter, MD[3]; John Brooks, MD[17]; Demetre C. Daskalakis, MD[17]; R. Paul McClung, MD[3]; Brett W. Petersen, MD[2]; Inger Damon, MD, PhD[2]; Christina Hutson, PhD[2]; Jennifer McQuiston, DVM[2]; Agam K. Rao, MD[2]; Ermias Belay, MD[2]; Andrea M. McCollum, PhD[2]; Monkeypox Response Team 2022 (View author affiliations)

View suggested citation

Photo 15.1   The CDC's Morbidity and Mortality Weekly Report (MMWR) is part of the U.S. public health system.

and 13) that climate change, as well as overpopulation (see **Chapter 14**), contribute to the problem of emerging diseases, we all share an imperative to move quickly toward supporting policies and practices that prepare the world for the inevitable pandemics that will follow in the footprints of COVID-19.

This chapter of the textbook departs from the previous ethic that most areas of expertise have much to contribute to public health practice (e.g., architecture, urban planning, marketing, law, and economics). Instead, this chapter offers you the conclusion that outbreak surveillance (conducted by epidemiologists) and vaccination campaigns require specialized expertise, thereby necessitating that governments employ full-time public health experts specifically to fortify preparedness. Moreover, the chapter will not focus on the United States. Pathogens can easily travel from one continent to another via human carriers, and thus the boundaries of any one nation mean nothing when it comes to ensuring the ongoing survival of the human race.

outbreak surveillance (conducted by epidemiologists) and vaccination campaigns require specialized expertise

Learning from the History of Smallpox and HIV

Occasionally, history can be our greatest teacher! This is clearly the case relative to smallpox. As a virus, smallpox could not be treated; it could only be controlled through increasingly more intense public health efforts. Similar to the early variants of COVID-19 (see **Chapter 1**), smallpox was transmitted through close contact with respiratory droplets from people with active cases. Thus, much like COVID-19, quarantine of infected people was common. In fact, in some nations that were highly committed to ending the spread of smallpox, a quarantine was legally enforced (armed guards routinely enforced the strict quarantine of active cases). Also like COVID-19, a vaccine was eventually developed. However, at this juncture, the parallels between the two diseases end. Although smallpox had been part of human history since the sixth century, the vaccine was "discovered" just prior to 1800 and not widely manufactured until another 100 years had passed. As the 1900s began, the new ability of humans to manufacture the vaccine was still not enough to control the rampant transmission of smallpox that occurred sporadically around the world (in local epidemics rather than an overall pandemic). It was not until 1952 that smallpox was declared **eliminated** on the North American continent, followed by Europe in 1953, South America in 1971, Asia in 1975, and Africa in 1977. In 1908, the World Health Organization (WHO) finally declared that smallpox had been successfully **eradicated** globally (see **Photo 15.2**). Note that disease **elimination** refers to "no remaining cases in a region" (i.e., North America), whereas disease **eradication** refers to no remaining cases anywhere in the world.

One important lesson from smallpox is that the creation of a vaccine has no real bearing on public health practice until that vaccine can be widely manufactured (and stored during shipping). Of course, this process no longer takes 100 years, as it did with smallpox. The incredibly fast pace characterizing COVID-19 vaccine development, manufacturing, and distribution was made possible by already-existing public health partnerships throughout the world.

A somewhat glaring lesson from smallpox, however, is that people were reticent to accept the vaccine: some individuals were willing to receive it only when an epidemic was occurring. Suspicions that the vaccine would cause smallpox or even lead to other diseases (including syphilis) were rampant in many parts of the world, including the United States. The lesson should be instructive in the future: vaccine availability is only one step in a chain of public health actions needed to control emerging diseases. **Figure 15.1** portrays this chain.

As shown in the figure, vaccine development must be followed by the rapid scaling up of vaccine manufacturing and distribution systems. Of course, this takes the vaccine to the people, but it does not mean the people will come to the vaccine! The next step has traditionally eluded public health practice: it requires localized vaccine promotion programs via face-to-face contact, social media, and education programs designed to dispel misconceptions and foster motivation for vaccine acceptance. Although this vaccine response seems thorough enough, the problem is typically that a large portion of the population does not receive the vaccine, thereby creating a need for the simultaneous public health functions of **case surveillance** (i.e., where, and among whom, are new cases of the disease occurring?) followed by a systematic routine of **contact tracing** (see **Chapter 1**) that begins with identified cases (i.e., people) to locate potential cases that may otherwise be left to spread unchecked throughout the population. Depending on the disease, it may be possible to provide treatment to infected persons – and this is a public health imperative. Also, as you know from living through the COVID-19 pandemic, quarantine (either self-imposed or forced) is an option for diseases that cannot be treated.

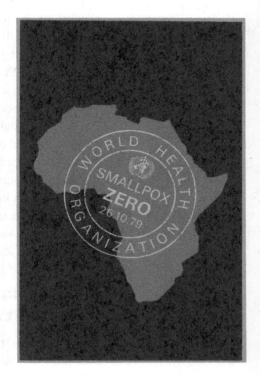

Photo 15.2   The eradication of smallpox occurred nearly 200 years after the discovery of a vaccine.

One important lesson from smallpox is that the creation of a vaccine has no real bearing on public health practice until that vaccine can be widely manufactured

A somewhat glaring lesson from smallpox, however, is that people were reticent to accept the vaccine

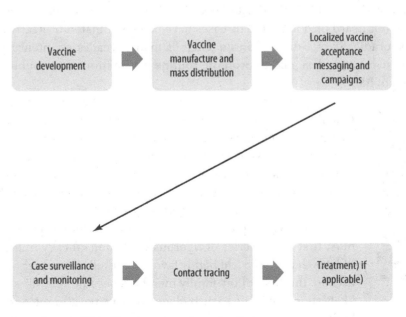

Figure 15.1   A necessary chain of public health actions to control emerging diseases

Fortunately, the smallpox virus did not mutate to the point of requiring new generations of the vaccine (thus necessitating a repeat of the top three steps shown in **Figure 15.1**). Indeed, smallpox was ultimately an "easy virus" when considered in the spectrum of diseases that have plagued humans. The nearly opposite example is HIV (see **Chapter 10**). For instance, although massive government investments were made to develop a vaccine as early as 1987, not one vaccine candidate has yet reached the stage of potential approval for use. Numerous vaccine candidates were tested at varying levels of safety and efficacy based on tightly defined protocols applied to all trials of a vaccine that could ultimately be approved for use. One candidate vaccine showed some very promising results at first; however, in the last leg of the multiple trial conditions required for approval, it was found to lack effectiveness, and the trial was ended in 2013. So, as of the date of this textbook, it has been 35 years (and at least $20 billion) since our nation's federal government first resolved to develop an AIDS vaccine. Moreover, it has been 25 years since President Bill Clinton announced his "new national goal for science" of developing an AIDS vaccine within one decade (Mitchell, 1997, p. 8). In his announcement, which was part of a commencement address, Mr. Clinton compared the quest for an AIDS vaccine to John F. Kennedy's goal of placing a man on the moon. Referring to Kennedy, Clinton remarked, "He gave us the goal of reaching this moon, and we achieved it ahead of time" (Mitchell, 1997, p. 8). As a student reading this textbook, your takeaway from this bit of political history is that some diseases have such a complex causative pathogen (in this case, the very illusive and rapidly mutating virus known as HIV) that **creating a vaccine is a less likely event than the first successful moon landing by U.S. astronauts**. The larger lesson is that the development and success of any future vaccines may or may not be as easily achieved as with the vaccine against COVID-19. In short, the future is **not** guaranteed to be one when vaccines are always possible.

Vaccines Have Already Eliminated Some Diseases in the United States

Recognizing that the United States is a nation with a small percentage (but nonetheless a sizable number) of people known as **anti-vaxxers** (see **Photo 15.3**), it is important to understand that the widespread success of vaccines is all too often taken for granted. For example, when was the last time you heard of a person in your community having the mumps? **Figure 15.2** provides an abbreviated list of diseases that most Americans either do not know about or have not heard of. That these diseases have been eliminated or nearly eliminated or occur only sporadically is a direct consequence of many decades of intense public health advocacy and legislation designed to promote routine vaccination of the public, often in the first few years of life.

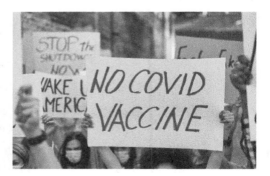

Photo 15.3   Anti-vaxxers typically have a long list of vaccines that they oppose.

Sadly, the passion and commitment of the anti-vaxxers is misplaced. One important function of public health thus becomes educating people so that misconceptions about vaccines can be dispelled. Amplified by social media, a typical anti-vaxxer message might read like this: "Vaccines are the real cause of disease – two of my family members became very ill after receiving the vaccines against the shingles, and my mother has had a sore arm for nine days since getting the flu vaccine." As you have already learned in this chapter, any vaccine approved for use in the United States must first pass a series of rigorous safety and efficacy trails: vaccine candidates that fail to yield highly favorable results will never be approved for use. So, the "two of my family members became very ill" statement most likely stems from the basic biology of a vaccine: it mimics an attack on the body to artificially stimulate an active immune response (see **Chapter 1**).

Without a doubt, a majority of people who claim that a vaccine made them ill are referring to the general malaise, fevers, and overall achiness that characterize an effective immune response. As for the "my mother has had a sore arm for nine days" statement, this probably resulted from how the vaccine was given (e.g., it was injected too far up on the arm and thus damaged shoulder tissue) rather than the vaccine itself.

From a more difficult viewpoint, public health practice must also contend with a history of medical mistrust (one that includes vaccines) among Black/African-American people in the United States. This history traces back to the tragic Tuskegee Study "experiments," which involved purposefully not treating Black men who had syphilis (this was a government-sponsored method of determining the long-term consequences of untreated syphilis). This Tuskegee-generated **medical mistrust** among African Americans remains an issue even now in terms of mistrust of vaccines (see **Box 15.1**). An in-depth treatment of the Tuskegee Study is available in an easy-to-read textbook (see Meyerson, Martich, & Naehr, 2008).

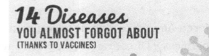

14 Diseases
YOU ALMOST FORGOT ABOUT
(THANKS TO VACCINES)

Routine vaccinations protect against these 14 diseases:

1. Polio	6. Rubella	10. Pneumococcal Disease
2. Tetanus	7. Hib	11. Rotavirus
3. Flu (Influenza)	8. Measles	12. Mumps
4. Hepatitis B	9. Whooping Cough (Pertussis)	13. Chickenpox
5. Hepatitis A		14. Diphtheria

Figure 15.2   For decades, the public had been receiving these vaccines during childhood

a majority of people who claim that a vaccine made them ill are referring to the general malaise, fevers, and overall achiness that characterize an effective immune response

---

BOX 15.1. THE HUMAN SIDE: AN EARNEST MISTRUST OF THE FLU VACCINE AMONG AFRICAN-AMERICANS

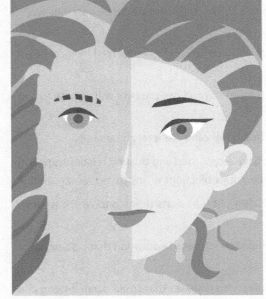

The word "legacy" implies a lasting memory of a positive part of the past. The **Tuskegee Experiment** created a lasting memory, but one that is very negative – even tragic. More than 50 years after Tuskegee, this blatant form of racism – committed in the name of science – continues to instill a well-earned distrust of the medical establishment among many African-Americans living in the United States. As an example, it has long been known that African-Americans are significantly less likely than White and Latinx Americans to receive an annual flu vaccine. This is a longstanding form of **vaccine hesitancy**, and it has a cultural overtone. One of many studies investigating why is worth learning about here.

By engaging people in what are known as **qualitative interviews** (these interviews have very broad and open-ended questions, with the goal of encouraging the people being interviewed to tell their story), behavioral science has much to offer public health practice. In qualitative interviews with more than 100 adults (African-American and White), a recent study produced some intriguing narratives from the African-Americans participants. These narratives were markedly different from those of their White counterparts in the study (Jamison, Quinn, & Freimuth, 2019). For instance, regarding vaccines, one African-American woman stated, "I don't trust the government for nothing that they're mixing up." Other African-Americans expressed similar sentiments, such as stating in regard to Tuskegee, "Different things have been done to us in the past. A certain portion of that is still holding true for a lot of us." A key point made by the authors of this study was that the older generation of African-Americans is prone to skepticism and mistrust regarding the medical establishment in general and vaccines more specifically. Of course, the degree to which this skepticism is attributable to the Tuskegee Experiment cannot be known, other than to say that Tuskegee was clearly a strong contributor. Thus, the human side here is that mistrust of vaccines is often deeply rooted in culturally inherited beliefs.

The concept of anti-vax beliefs is only one of several barriers to the efficient vaccination of entire populations. Other barriers include a lack of easy access, a lack of "remembering," and a general sense of not needing the vaccine until sickness becomes an obvious reality. Even in a high-income nation like the United States, a highly trusted system for vaccine distribution is often fraught with issues relative to compliance by the public. That trusted system is our schools: particularly elementary schools, but also secondary schools (see **Box 15.2**).

BOX 15.2. PUBLIC SCHOOLS AS A LEADER FOR VACCINATING THE PUBLIC

Advocated and guided by the Centers for Disease Control and Prevention, the U.S. public school system is one that offers an ideal public health advantage: vaccinating large numbers of children, adolescents, and teenagers. Perhaps more than any other reason, the primary factor making schools this ideal venue is convenience. Given that students attend school 180 days (or more) each year, it is easy to see how the convenience factor transforms schools from a place of learning to a place that advances public health.

When a school, or an entire school system, decides to engage in the public health responsibility of vaccinating young people, the result is known as a **school-located vaccination clinic** (SLVC). These clinics typically exist in partnership with local health departments. This partnership is advantageous for several reasons:

- Local health departments receive funding from state health departments to purchase and dispense vaccines to the community.

- In addition to school nurses giving vaccinations at school-located vaccination clinics, nurses employed by local health departments can also fill this role.

- Local health departments may have budgets and resources that can be used to promote parent's willingness to consent to the vaccination of their child/adolescent.

From the perspective of a local health department, the partnership with schools offers several advantages:

- School personnel who administer vaccines (typically, "the school nurse") have established and trusting relationships with students and their parents. This relationship often minimizes the odds of parental objections to any particular vaccination.

- School nurses are skilled in record-keeping, thereby creating a type of safety net that alerts them as to which students may be overdue for any given vaccine.

- School nurses working in schools with SLVCs are well-positioned to provide school-based education that dispels prevalent myths about particular vaccines.

As emerging infections continue to add to an already large burden of infectious diseases that could occur among children and adolescents, schools provide a frontline defense in the human struggle to remain disease-free. Thus, in addition to a large number of typical vaccinations that can be provided by SLVCs, newer vaccines (e.g., the COVID-19 vaccines and the Gardasil vaccines that protect against a virus that can lead to cancer) are excellent examples of magnifying prevention efforts through the use of no-cost and pre-existing infrastructures (i.e., the public schools). Without question, as new diseases emerge that can infect children and adolescents, our public health efforts will increasingly rely on SLVCs to efficiently protect the health of the public by providing newly developed vaccines to enrolled students.

Emerging Diseases of Concern

Now that you have a basic appreciation for both the value of and issues related to relying on vaccines to protect humanity against emerging diseases, it is time to learn about the threats we may soon face from these various pathogens. First, however, a bit of terminology is important here. The term **emerging diseases** includes the re-emergence of a past disease (such would be the case, for instance, if smallpox were to somehow be released from one of the two laboratories holding the remaining virus – one in the United States and one in Russia). The term also embodies bacterial diseases that have previously been held in check by antibiotics. Thus, the prospect of currently known microbes developing **antibiotic resistance** is a valid concern for the future of public health. Antibiotic resistance occurs when a species of bacteria mutates beyond the ability of all previously used antibiotics to prevent the replication of the bacteria. Currently, in the United States, an example of this is the sexually transmitted disease gonorrhea. As of 2022, only one antibiotic in a previously large arsenal of treatment options is effective against the gonorrhea bacterium.

To begin understanding the control of emerging diseases, it is vital to grasp the concept of emerging diseases as a global concern. This principle is why surveillance and forecasting are entrusted to a widely respected and supported organization known as the **World Health Organization** (WHO). Based on financial support from nations around the world and the United Nations, the WHO has been the global leader in issuing warnings relative to emerging diseases since its inception in 1948. Moreover, the WHO plays an ongoing and active role in controlling disease outbreaks and the prevention efforts (including vaccination) that must be widely implemented to avert pandemic spread. For example, the WHO led the global response that ultimately resulted in eradicating smallpox. In 2015, the WHO issued a report describing the top eight emerging diseases of concern for the human race (Pizzi, 2015). To help you understand at least some of the basic threats posed by these eight diseases, think of them as falling into three categories. As you might guess, the categories include infections that attack the most essential systems in the body: the cardiovascular system, the respiratory system, and the brain. To be clear, other emerging diseases impact less vital systems in the body; however, it is likely that most emerging diseases will fall into one of these three categories:

> **Category 1: Hemorrhagic fevers** – Diseases characterized by heavy internal bleeding, often leading to death.
>
> **Category 2: Severe respiratory syndromes** – Broadly classified as various types of severe acute respiratory syndrome (SARS). These diseases have a high fatality rate due to loss of lung function.
>
> **Category 3: Swelling of brain tissues** and the tissue covering the spinal cord.

Hemorrhagic Diseases

To understand this category of disease, it is important to first understand that every tissue in the human body has a blood supply. That blood supply comes from **capillary beds**. You may remember learning in high school about oxygenated blood (often shown in red) and venous blood (often shown in blue). In a nutshell, oxygenated blood delivers oxygen to tissues in the capillary beds. At the same time, the capillary beds use the red blood cells as vehicles for transporting the waste product from oxygen use (that is, carbon dioxide) back to the lungs, where it is expelled into the atmosphere. As you can imagine, capillary beds are highly efficient and, of course, vital to life. It is the very tiny blood vessels and veins of the capillary beds that inflame and rupture during any type of hemorrhagic illness. This leads to internal bleeding and compromises the body's immune response. In typical cases of death, the person loses most of their

it is vital to grasp the concept of emerging diseases as a global concern

Sadly, even the disposal of deceased bodies is a risk factor for continued disease transmission

blood volume to the spaces in between various tissues of the body. Sadly, even the disposal of deceased bodies is a risk factor for continued disease transmission because the contaminated blood may leak out of body orifices and represent a biohazard for people handling the body (this is one reason bodies may be cremated as soon as possible after death).

As just a bit of public health history, CDC workers responding to an outbreak of Ebola virus disease in the late 1970s in Zaire quickly discovered a primary route of person-to-person transmission of that virus. They learned about a sacred funeral custom that included a family member of the deceased manually evacuating the rectum and colon of feces before burial. As you can imagine, blood from the action of inserting a hand, wrist, and lower arm into a rectum and colon could easily enter a family member's body through even the smallest of tears, abrasions, or cuts – thereby transferring the virus from the deceased person to the family member. And, as you might guess, the family member might die from Ebola, and yet another family member would perform the burial ritual, sadly perpetuating the cycle of infection and death.

In their listing of eight high priority emerging diseases, the WHO includes four that are hemorrhagic: (1) Crimean-Congo hemorrhagic fever, (2) Ebola virus disease, (3) Marburg virus disease, and (4) Lassa fever (Pizzi, 2015). Rather than drawing distinctions between these four emerging diseases, it is sufficient for you to know that these – and a number of other types of hemorrhagic fevers – are typically spread by the bite of ticks, infected animals, or person-to-person contact that involves exposure to the infected blood or body fluids of one person to another person, who then becomes infected. Although airborne transmission is highly unlikely, public health professionals who respond to outbreaks such as the 2014 West African Ebola epidemic (which claimed more than 11,000 lives) wear protective clothing that includes protection for the eyes and respiratory system (see **Photo 15.4**).

With the exception of yellow fever and Argentine hemorrhagic fever, vaccines for this disease category have not yet been developed. This translates into a massive public health need to engage in the ecological control of the vectors that spread the viruses (e.g., ticks and other insects, rodents) and install regulations – including educational policies – that help curb person-to-person transmission through the exchange of body fluids. These regulations must also include a simple commodity that is often taken for granted and thus overlooked by high-income nations: ample availability of new needles and syringes for medical use.

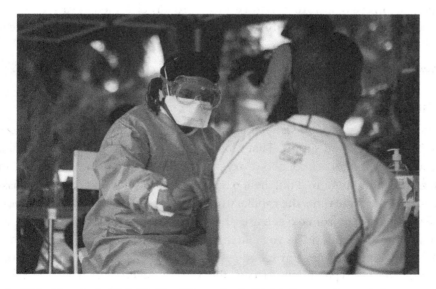

Photo 15.4   A public health worker during the 2014 West African outbreak of Ebola is shown wearing standard protective gear.

Indeed, the hemorrhagic fevers highlight a longstanding shortcoming of global public health practice: the lack of ample availability of the most basic tools (new needles and syringes) for medical care and vaccination campaigns. To illustrate this, consider that in 2000, a global estimate of the percentage of unsafe injections (i.e., lack of both new needles and syringes) was 38.5%. Although this percentage was dramatically reduced by 2010 to just 5.5%, even this seemingly small value equates to millions of unsafe injections (Hayashi, Hutin, Bultery, Altaf, & Allegranzi, 2019). During outbreaks of hemorrhagic diseases, a primary public health response is to be sure that all medical injections given in the affected geographic area are safe injections, thereby avoiding the unfortunate outcome of medically transmitting the causative virus.

Respiratory Syndromes

SARS was first identified in 2004 during an outbreak in China that spread to four other nations. It is important to understand that the coronavirus humans now know so much about is the cause of SARS (remember from **Chapter 1** that the medical designation for COVID-19 is SARS-CoV-2). The physiology of SARS involves the air sacs of the lungs (known as **alveoli**) being destroyed by the infection, as well as an often overwhelming immune response that wreaks havoc in its own right. The result is massive destruction of alveoli, along with inflammation of lung tissue and a build-up of fluids that further suppress the remaining lung function. In short, this rapid loss of lung function leads to a lack of oxygenation to vital organs (including the heart) and, ultimately, to a person's death.

In the WHO 2015 listing of the top eight diseases of global priority (Pizzi, 2015), two are SARS viruses: (1) Middle East respiratory syndrome coronavirus (MERS-CoV) and (2) SARS, along with its variants (including COVID-19). As an interesting side note, this 2015 WHO list was published more than four years prior to the emergence of COVID-19. Thus the warning issued by the WHO carried a great deal of credibility, and such warnings should always be a cause for concern and public health action.

Diseases Leading to Swollen Brain Tissue

The remaining two diseases in the 2015 WHO list are (1) Nipah virus disease and (2) Rift Valley fever. Both are primarily zoonotic (see **Chapter 1**) in terms of transmission. For instance, bats and bat dung (known as guano) are common vectors in transmitting the Nipah virus to humans. This zoonotic transmission is broadly defined in that, for instance, any human contact with the body fluids of an infected fruit bat — such as the common practice in some areas of eating the raw sap of palm trees that are also a feeding ground for the bats — can lead to human infection. The fear is that either or both of these emerging viruses could someday mutate to be spread by human-to-human contact. If that scenario developed, the contact needed to acquire the disease from an infected person could be as simple as a kiss. Clearly, it is not prudent to simply wait for this to happen and thus act far too late. An ethical and moral imperative exists to anticipate this level of mutation and invest massive funding resources into the development of vaccines (none exist currently).

The Nipah virus causes **encephalitis**: a swelling of the entire brain. Conversely, Rift Valley fever causes **meningitis**: a swelling of the outer layer (i.e., the covering of the brain, known as the meninges, and the covering of the spinal cord). In either instance (encephalitis or meningitis), the swelling can lead to mental confusion, cognitive deterioration, coma, and death.

hemorrhagic fevers highlight a longstanding shortcoming of global public health practice: the lack of ample availability of the most basic tools (new needles and syringes) for medical care and vaccination campaigns

a primary public health response is to be sure that all medical injections given in the affected geographic area are safe injections

SARS was first identified in 2004 during an outbreak in China that spread to four other nations

An ethical and moral imperative exists to anticipate this level of mutation and invest massive funding resources into the development of vaccines

What Can Be Done?

As time goes by, the list of high-priority emerging diseases will doubtless change and expand. Moreover, these eight diseases and others that have existed for decades will mutate, creating the sobering possibility of the pathogens "outwitting" humankind. It is entirely appropriate to think about humans and pathogens being engaged in the ultimate battle – one that humans never win – instead, the game is too close to predict a winner. As science writer Laurie Garret has so eloquently stated, we live in a world that is ecologically "Out of Balance" (see **Photo 15.5**) and therefore highly vulnerable to the continued emergence of deadly infectious diseases. Thus, once again, you can imagine that critical public health practices must center on actions that seek to restore a balance between humans, the environment, animals, insects, and so on. These actions, for example, could be designed to control the bat population or eliminate the virus from the bat population (which is possible via genetic engineering). The seemingly mundane task of rodent control is also an example of a vital public health function that has been part of public health practice for centuries! Designing chemical methods of rendering rats sterile or infertile, for instance, is a form of laboratory work that may ultimately save millions of human lives. The housing and proximity of swine (i.e., pigs), cattle, sheep, and goats to people – as well the safety of people such as farm workers exposed directly to these animals – is another critical horizon for the focus of public health efforts pertaining to the elimination and control of emerging diseases.

think about humans and pathogens being engaged in the ultimate battle – one that humans never win

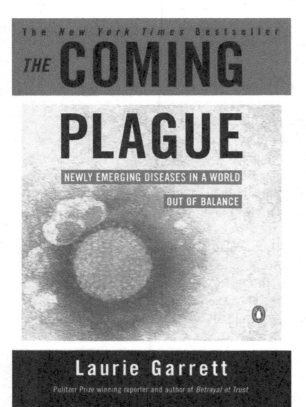

Photo 15.5   In her detailed introduction to the global problem of emerging diseases, Laurie Garret provides a riveting summary.

As described by Garrett (1994), a key aspect of controlling epidemics (referring only to infectious diseases) is rapidly deploying highly trained public health workers to quickly engage in the process of diagnosing the causative agent, understanding how this pathogen spreads, and using the most expedient means available to interrupt the chain of transmission (see **Chapter 1**).

Examples of Effective Public Health Systems

As with all warnings (e.g., "winter is coming"), the world has rallied to escalate the human response to threats of existing disease endemics that could become epidemic (please recall that **endemic** implies low but steady rates of new occurrences of infectious disease, whereas **epidemic** implies record rates of a disease in terms of how quickly new cases are diagnosed and reported to public health authorities). For example, a key mission of the U.S. Peace Corps involves an aggressive global malaria control program (see **Photo 15.6**). Unfortunately for humans, malaria has been a consistent winner in terms of yearly new cases diagnosed around the world. Fortunately for humans, malaria generally is not lethal – instead, its sequelae (**sequelae** is a term used to denote clinically observable effects of a disease) center around long-term fatigue and weakness caused by the lack of red blood cells that typifies malaria infections (which may last for several months).

An incredibly powerful public health organization that has a tremendous track record of success in controlling the spread of infectious diseases (including emerging pathogens) is the **Carter Center**, located in Atlanta, GA. Founded by President Jimmy Carter, the mission of the Carter Center is to eliminate infectious diseases that otherwise are largely not focal points of

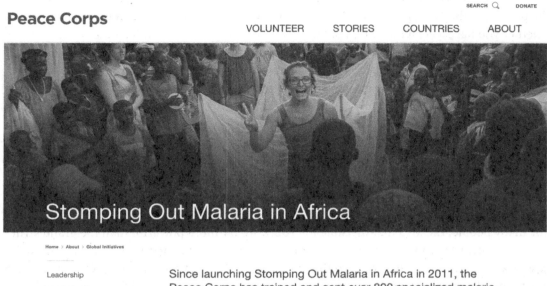

Peace Corps

SEARCH   DONATE

VOLUNTEER   STORIES   COUNTRIES   ABOUT

Stomping Out Malaria in Africa

Home > About > Global Initiatives

Leadership

Agency Priorities

Since launching Stomping Out Malaria in Africa in 2011, the Peace Corps has trained and sent over 800 specialized malaria prevention Volunteers to serve in communities across Africa.

Photo 15.6   The Peace Corps has been devoted to improving public health since its inception in 1961.

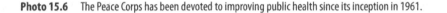

the WHO, the CDC, or other global agencies dedicated to controlling epidemics. For instance, the Carter Center is well known for its outstanding record in the elimination of **Guinea worm disease**. As a parasite, the guinea worm enters the human body in its egg stage. Within 12 months, the female maturing parasites grow to a length of up to one meter. This very long worm ultimately creates an exit wound from the human host. That exit wound allows the parasite to emerge, and as you can imagine people are tempted to pull it all the way out – but it is not so simple. The slow exodus of the worm (perhaps one or two centimeters per day) creates an excruciating feeling of burning pain, and pulling on the worm only breaks it and causes more damage inside the body of the host. The solution is typically to slowly (i.e., day by day) wrap the worm around a stick or similar object until it is completely extricated from the body. To avoid this debilitating experience, the Carter Center has been successful in preventing the larva (i.e., the worm in its egg stage) from entering the human body through drinking water. The public health solution preferred by the Carter Center is focused on providing water filters – along with intensive community-level education about how to use them and the importance of doing so – to entire populations residing in areas that rely on larva-contaminated drinking water for their daily needs.

As most Americans learned during the first two years of the COVID-19 pandemic, the **Centers for Disease Control and Prevention** (CDC) is another invaluable part of our public health readiness regarding emerging infectious diseases. For example, the CDC sponsors and manages a monthly professional journal known as *Emerging Infectious Diseases*. This professional journal serves as a central point of communication among virologists, microbiologists, epidemiologists, and other disciplines involved in controlling emerging epidemics. Also, for example, in August 2022, the CDC organized and hosted the 11th International Conference on Emerging Infectious Diseases, held in Atlanta, GA. As emphasized previously in this chapter, the prevention and control of emerging infectious diseases, by necessity, must be a coordinated global effort. To punctuate this point, it is important to note that the CDC-sponsored conference was held in cooperation with the **Task Force for Global Health**, thereby making the proceeding truly global instead of focusing solely on the United States.

the prevention and control of emerging infectious diseases, by necessity, must be a coordinated global effort

Also highly notable relative to the CDC's contribution to controlling emerging diseases is the point that the CDC plays a key role in the **Global Health Security Agenda**. Regardless of whether you have a keen interest in public health, it is important to understand the most basic function of this agenda. That function is nicely summarized by the term **security** that is part of its name. Security refers to everything people need to live, ranging from medical care to food to a sound economic infrastructure. As stated eloquently by CDC, "Global outbreaks not only cause illness and death, they can also lead to a decrease in demand for U.S. services and exports, jeopardizing the economy and American jobs (CDC, 2022b)". Thus, for instance, if your career takes you into a business profession (e.g., banking, financing, real estate, manufacturing, or retailing), you have an inherent interest in at least this one aspect of public health.

The Delicate Balance of Life

For many people, the idea that invisible microbes are far more powerful than the grand structures created by humans is not something they can understand or accept

Vaccines are the leading "best hope" for the long-term security of the human species

For many people, the idea that invisible microbes are far more powerful than the grand structures created by humans is not something they can understand or accept. But this is indeed the case – as was dramatically shown to the world by the COVID-19 pandemic. Climate change creates conditions that favor emerging microbes, as do war, poverty, and food insecurity. With these advantages growing each year, it is incumbent on humans to expand our ability to prevent and control the emergence and spread of microbes. This can be achieved largely through a greatly enhanced global infrastructure relative to vaccine development, manufacturing, and distribution. Vaccines are the leading "best hope" for the long-term security of the human species. However, that security also relies on several other public health functions.

Figure 15.3 depicts the necessary public health functions that must be firmly in place to avoid the balance of power ultimately favoring microbes over humans. Starting at the top, consider first how vital environmental regulations are to maintaining an advantage over microbes. With nearly continuous deforestation, for example, our planet becomes progressively more hospitable to microbes that were once held in check by a sophisticated ecologic system of plant

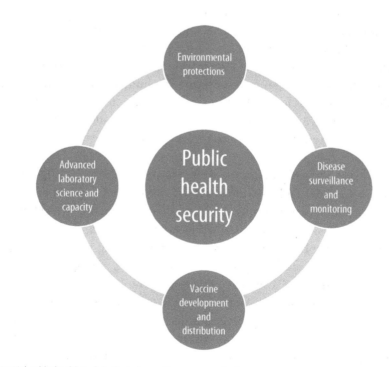

Figure 15.3   Essential public health tools in the balance of power over microbes

and animal species. Regulations of water supplies are similarly vital given that stagnant, polluted, and ecologically imbalanced (meaning a lack of biodiversity that favors microbes) water supplies are a significant problem worldwide (including in the United States). Even regulations as seemingly inconsequential as protecting environments against invasive plant and animal species are crucial to at least preserving the current standoff in the balance of power between microbes and humans.

Moving clockwise in **Figure 15.3**, consider how all the nations on the planet must set aside geopolitical differences and work in a coordinated manner to create and manage systems that sound an early alarm when an emerging disease may be occurring. As noted previously, these global systems already exist. However, the rapid advance of emerging microbes requires that these systems be greatly expanded and centrally coordinated. For instance, an outbreak of Lassa fever in South Africa today should become known to public health authorities in other African nations, as well as those in nations where travelers from the region having the outbreak may be found. Surveillance implies monitoring. Monitoring, in turn, implies that any one region or nation detecting an outbreak can sound the alarm for all other nations that may be impacted by what could become the rapid spread of the microbe – escalating it to epidemic levels or even to a full-blown pandemic.

Again moving clockwise in the figure, consider next the stellar track record of vaccines you have learned about in this chapter! It is important, however, to transcend the idea that humans can quickly make a highly efficacious vaccine following the detection of a new epidemic. The rapid development of the vaccines against COVID-19 masks the fact that decades of virology and vaccinology research laid a foundation that greatly facilitated the speed of this process. Again, as "we the people" proceed into an uncertain future, it is our task to be sure the U.S. government is well-funded to continue and expand an ambitious agenda of virology and vaccinology research.

Moving next to the final component, it is – as you might suspect – no simple task to isolate and sequence the genes of a virus, bacterium, protozoan, or other form of pathogen. Moreover, because so many nations in the world lack the capacity for advanced laboratory science relative to this daunting task, high-income counties such as the United States must play a leading role in terms of readiness to identify emerging pathogens. Once the "identification" stage is complete, laboratories in high-income countries must be amply staffed and equipped to develop and test (in animals) potentially efficacious treatments for emerging diseases. Potentially efficacious treatments must become the subject of a planned series of clinical trials that can be thought of as a pipeline, constituting an entirely separate and different branch of health science. **Clinical trials** involve several prescribed phases. Given the complexity and time-consuming nature of these trials, any future emerging disease will most likely be victorious over humans for a (hopefully) short period of time, at best. Thus, this final component only complements, rather than dominates, the public health preparedness that must be firmly in place. Noteworthy here is that although treatment is not a prevention practice with respect to the person receiving it, treating infectious diseases that efficiently spread through human-to-human contact reduces the odds of people encountering someone who transmits the pathogen to them. In short, as fewer and fewer people have active infectious, the odds of transmission drop correspondingly.

> Potentially efficacious treatments must become the subject of a planned series of clinical trials that can be thought of as a pipeline

The model shown in **Figure 15.3** warrants a caveat: fortifying our public health infrastructures against emerging microbes must also involve a parallel and ongoing effort to gain the trust, support, and cooperation of the public. So, this chapter ends where the first few chapters of this textbook began – by suggesting that your role in public health is no less valuable or vital than your traditionally civic-minded role as a registered voter in our longstanding democracy. Specifically, your role in maintaining a human advantage over emerging microbes is to support

> fortifying our public health infrastructures against emerging microbes must also involve a parallel and ongoing effort to gain the trust, support, and cooperation of the public

funding, regulations, and legislation necessitated by the components shown in **Figure 15.3** while also being an active part of your community effort to fully gain that very important trust and cooperation from people who may be less informed than you about the ultimate value of preventing and controlling emerging diseases.

Review and Key Terms

This final chapter began with a quote from the *Game of Thrones* character Ned Stark, warning his people that "winter is coming." That metaphor describes how a civic-minded person should view the threat of emerging infectious diseases. Although areas of the world have had wonderful success in the **elimination** of some infectious diseases, the global **eradication** of infectious diseases remains one of the greatest challenges facing humans in general and public health in particular. Through the lens of history (e.g., smallpox), many standard public health practices have been widely applied in the United States and throughout much of the world. One crucial practice is the use of **case surveillance** to carefully monitor populations for any signs that an outbreak of infectious disease may be occurring. In the United States, for example, this approach was applied to six cases of unexplained illness among gay men in 1981. That initial case surveillance of six people was the first alarm for the emergence of what later became known as HIV/AIDS.

A second crucial practice is **contact tracing**. When the transmission of an emerging disease occurs through human-to-human contact, a front line of public health defense is to quickly locate new cases, interview the people infected to determine who else they may have infected, and then find the named contacts to continue this chain of inquiry. These two time-honored public health practices will certainly be used, as our world appears to be more rapidly favoring the emergence of microbes that have never before been known as human pathogens. The threat of rapidly emerging infectious diseases requires a globally coordinated response. The leading global agency for this response is the **World Health Organization** (WHO).

A feature of this chapter is a WHO list of the top eight emerging diseases – those that pose the greatest threat to the human species. To simplify this list, the chapter organized these diseases into three broad categories. The first is the **hemorrhagic diseases**, which lead to a breakdown of the integrity of an integral part of the circulatory system: the **capillary beds**. The second category is broadly known as **severe respiratory syndrome**. This category contains the emergence of coronavirus. The third category involves the central nervous system, primarily (but not exclusively) the brain. Some of the emerging diseases lead to dangerous swelling of the entire brain (**encephalitis**), while others lead to inflammation of the outer layer of the brain, known as the meninges (**meningitis**).

Beyond the work of the WHO, the United States and other high-income nations currently have a reasonably functional set of organizations capable of responding to emerging diseases of the future. For instance, both the U.S. Peace Corps and the **Carter Center** have a distinguished history of working to resolve epidemics. The Carter Center is somewhat of a model in responding to epidemics; this is particularly demonstrated by its great success at what could soon be the eradication of **guinea worm disease**. The U.S. **Centers for Disease Control and Prevention** (CDC) has traditionally played a strong role in the global response to the threat of emerging diseases.

This chapter also brought to the surface a number of vaccine-related issues that you may have experienced personally or via family members: the lack of public willingness to receive vaccines. The epitome of this unwillingness is a movement known as **anti-vaxxers**. But the anti-vaxxers are only a small part of the larger problem in nations such as the United States. That larger problem involves either a form of **medical mistrust** toward clinics and vaccines or complacency among the public that keeps people from taking proactive measures against life-threatening diseases. Partly because of this mistrust and/or complacency, one of the most successful public health approaches to vaccination involves childhood vaccines that are given as part of standard pediatric care.

As the chapter reached a climax, you became aware that we, as humans, exist in what is best characterized as a delicate balance of power between microbes and public health. The microbes have enjoyed several advantages created by a combination of climate change, poverty, food insecurity, and so on. However, the human response can be greatly escalated! The last section of the chapter provided you with a model (**Figure 15.3**) of an integrated response to the threats posed by emerging microbes. You learned, for example, the value of supporting an expanded domestic and global infrastructure relative to vaccine development and distribution. You also learned that research infrastructures for treating emerging diseases are necessary for prevention (at least in the case of infections that are spread by human-to-human contact). You also learned that **clinical trials** of new treatments can be time-consuming. This reality suggests that most emerging epidemics may take an unfortunate toll on human life during times prior to the development and widespread distribution of effective treatment regimes.

For Practice and Class Discussion

Practice Questions (answers are located in the appendix to this textbook)

1. As shown by history, simply creating vaccines and making them available may:
   a. Be ample to create near elimination of the diseases
   b. Be ample to create near eradication of the diseases
   c. Fail as a public health response due to the unwillingness of people to be vaccinated

2. Hemorrhagic fevers lead to death by:
   a. Causing a loss of blood internally
   b. Causing the sudden and severe loss of lung function
   c. Creating dangerous swelling of the meninges

3. In thinking about the threat of emerging epidemics as a call for the public health system to be prepared, what role is played by case surveillance systems?
   a. These systems quickly determine the causative agent of the disease.
   b. These system act as a first alarm to trigger a more intensive public health response.
   c. Case surveillance is a logical conclusion to the public health practice of contact tracing.
   d. All of the above

4. Which organization is **not** exclusive to the U.S.-based infrastructure of preparedness for emerging diseases?
   a. The Peace Corp
   b. The CDC
   c. The WHO
   d. The Carter Center

5. Which one of the following diseases can be considered eradicated, as opposed to eliminated?
   a. Smallpox
   b. Measles

      c. Mumps

      d. Rubella

6. Rhonda is a 41-year-old who normally neglects to have an annual flu shot. She also was never vaccinated against COVID-19. Her three children have all attended school and received the entire childhood vaccination series. Which phrase **best** characterizes Rhonda?

      a. Anti-vaxxer

      b. Not concerned about the threat of disease

      c. Unwilling to comply with public health guidelines

7. Vaccines are capable of being the only public health tool in the likely event of an epidemic caused by an emerging disease.

      a. True

      b. False

8. Emerging diseases also include the prospect of currently known microbes developing antibiotic resistance.

      a. True

      b. False

9. As a candidate for president of the United States, Senator X stated, "We must fortify our borders and focus all of our disease prevention efforts on only the citizens of this great nation." What is wrong with this statement?

      a. It ignores the fundamental principle that the control of emerging infectious diseases must occur at a global level.

      b. It misses the point that the only way to control emerging infections is to end all travel into the United States.

10. How is it possible that deforestation is a cause of emerging diseases?

      a. It leads to starvation, which then makes people vulnerable to disease.

      b. It destroys plant and animal species that previously held some microbes in check.

      c. Deforestation is a direct cause of bacterial-related drug resistance.

Discussion Questions

11. Go to the WHO website to determine the most recently released list of the top threats in terms of emerging infectious diseases. Compare the list you find there to the one described in this chapter. What diseases have remained on the list? What diseases have emerged most recently in your lifetime?

12. Unless you were raised in an anti-vax family, chances are that you have had most of the vaccines shown in **Figure 15.2**. Chances are also good that you do not have a personal record of which vaccines you have – and have not – received in the past. Use any resource available to you to construct what can become "My Personal Vaccine History."

13. As much as vaccines have previously rescued humans from massive death, nations (including the United States) still debate whether adult vaccines (e.g., COVID-19) against emerging diseases should be mandatory. In two pages of double-spaced font, take a stand on this issue. Be very clear in your argument, and back up what you state with principles, facts, and so on, taken from this chapter. When you are finished, post this to an electronic location used by your class. It is likely that your instructor for this course will enjoy moderating this type of organized written debate among people taking this course.

References

Centers for Disease Control and Prevention (2022a). Vaccines for your children. https://www.cdc.gov/vaccines/parents/diseases/forgot-14-diseases.html

Centers for Disease Control and Prevention (2022b). Protecting Americans from the threat of infectious disease. https://www.cdc.gov/globalhealth/security/ghsareport/2018/protecting-americans.html

Centers for Disease Control and Prevention (2022c). Considerations for planning school-located vaccination clinics. https://www.cdc.gov/vaccines/covid-19/planning/school-located-clinics.html

Hayashi, T., Hutin, Y., Bultery, M., Altaf, A., & Allegranzi, B. (2019). Injection practices in 2011–2015: A review using data from demographic and health surveys. *BMC Health Services Research*, *19*, 600.

Meyerson, B. E., Martich, F. A., & Naehr, G. P. (2008). *Ready to Go: The History and Contributions of the U.S. Public Health Service*. Research Triangle Park, NC: The American Social Health Association.

Mitchell, A. (1997). Clinton calls for AIDS vaccine as a goal. *The New York Times*, May 19. https://www.nytimes.com/1997/05/19/us/clinton-calls-for-aids-vaccine-as-goal.html

Pizzi, R. (2015). WHO identifies top emerging diseases. *MDedge*, December 18. https://www.mdedge.com/chestphysician/article/105289/emerging-infections/who-identifies-top-emerging-diseases

Chapter 1

1. Which one of the following terms is **not** applicable to understanding how vaccines work?
   a. Memory cells
   b. Antibodies
   c. **Neurotransmitters**
   d. Surface proteins
   Recall that you learned how a vaccine stimulates antibody production and that the blueprint for these antibodies is stored in memory cells. You also learned that some (even most) vaccines work by simulating the surface proteins of the pathogen.

2. The most common portal of entry for the COVID-19 virus is:
   a. **The olfactory system**
   b. The lower eyelids
   c. Ingesting the virus via contaminated foods
   d. The mouth
   Remember that this is why inhaling aerosolized droplets of COVID-19 is so efficient at transmitting the virus – the olfactory system is in the nose.

3. The concept of corporate interests taking precedence over public safety from COVID-19 is **best** illustrated by which example?
   a. Increasing taxes for middle-class Americans
   b. **A rush to return to retail sales and dining in indoor restaurants**
   c. Mandatory vaccination of all employees
   This was seen over and over again within the first few years of the pandemic.

4. Regarding the history of COVID-19, which statement is **true**?
   a. The virus entered the United States almost one year after it first appeared in China.
   b. **The Trump administration engaged in prolonged denial about the severity of this virus.**
   c. The U.S. Department of Defense quickly vaccinated all members of the military, even before the American public began receiving the vaccines.
   d. The COVID-19 pandemic was inevitable – it could not have been any less devastating in terms of cases or human lives lost.
   The chapter gives several very clear examples of how government self-interests (especially the Trump White House) downplayed the epidemic in hopes of reopening the economy and getting people to focus on other things.

Understanding the Science and Practice of Public Health, First Edition. Richard Crosby.
© 2023 John Wiley & Sons, Inc. Published 2023 by John Wiley & Sons, Inc.

5. Which part of the chain of infection for COVID-19 pertains to white-tailed deer?
    a. **Reservoir**
    b. Portal of exit
    c. Acquired immunity
    d. Mutation of the pathogen
        Having found that about 30% – or more – of the white-tailed deer population harbors COVID-19 was a terrible turn in this epidemic because it implied that the virus (unlike smallpox) could always re-emerge by zoonotic transmission.

6. The difference between an **epidemic** and the term **endemic** is:
    a. All epidemics begin as endemics.
    b. Only endemics occur on a global scale.
    c. Epidemics are not controllable.
    d. **Epidemics are characterized by massive case rates; when these fall to a low and stable level, the term endemic applies.**
        It is always the hope and the goal during an epidemic to quickly reduce the case rate to a very low level – one that stays low (it is unusual to eliminate or eradicate a disease entirely).

7. Which example **best** illustrates the principles of a propagated disease?
    a. A common source serves as a point of infection for most new cases.
    b. An animal-to-human mode of transmission becomes dominant.
    c. **Human-to-human transmission of the pathogen is favored by environmental conditions such as overcrowding.**
    d. After several successive mutations, the pathogen develops memory cells.
        The term **propagate** literally means going from one person to the next. This is how some (not all) infectious diseases spread – especially those that spread by exhaled airborne particles, such as the flu, tuberculosis, and COVID-19.

8. Which statement is **most** applicable to understanding the health disparities of COVID-19?
    a. **The protective behavior of sheltering in place was less possible for essential workers.**
    b. Black Americans lacked health insurance needed to receive the vaccine.
    c. Latinx Americans were often refused hospital care.
        Unfortunately, history will show this as a major cause of huge disparities between the classes, with low-income people typically having jobs that demanded being onsite. Remote working was not an option for millions of low-income people.

9. Which organization has the **most** influence relative to controlling pandemics?
    a. The U.S. Advisory Committee on Immunization Practices
    b. **The World Health Organization**
    c. The Centers for Disease Control and Prevention
        You may have been tempted to choose answer **c** here, but the key to this question lies in the word **pandemic**. Remember that this term implies a global response, and the CDC is a U.S. organization.

10. Which statement about COVID-19 is **false**?
    a. Immunity can be acquired by having the disease.
    b. Although the vaccine is extremely safe, there is a very small risk of Guillain-Barré syndrome.
    c. The virus can enter the body through the eyes.
    d. **Fully vaccinated people cannot transmit the virus to others.**

If you missed this one, go back into the chapter and read again about acquired immunity, the slight risk of Guillain-Barré Syndrome, and the eyes as a portal of entry. Also remember that the vaccine only prevents moderate to severe illness.

Chapter 2

1. Which example **best** illustrates primary prevention?
   a. Having a mammogram
   b. Being treated for early-stage cardiovascular disease
   c. **Good oral hygiene**
   d. Annually checking your blood cholesterol levels
   This is the only option that is intended to avert the disease process entirely.

2. The elimination of health disparities is **most** dependent on:
   a. Constantly improving clinical interventions
   b. Making health-related counseling and education widely available
   c. Creating highly effective interventions designed for individuals
   d. **Changing inequitable socioeconomic conditions**
   Remember that health disparities are ultimately rooted in the larger socioeconomic disparities that plague our nation.

3. Which example **best** illustrates how public health averts infectious disease?
   a. Regulating the tobacco industry
   b. Regulating carbon emissions
   c. **Allowing needle/syringe exchange programs to function legally**
   d. Taxing alcohol sales
   This is the only option that does not describe a chronic disease.

4. Which example **least** illustrates a public health program?
   a. **A program that helps diabetics control their disease**
   b. A social media campaign designed to motivate less use of sodium in cooking
   c. Reducing the costs of organic produce
   d. Adding fluoride to drinking water
   This is a medical "after the fact" approach to health. It is also a "one person at a time" approach.

5. Which public health tool applies to the process of providing highly relevant and specific information to legislators?
   a. **Education**
   b. Regulatory/Policy changes
   c. Making structural-level changes
   d. All of the above
   Remember that education for people who make policy and laws is also an important function of Block 1 in Figure 2.2.

6. Which public health tool applies to the process of creating sustainable interventions?
   a. Education
   b. Regulatory/Policy changes
   c. **Making structural-level changes**
   d. All of the above
   Structural changes are typically highly sustainable, lasting for years or even decades.

7. Why is a pump handle such an important part of this module?
   a. **Removing the handle from just one pump was the key part of John Snow's intervention to prevent cholera.**
   b. It was shown that these handles were a source of transmitting cholera.
   c. The old-fashioned water pump (used by hand) is a symbol of how easy it was to die of a water-based illness in the 1800s.
   d. This was the centerpiece of germ theory and the start of medicine.
   This was the founding of the science of epidemiology.

8. Which one of the following is **least** illustrative of a risk condition?
   a. Social customs and practices that encourage and support ongoing behaviors that are harmful to the body
   b. Climate change
   c. Income inequality and socioeconomic disparities
   d. **Having diabetes develop before age 40**
   Risk conditions are part of the social, physical, and economic environments that surround the lives of the public. Having diabetes at a young age is a risk factor rather than a risk condition.

9. As the science of public health, epidemiology serves multiple functions. Which one of the following examples is **least** related to the science of epidemiology?
   a. A restaurant chain is investigated for causing an outbreak of hepatitis A.
   b. A long-term study of factory workers identifies risk factors for chronic back pain.
   c. **The role of political support is assessed regarding a program designed to control second-hand tobacco smoke.**
   Epidemiology investigates factors that lead to disease – it is not concerned with the factors (such as political support) that relate to policies.

10. As a share of the gross domestic product, U.S. medical care costs greatly exceed expenditures for the entire U.S. Department of Defense.
    a. **True**
    b. False
    In fact, they exceed the national defense budget by nearly five times!

Chapter 3

1. The plague would have been much worse had it not been for the public health efforts of Chadwick. Which one of the following was **not** included in these efforts?
   a. Cleaning public streets
   b. **Installing fire hydrants**
   c. Removing garbage on a regular basis
   d. Removing human waste from public spaces
   Even city water was an issue at this time in history. Fire hydrants came later.

2. Which one of these early public health actions was responsible for the control of smallpox?
   a. **Vaccination of entire populations**
   b. Pasteurization of milk
   c. Improved public sanitation services
   d. Improved health education
   Remember that it took more than a decade to finally vaccinate the human population of the world. This lesson was too easily ignored when COVID-19 vaccines were finally approved.

3. All of the following terms except one apply to VD control in the middle of the 20th century. Which term does **not** relate to this set of public health actions?

   a. Antibiotics

   b. Public health advisors

   c. **Vaccination**

   d. Contact tracing

   Even now, vaccines against sexually transmitted infections are limited to the human papillomavirus (a rather harmless infection compared to the syphilis and gonorrhea epidemics that were fought by public health advisors).

4. As pathogenic diseases subsided and chronic disease became the leading causes of morbidity and mortality, health education became a job of local and state health departments.

   a. **True**

   b. False

   This is still the case today. Local and state health departments are highly committed to education campaigns that are disease-specific.

5. The Health Belief Model relies on two main concepts. These are:

   a. Perceived susceptibility and perceived severity

   b. **Expected net gain and perceived threat**

   c. Perceived threat and modifying factors

   d. Social contagion and cues to action

   If you struggled with this one, please go back and notice that these are keywords (shown in bold) and described as the primary drivers of whether people adopt health-protective behaviors.

6. Kidney failure is increasingly common in the United States. Of the options listed, which would be the most significant in terms of a root cause?

   a. Hypertension

   b. Inadequate health care

   c. Poverty

   d. **Sodium consumption**

   You may have answered **a**; if so, recall that a primary cause of hypertension is sodium. The overconsumption of sodium, by the way, is shared among people of all socioeconomic conditions.

7. Public health practice cannot do everything. Instead, it must prioritize its efforts. This occurs by:

   a. Selecting actual causes of morbidity and mortality that can be changed through population-level intervention

   b. Following the advice and wisdom of congressional mandates

   c. Targeting only the leading forms of death

   d. **Selecting health behaviors that can be altered by policy changes**

   The answer serves as a great review – be sure you understand it.

8. Shifting the mean implies all of the following **except**:

   a. Creating a population-level impact

   b. Upstream thinking

   c. **Focusing on those most at risk**

   d. Targeting actual causes of morbidity and mortality

   Remember that public health is distinct from medical care in that everybody is a target of health promotion efforts.

9. Which action is the **least** upstream in terms of public health practice?
    a. Taxing tobacco
    b. **Providing free childbirth services to teens**
    c. Regulating the food industry's use of sugar and sodium
    d. Using massive social media campaigns to promote daily walking for all people
    The action in answer **b** is very much characterized by downstream thinking.

10. All of what forms public health practice is global in terms of the actions needed to create conditions that avert morbidity and mortality.
    a. True
    b. **False**
    Although global cooperation is essential for controlling infectious disease and stemming the progress of climate change, public health actions are largely shaped and limited by the culture, economics, politics, and laws of any given nation.

Chapter 4

1. Which one of the following is **not** true about nicotine?
    a. It is at least as addictive as cocaine.
    b. It is extracted from tobacco for use in e-cigarettes.
    c. **Nicotine is carcinogenic, especially in the trachea and lungs.**
    d. It stimulates vasoconstriction and increases the adhesiveness of blood platelets to artery walls.
    Recall that it is the tars in cigarettes that act as carcinogens (nicotine is the drug).

2. A true public health approach to preventing death from tobacco would involve each of the following actions **except**:
    a. **The widespread distribution of brochures in clinics and doctor's offices**
    b. Funding community-based organizations to pass ETS policies/laws
    c. Changing entire cultures relative to smoking and other forms of tobacco use
    d. Taxing all tobacco products
    This is not a public health approach (and it is not effective).

3. In a few words, the concept of price elasticity refers to:
    a. **A degree of tolerance in price that, when exceeded, translates into a decrease in demand**
    b. The price point at which a company no longer makes a profit on the product
    c. A method of keeping consumers happy by placing limits on tax increases for any given product
    This is an important principle that public health has adopted from the field of economics.

4. The state of New Hampshire would like to mimic the California Tobacco Control Program. This state, however, has limited funds and wants to begin with an effort that will yield the greatest impact for the amount of funds allocated. Which one (**best**) approach should the state use?

   a. Provide funding to support the costs of the nicotine patch for people on Medicare who want to end their dependence on tobacco.

   b. **Adopt the Truth Campaign as part of the statewide health curriculum for high school students and even middle school students.**

   c. Train high school teachers to teach students basic facts about the harmful effects of tobacco and vaping.

   d. Develop and fund a statewide network of social media experts who can then build websites that teach teens the harmful effects of tobacco use and vaping.

   A key lesson of the California Tobacco Control Program was that knowledge about smoking did not change teens' minds. However, insights about the corrupt practices of the tobacco industry worked nicely!

5. Given the high costs associated with paying for employees' healthcare expenses, a large company has recently created an employee education-based program designed to help people end tobacco dependence. Which one company policy would be **best** suited to also help this effort by its influence on social norms?

   a. Provide smoke-free break rooms

   b. Refuse to pay for health insurance for employees who smoke

   c. Provide the nicotine patch at no cost, upon request

   d. **Prohibit tobacco use and vaping on all company property**

   The chapter taught you that ETS laws are highly influential in terms of altering social norms.

6. The California Tobacco Control Program relies **least** on which level of intervention?

   a. **Intrapersonal**

   b. Interpersonal

   c. Institutional

   d. Community

   e. Policy/law

   Take another look at Figure 4.1. You will see that this is not a big part of the approach.

7. When a pregnant woman inhales secondhand smoke, several effects occur on the fetus. These effects can all lead to issues with fetal development. Which of the following is the **least** likely of these issues?

   a. Premature birth

   b. Low birth weight

   c. **Compromised fetal immunity**

   d. Subsequent childhood risk of asthma

   You learned about **a**, **b**, and **d** in the chapter. All three are prominent outcomes of maternal smoking. Option **c** is simply a distractor here.

8. The Master Settlement Agreement currently provides states with millions of dollars, yet only a small portion is used to fund tobacco use prevention programs.
    a. **True**
    b. False
        In fact, it is less than 3%!

9. A key philosophy of the Truth Campaign is:
    a. Teens need to know the facts about how smoking harms their bodies.
    b. All people deserve access to medically accurate information about tobacco.
    c. **The hidden injustices of the tobacco industry must be exposed.**
    d. Taxing tobacco products will greatly reduce teen smoking.
        This also has tremendous implications for the control of other industries that create and distribute products that are antithetical to public health.

10. The public health approach of making health-compromising products – such as nicotine – too expensive for people to easily afford is based on the economic principle of:
    a. Supply and demand
    b. **Price elasticity**
    c. Market justice
    d. A comprehensive approach
        Again, this is a vital form of public health practice!

Chapter 5

1. Which one of the following is **least** relevant to metabolic syndrome?
    a. Built environments
    b. Triglycerides
    c. Body mass index
    d. **Prevalence rates**
        Remember that prevalence rates simply measure how common (or uncommon) any given health condition may be at a given time in an entire population.

2. Which term is the **least** consistent with the tenets of the farm-to-table movement?
    a. Organically grown
    b. **Low to moderate use of mild antibiotics**
    c. Smaller carbon footprint
    d. PBWF friendly
        Even small amounts of antibiotics are unnecessary when rapid mass production of milk or meat is not the goal.

3. The concept of wellness implies all of the following **except**:
    a. Any given population will have relatively equal numbers of people at either extreme of a bell-shaped curve.
    b. **Normal is represented by the entire area to the left of the mean in the bell-shaped curve.**
    c. As a rule, lower numbers are always better when it comes to blood pressure, heart rate, and lipid levels.
        Although the paradigm in medical care would classify all people to the left of the bell curve's highest point as normal, it is clear that tremendous variation in levels of wellness exist.

4. In terms of METS, which statement is true?
   a. Even 1.5 METS is enough to qualify as moderate to vigorous physical activity (MVPA).
   b. METS must exceed 4.0 to truly count movement as a benefit to health.
   c. **METS of 1.5 to 3.0 represent healthy movement and qualify as MVPA.**
   d. METS are a measure of sodium intake and do not relate to movement or exercise.

   Movements as simple as walking or cleaning a home typically consume 1.5 to 3.0 METS; this is moderate exercise.

5. Arnold is currently overweight but not yet obese. He is 15 years old and consumes a heavily animal-based diet. Barring public health intervention or independent behavior change, how likely is Arnold to become an obese adult?
   a. **Extremely likely**
   b. Somewhat likely
   c. It is unpredictable.
   d. Not likely because most teens grow out of this overweight phase

   A key learning objective of this chapter involved understanding that the behaviors and conditions that lead to obesity begin early in life, thus highlighting the need for public health intervention during childhood and the teen years.

6. Which food is **least** likely to lead to chronic hypertension?
   a. Commercially canned tomatoes
   b. A GMO-free product used to make cornbread
   c. A sodium-free hamburger
   d. **Red beans and rice made from scratch**

   Bear in mind that both sodium (choices **a** and **b**) and animal fats (choice **c**) create the condition known as **hypertension**.

7. Which example **best** illustrates the concept of a built environment?
   a. **A city closes off entire downtown streets to all vehicles between 8:00 a.m. and 6:00 p.m. every weekday. Only pedestrians and cyclists are allowed to enter and use these streets.**
   b. A workplace begins to offer all employees a 30-minute break between their lunch hour and the end of the shift at 5:00 p.m. Management constantly posts reminders that this added time should be used for vigorous movement.

   The term **built environment** does not always imply "building something" – instead, city policies may repurpose existing space to promote movement.

8. Which term/phrase is **least** related to the concept of wellness as applied to CVD?
   a. Subsidizing corn
   b. **Subsidizing farm-to-table movements**
   c. Food labeling laws
   d. Regulating the fast-food industry

   Do not be fooled into thinking that corn is a valuable plant-based food. Most corn is a GMO, and its refined products are largely used to make sugar (i.e., high fructose corn syrup).

9. The China Study pertains to all of the following **except**:
   a. Metabolic syndrome
   b. Cholesterol
   c. Triglycerides
   d. **Sustained daily movement**

   This landmark study was entirely devoted to understanding the role of a PBWF diet in preventing CVD and obesity.

10. Which factor of metabolic syndrome tends to be socially contagious?
    a. Comfort eating
    b. **Obesity**
    c. Hypertension
    d. Inactivity physiology
    Only options **b** and **c** are part of metabolic syndrome – and of the two, only **b** has been demonstrated as being linked to social ties and clusters or friends.

Chapter 6

1. Which one of the following terms is **least** relevant to Type 2 diabetes?
   a. Glycemic load
   b. Glycogen
   c. **Neurotransmitters**
   d. The pancreas
   Remember from Box 6.4 that neurotransmitters are chemicals in the brain.

2. In general terms, the trajectory of the U.S. diabetes epidemic is:
   a. **Doubling every 10 years**
   b. Staying relatively stable
   c. Increasing only slightly each year
   d. Decreasing as a result of lifestyle interventions
   This is shown visually in Figure 6.2 and explained in the accompanying section of the chapter.

3. The concept of behavioral economics, applied to the prevention of diabetes, implies that:
   a. **Increasing taxes on sugar-laden foods and eliminating subsidies to sugar producers can greatly reduce sugar consumption.**
   b. Sugar can become an inelastic market product.
   c. The National School Lunch Program should be significantly revised.
   Recall that behavioral economics is a field of study that explores how changes in price influence consumer behaviors (including health behaviors).

4. Regarding the Sugar Research Foundation (SRF), which statement is true?
   a. The research produced by the SRF is vital to public health.
   b. **The SRF has engaged in practices designed to protect the "good food" image of sugar.**
   c. Supported by the U.S. Department of Agriculture, the SRF administers the WIC program.
   d. The SRF has produced research supporting the role of sugar in the development of Type 2 diabetes.
   This "good food" image was indeed engineered and purchased by the SRF.

5. Which food item would be **allowed** for purchase using a SNAP debit card?
   a. Hot baked chicken held in a roaster and ready to eat
   b. Dry wine with no added sugar
   c. An herb that curbs the appetite for refined carbohydrates
   d. **A marshmallow Easter bunny coated with milk chocolate**
   As a professor of public health, I was shocked when I did this research to write the chapter. The level of insanity in this federal program is simply unbelievable.

6. Which statement about sugar subsidies is accurate?
   a. These subsidies are a way to return funding to the states.
   b. Subsidies only apply to producers of organic sugar.
   c. These subsidies no longer exist. Congress has repealed the 1981 Farm Bill.
   d. **Sugar subsidies go directly to the sugar producers.**
   Yes, the U.S. government pays for the production of sugar!

7. Which example **best** illustrates the concept of a downstream approach to controlling Type 2 diabetes?
   a. **Lifestyle interventions**
   b. Life insurance companies offering discounts on yearly premiums to people with test results indicating normal A1c levels

   Option **b** is something that could exist someday – if so, it would apply at a population level and might greatly reduce sugar consumption. However, option **a** is the very essence of a downstream approach because these programs are typically applied after issues with A1c levels have already surfaced and because the approach is implemented at the individual level.

8. The National School Lunch Program regulates:
   a. Sugar content
   b. **Minimum calorie content**
   c. Maximum fiber content
   d. Minimum sodium content

   An interesting point in this chapter was that sugar is often used to bump up the calorie count so the lunch being served meets the minimum calorie requirement.

9. The role of culture is important to consider relative to sugar consumption. Which one of the following examples is **least** illustrative of this principle?
   a. **Chocolate is often loaded with sugar even though its value as a way to stimulate endorphins is compromised by diluting the cocoa content.**
   b. Halo foods such as pie and ice cream continue to be American favorites.
   c. Sugar is relatively price inelastic: people buy it no matter what.
   See Box 6.4 – fascinating!

10. Which food has the **least** sugar per gram?
    a. Organic ketchup
    b. Commercially made baked beans
    c. **Canned tuna (in water rather than oil)**
    d. Canned fruit (not in water or its own juice)

    You may have been tempted to choose option **d**, but that is not correct because the juice used in canned fruit products is often loaded with added sugar. Also, just so you know, commercially prepared baked beans are typically made with sugars. Ketchup, of course, is a primary source of sugar in terms of sugar content per gram of the product.

Chapter 7

1. Which one of the following terms is **least** relevant to a Hygeia-based approach to cancer prevention?
   a. Protective factors
   b. **Frequent cancer screenings**
   c. Antioxidants
   d. The HPV vaccine
   Remember that screening is the realm of medical care.

2. The standard American diet lacks this vital protective factor against colorectal cancer.
   a. Antioxidants
   b. Antibodies
   c. **Vegetable fiber**
   d. Iodine
   Incredibly, vegetable fiber could save millions of people from colorectal cancer.

3. The concept of primary prevention as applied to breast cancer is best represented by which term?
   a. **A PBWF diet**
   b. Removing sugar from the standard American diet
   c. The use of mammography
   d. Preventing BRCA1 from reproducing
   To date, the best-known primary prevention practices for breast cancer all involve a shift toward plant-based diets.

4. Regarding breast cancer prevention, which statement is **false**?
   a. **Obesity is only a potential risk factor; more research is needed.**
   b. The consumption of berries is a protective factor.
   c. Mammography is important because not all breast cancers grow slowly.
   d. The presence of BRCA1 or BRCA2 is a known risk factor.
   Obesity later in life is now a well-established risk factor for breast cancer.

5. Which term is most implicated in the etiology of cervical cancer?
   a. Nicotine
   b. Polysaccharides
   c. **Persistent HPV**
   d. Cellular deregulation
   HPV is very common! Only when it becomes an ongoing infection does the true risk of cervical dysplasia begin.

6. Which statement about cervical cancer is accurate?
   a. **Virtually every case of this cancer is entirely preventable.**
   b. The HPV vaccine is 100% effective.
   c. The cervix of middle-aged women is particularly susceptible to HPV.
   d. Even stage 3 cervical cancer is relegated only to the os.
   It has been said that cervical cancer is a **sentinel event** in public health, meaning cases signal a need to improve public health practices.

7. Condom use does have a place in the prevention of cervical cancer. This is true more so from a public health perspective than the medical paradigm.
   a. **True**
   b. False
   Despite the bravado of the medical establishment, population-level reductions in HPV infections – and thus cases of cervical cancer – can be achieved through condom use.

8. Which screening test also serves as a method of primary prevention?
   a. Pap testing
   b. Mammography
   c. **Colonoscopy**
   d. Genetic testing for BRCA2
   This is because the procedure can surgically remove polyps before they become cancerous.

9. The role of culture is important to consider relative to cancer prevention. Why is this true?
   a. **People do not want to invest in daily tasks to prevent something they believe can be fixed someday by a doctor.**
   b. Medical doctors are profit-driven and actively discourage prevention.
   c. Most people are ready to change their diets; they just need guidance.
   Cancer prevention is not going to be easy!

10. Which general statement best summarizes this chapter?
   a. **Some cancers are highly preventable if public health practice creates the conditions that allow protective actions.**
   b. Thanks to chemoprevention, cancer is becoming a thing of the past.
   c. A PBWF diet is the best defense against cervical cancer.
   d. Mammography is an important form of primary prevention.
   This is the most valuable point you should remember from reading this chapter: the cure is prevention.

Chapter 8

1. Joe, a big drinker, is also an athlete. Joe read this chapter and now knows that acetaldehyde is probably negatively impacting his cardiovascular endurance. What advice is best for Joe (who will not abstain or reduce his consumption)?
   a. To minimize the time it takes to convert acetaldehyde to acetate, Joe should drink very slowly.
   b. To minimize the time it takes to convert acetaldehyde to acetate, Joe should only drink when eating a decent-sized meal.
   c. **To minimize the time it takes to convert acetaldehyde to acetate, Joe should drink very slowly, and he should only drink when eating a decent-size meal.**
   d. Joe should be screened for cirrhosis and alcohol-induced myopathy.
   Remember that acetate is harmless, and the liver can only work at a set pace to make this safe conversion.

2. On a rose curve, about what percent of the U.S. population would be located at the far-right end in terms of alcohol consumption levels?
   a. Nearly 30%
   b. About 50% of all adults
   c. **Less than 10%**
   d. Between 30% and 50%

   The estimate from the CDC is actually that 8% of the population consumes just 50% of all the alcohol sold in the United States.

3. "Alcohol is the new tobacco" implies that:
   a. **State and federal government-based regulations have not yet reduced the sales capacity of the alcohol industry.**
   b. ABC commissions are functioning well; therefore, alcohol use will soon decline (just as occurred for tobacco).
   c. Science is just now learning about the negative effects of alcohol on the body.

   As this chapter emphasizes, the past approaches to reducing U.S. alcohol consumption have not been effective. A greatly enhanced set of regulations on alcohol sales will be needed (just as was done with tobacco).

4. Manufacturers of whiskey may or may not be fully aware of the billions of U.S. dollars needed every year to pay for the large share of medical costs resulting from alcohol-induced chronic diseases such as cardiomyopathy, alcohol-induced hepatitis, and cirrhosis. This taxpayer-absorbed cost is known as:
   a. A form of reciprocal causation
   b. **A negative externality**
   c. The distributive law
   d. The density principle

   Think of this as applying to far more than just alcohol – the concept applies to dozens of public health hazards caused by various types of industries.

5. After several decades of research, it is now known that a highly effective strategy to reduce overall (population-level) alcohol consumption is to increase the MLDA in all 50 states.
   a. True
   b. **False**

   Many studies have shown that lowering the MDLA has no effect whatsoever.

6. Alcohol sales in the United States increased at the height of the COVID-19 pandemic.
   a. **True**
   b. False

   This was the subject of Box 8.1.

7. Which effect of excess alcohol use is also a risk factor for adult-onset diabetes?
   a. Hypertension
   b. **Obesity**
   c. Congestive heart failure
   d. Cardiac myopathy

   Think of alcohol as refined carbohydrate – it leads to obesity and elevated blood sugar levels (both of which greatly increase the odds of developing diabetes).

8. As a long-time heavy drinker, Juan often finds himself feeling weak and lethargic. He complains that he "has no strength left in his body." This is most likely a consequence of:
    a. Alcohol-induced hepatitis
    b. Deregulation of acetate
    c. **Myopathy**
    d. Neurological deterioration
        Myopathy is a general weakening of the skeletal muscles.

9. Of the following possible public health strategies, which one has the **least** chance of reducing population-level alcohol consumption?
    a. **Warning labels on all alcoholic beverage containers**
    b. Large increases in state excise taxes on alcohol
    c. Creating zoning regulations to reduce the density of sales outlets
    d. Social movements that support reduced consumption
        The idea of consumer education did not work with tobacco and has not worked with alcohol.

10. The concept of social contagion relates to:
    a. **Density of alcohol sales outlets**
    b. The distributive law
    c. Reciprocal causation
    d. Social cognitive theory
        Recall that a **neighborhood effect** exists, and this effect can support or discourage excess use.

Chapter 9

1. Harm reduction, as applied to the opioid crisis, is best described as:
    a. Changing the demand side of the equation relative to the supply and demand of opioids
    b. Altering the strength of opioids by reducing potency with fentanyl
    c. **Providing people with OUD with access to SSPs and OST**
        Recall that both of these programs are vital to reducing the crisis.

2. Which disease has become the largest epidemic of the opioid crisis?
    a. Hepatitis B
    b. **Hepatitis C**
    c. Human immunodeficiency virus
    d. Soft tissue infections
        Hepatitis C rises in direct correspondence with an increase in the number of Americans injecting opioids.

3. Tracing the history of the opioid crisis back to its origin, what term best captures the initial cause?
    a. **The fifth vital sign**
    b. Fentanyl
    c. Hepatitis
    d. The First Commission
        Remember that this was about pain: i.e., that people could always be helped to manage their pain through drugs.

4. Evidence supports the value of both SSPs and OST relative to harm reduction. Of these two options, however, the evidence is much stronger relative to OST.
   a. **True**
   b. False
      As SSPs evolve, they may become more effective; OST programs have evolved more rapidly and are more effective relative to harm reduction.

5. Of the following professions, which one has the greatest potential to mitigate and resolve the opioid crisis?
   a. Police officers
   b. Parole officers
   c. Public health social workers
   d. **Pharmacists**
      This chapter provides you with a host of possibilities for the role pharmacists can play in turning back the tide of the crisis.

6. SSPs are also thought of as distribution programs for syringes and needles. This is particularly the case when:
   a. **The exchange is greater than a 1 to 1 ratio**
   b. These programs are co-located in pharmacies
   c. PWID can receive their injection equipment anonymously
   d. Law enforcement supports the exchange efforts
      When this ratio is greater than a simple one-to-one exchange, the hope is that people using SSPs will then provide clean equipment to PWID not using SSPs.

7. Which one of the following is not a BBI?
   a. Staph aureus
   b. Hepatitis B
   c. **Needle tracks**
   d. Hepatitis C
      Needle tracks are unhealed puncture wounds where PWID have injected.

8. OxyContin is no longer the main driver of the opioid crisis. Instead, the more recent drivers are:
   a. Fentanyl and heroin
   b. **Fentanyl and other synthetic opioids**
   c. Heroin and methamphetamines
   d. Narcan and methadone
      Fentanyl was the first synthetic opioid. Other synthetics have followed in its wake.

9. The public health response to the overdose death rates caused by the opioid crisis has largely been characterized by:
   a. An equal mix of tertiary and primary prevention
   b. Mostly tertiary prevention in the form of harm reduction
   c. **Mostly tertiary prevention in the form of Narcan**
   d. Mostly primary prevention based on the use of BBI inhibitors
      Bear in mind that overdose is only the tip of the iceberg relative to the health effects of the opioid crisis.

10. One great public health success of the opioid crisis has been that SSPs are now implemented and conducted using a universal system overseen by the Joint Commission.
    a. True
    b. **False**

    Unfortunately, SSPs are not well coordinated. These programs are implemented from a range of perspectives, many of which limit effectiveness.

Chapter 10

1. Which one of the following prevention options was developed and is intended primarily for people who are HIV-uninfected but at high risk of HIV acquisition?
    a. **PrEP**
    b. TasP
    c. The information-motivation-behavioral skills model
    d. HIV testing and counseling

    Keep in mind that PrEP is taken by healthy people who are at high risk of HIV acquisition.

2. The cascade regarding the continuum of care refers to:
    a. The event of seroconversion that happens soon after HIV acquisition
    b. **"Falling out" of care, which results in only a small percentage of people having the full benefit of antiretroviral therapies**
    c. A lack of medical attention to the condom use needs of PrEP users

    The cascade, of course, is the main reason public health practice must strive to find ways to keep people on the continuum.

3. In regard to PrEP, risk compensation refers to:
    a. People who begin using condoms after they acquire a sexually transmissible infection
    b. **People giving up on condom use because they begin PrEP use**
    c. The use of condoms in the context of seropositioning
    d. The use of condoms in the context of serosorting

    This is all too common, especially among people who are at risk of STIs.

4. In a monogamous male couple where one person is not living with HIV and the other is a PLWH, which sexual behavior of the HIV-uninfected partner is the most likely to lead to HIV transfer?
    a. Receiving oral sex (no condom)
    b. Receiving vaginal sex
    c. Being an insertive partner (top) in anal sex and not using a condom
    d. **Being a receptive partner (bottom) in anal sex and not using a condom**

    As you learned in this chapter, this is by far the most risk-prone behavior for the bottom partner who is HIV-uninfected.

5. The United States has experienced record levels of STI incidence in recent years. This may be partly attributable to PrEP.
    a. **True**
    b. False

    Other factors have also contributed to the increase in STIs.

6. Lowering community viral load, promoting adherence to ART, and averting the ART cascade are critical to:
   a. The CDC's compendium model of HIV prevention
   b. **TasP**
   c. Reducing racial and sexual minority HIV disparities
   d. PrEP
   The idea of TasP is indeed global and very well-funded. Its theory is outstanding – the challenge is fully realizing the potential of this strategy.

7. Which of the following does not apply to the concept of prevention case management?
   a. Counseling for PrEP
   b. Housing assistance
   c. **Assistance with low literacy issues**
   d. Education and distribution of condoms
   Refer to the bulleted list of items shown in the chapter.

8. PrEP is designed to avert the acquisition of HIV from an HIV-infected sex partner, whereas TasP is designed to avert HIV transmission for the person taking it.
   a. **True**
   b. False
   The twin approaches of PrEP and TasP form the entire medical arsenal of HIV prevention.

9. Jerri is a male who has a chancre on his penis. He is also living with HIV. To avoid transmitting the virus to his male sex partner while still having a sex life with him, they determine that Jerri should be the bottom partner in anal receptive sex. What level of risk does this pose to his HIV-uninfected partner?
   a. The risk is the highest possible because of syphilis.
   b. As long as Jerri is the receptive partner only, there is no risk to his partner.
   c. **This seropositioning only reduces the risk for the partner – risk still exists.**
   Because Jerri is an insertive partner in anal sex, his boyfriend has at least five times less risk than he would in the receptive position (probably much more, given the chancre).

10. A potential harbinger of HIV medication resistance is:
    a. **The rapid emergence of drug-resistant gonorrhea**
    b. The fact that PrEP use is becoming far less protective than it used to be
    c. The observation that HIV seroconversion is happening before the window period
    Just as gonorrhea developed resistance, so too will HIV.

Chapter 11

1. Which of the following terms is **least** implicated as a root cause of homicide caused by gun violence?
   a. Toxic masculinity
   b. Superstructure of the media
   c. **America's mental health crisis**
   d. American narratives about guns
   Remember that mental health issues are only a small part of the reasons behind homicides from gun violence.

2. Which safety feature of a car is the best example of a mitigating device?
   a. **Collapsible steering column**
   b. GPS sensor that warns of an impending collision
   c. Raised reflectors on four-lane highways
   d. Grooved pavement that warns drivers of an impending road hazard
   To **mitigate** implies that the accident will occur, so the goal is to reduce the severity of injuries.

3. One common American narrative is that "the government wants to take away our guns." Which statement is **false** in this regard?
   a. Buy-back programs will pay people for guns.
   b. **People who own assault weapons purchased under the background check system would be exempt from any ban.**
   c. Federal and state proposals to ban weapons are not focused on guns designed to hunt game.
   d. These programs have been very successful in other high-income nations.
   Nobody would be exempt.

4. Although mass shootings garner a considerable amount of coverage by the media, they represent a very small portion of the total gun deaths that occur annually in the United States.
   a. **True**
   b. False
   Remember that the vast majority of the more than 100 gun deaths occurring each day are not attributable to mass shootings. Mass shootings are only the tip of the iceberg.

5. The dual actions of surveillance and monitoring are best exemplified in this chapter by the:
   a. Gun buy-back program
   b. Brady Handgun Prevention Act
   c. **Fatality Analysis Reporting System**
   d. Regulation of the auto industry
   This system works eloquently to capture data that is then used to judge the value of new regulations.

6. Which statement relative to passing federal laws banning assault weapons is true?
   a. **As of 2022, Congress had yet to pass any legislation on to the executive branch (i.e., the White House).**
   b. Presidential bills that ban assault weapons have been vetoed by Congress.
   c. Laws banning assault weapons constantly change with each new White House administration.
   d. Only the Brady Act has ever been used to successfully ban assault weapons.
   A key take-home point in this chapter is that the U.S. Congress has historically ignored its responsibility to pass protective legislation that saves lives.

7. Which issue is **not** characterized by a racial disparity that favors White Americans?
   a. Long-term injuries from gun violence
   b. Deaths from gun violence
   c. **Daytime deaths from auto collisions**
   d. Being the victim of gun violence
   This is one of the few public health problems that significantly impacts White Americans.

8. One solution that may contribute to reducing gun violence involves the use of manufacturing technology so that guns can be used only by their licensed owner. These are:
   a. Safe guns
   b. **Smart guns**
   c. Registered guns
   d. Non-repeating weapons
      Smart guns use various technologies that prevent anyone except the registered owner from firing the gun.

9. As you learned from reading this chapter, the general decline in auto fatalities is a product of engineering based on research, with federal mandates used to make innovations mandatory. The current trend is for this same pattern to be applied to controlling gun violence.
   a. True
   b. **False**
      In an ideal America, this would be true – but sadly, it is anything but true.

10. If guns, gun purchasing, and gun carrying were regulated along the same lines as current regulations for cars and other vehicles, all of the following would be likely to occur except:
    a. Sales may be limited to non-felons
    b. The speed at which guns can fire multiple rounds of bullets could be regulated
    c. **The Second Amendment would be revised by the U.S. Congress**
    d. Assault weapons would only be sold to persons trained and certified (annually) in using these weapons.
       There is no limit on the options that could be used to regulate guns. To date, however, no U.S. Representative to Congress has publicly suggested revising this amendment.

Chapter 12

1. A natural form of annual water storage takes the form of:
   a. **Snowpack**
   b. Greywater reuse systems
   c. Desalination systems
   d. Potable greenhouse effects
      Snow is much more than something for winter sports!

2. Which human action leaves the largest water footprint?
   a. Eating a serving of oatmeal
   b. **Eating beef**
   c. Consuming organic vegetables as an entire meal
   d. Drinking a glass of wine
      Always remember that animal products leave a far larger water footprint than plant-based food products.

3. Which human adaptation would most reduce the amount of methane gas entering the atmosphere and also conserve water?
   a. Less use of gasoline-powered cars
   b. **Using electric heat and ovens rather than heating and cooking with natural gas**
   c. Reusing greywater for vegetable gardens
   d. Enforcing the Clean Water Act such that all industries must fully comply
      Recall that fracking natural gas releases huge amounts of methane from the earth and that fracked wells use upward of one million gallons of water per well.

4. Which term represents the **least** advanced technology for adapting to the water crisis at this time in history?

   a. Fracking
   b. Public health engineering
   c. **Desalination**
   d. Reverse photosynthesis

   The science for this technology has not yet advanced to a point that massive quantities of potable water can be produced cost-effectively.

5. The Flint water crisis was mostly a problem caused by a heavy metal: lead. The contamination of water with excess heavy metals also comes from:

   a. **Stormwater that enters treatment plants**
   b. Acid rain
   c. Greywater recapture and use
   d. Microplastics

   You learned that stormwater on pavements collects heavy metals.

6. A large industry located on the banks of the Ohio River produces soaps and other products that all contain POPs. The company was fined for dumping some of its industrial run-off into the river. The POPs will:

   a. Ultimately dissolve and thus become harmless to humans
   b. Be completely removed from any water used for humans when it is processed at water treatment plants
   c. **Enter the food chain via the use of this water for agriculture**

   The word **persistent** in the term **POPs** should be taken to heart – these do not ever dissolve and can easily enter the food chain.

7. The industry described in Question 6 is an example of:

   a. **Point source pollution**
   b. Common source pollution
   c. Microplastic poisoning
   d. The need for improved public health engineering

   Sadly, point source pollution from industry is sometimes punished with just a monetary fine rather than closure.

8. Building codes are used to conserve water! The best example listed here is:

   a. **Mandating the use of WaterSense-labeled toilets**
   b. Offering incentives for people to install greywater recapture systems
   c. Using green space to reduce the amount of stormwater running into streets
   d. Calculating the average water footprint of a newly constructed home

   Building codes only apply to the structures, so **c** is not a plausible option. Option **b** may have been an attractive option to you, but building codes and incentives are not the same.

9. The Johnson family has owned and operated a 2,000-acre cattle ranch in Utah for more than 100 years. None of the family members ski or care about snow-related recreation activities. However, every year they measure the snowpack depth in the Colorado Rockies. Why?

    a. **Snowpack in the Colorado Rockies supplies the Colorado River with most of its water. The river, in turn, supplies water to much of the southwestern United States, including parts of Utah.**

    b. Snowpack is an organic pollutant that may carry heavy metals into waterways that eventually are used to provide water to the family's cattle. This creates beef that will not pass standards setting limits on heavy metals in human food.

    The opening photos in this chapter provide a visual lesson in why snow in the Colorado Rockies is vital to people in the southwestern U.S.

10. Sludge is a solid substance that the Clean Water Act mandates must be safely disposed of in state-operated landfills.

    a. True

    b. **False**

    Public health law is lacking in this regard. Sludge can legally be used as what is known as **biosolid compost**.

Chapter 13

1. A key point in this chapter was that small changes can add up to make large differences. Of course, this depends on a sufficiently large number of people making these small changes. Which bolded term in the chapter is **most** applicable in this regard?

    a. **Diffusion of innovation theory**

    b. Subsidies

    c. Pollinators

    d. Agribusiness

    DOI theory is focused on the idea that large populations can make seemingly small adaptations.

2. Which food has the most efficient feed conversion ratio?

    a. Farm-raised trout

    b. Lamb

    c. **Walnuts**

    d. Organically raised chicken

    A simple rule to remember is that all plant-based foods have far more favorable conversion ratios.

3. Clearly, the U.S. government can up its game to increase the food supply and reduce climate change caused by agribusiness. Which regulatory target is **not** within the realm of the federal government?

    a. The SNAP

    b. **Deforestation of the Amazon rainforest**

    c. Neonicotinoids

    d. Beef subsidies

    Options **a** and **d** are government programs you learned about in this chapter, and option **c** is part of the larger regulatory power of the EPA. However, option **d** will require a coordinated global effort.

4. Cover crops add nitrogen to the soil. This is important to humans because:
   a. **It is the source of amino acids.**
   b. It averts erosion.
   c. Nitrogen is vital to the lives of pollinators.
   d. It gives improved feed conversion ratios

   Nitrogen is the basis for what will become any type of protein.

5. Which food has the **least** efficient feed conversion ratio?
   a. Lean white pork
   b. Chicken breasts
   c. **Roast beef**
   d. Legumes

   The same rule used to solve question 2 also applies here in ruling out option **d**. Of the remaining options, you learned that beef is by far the most costly to the environment and has the least favorable conversion ratio of any animal-based food.

6. A young farmer in Nebraska makes this post on social media: "I will be changing 30% of my operation next year to no-till farming." Imagine that most other nearby farmers reading this post react by saying something like, "What is he talking about?" Applying DOI theory to this scenario, the young farmer making the post is **best** described as:
   a. **An innovator**
   b. Part of the early majority
   c. A laggard
   d. A spokesperson for agribusiness

   DOI is highly reliant on innovators engaging in peer modeling.

7. An entire community is devoted to redistributing excess farm produce. This is a practice known by the general name of:
   a. Early adoption
   b. Peer modeling
   c. Food miles
   d. **Food rescue**

   It is likely that a progressively greater number of U.S. communities will adopt the practice of food rescue in the coming years.

8. Sometimes, small things can be the reason for big problems. With that in mind, which term is actually no small thing relative to addressing the food crisis?
   a. Conventional farming
   b. **Pollinators**
   c. Soil contamination
   d. Omnivores

   Insects such as bees may seem small, but without pollinators, the human race would be in grave danger of massive starvation.

9. Although meat is a superior source of dietary protein, plant-based sources rank a very close but clear second place.
   a. True
   b. **False**

   Remember that you learned about the great protein myth in this chapter. Plants provide all the amino acids your body needs.

10. Imagine you have the power to suddenly change only one federal regulatory policy regarding food. Which action would produce the **greatest** return in terms of food causing climate change?
   a. **End the practice of subsidizing beef production.**
   b. Make more people eligible for SNAP.
   c. Educate American farmers about no-till practices.
   d. Genetically modify beans to produce greater levels of amino acids.

   The one lesson from this chapter that most students never forget is that the beef industry is a major cause of climate change. Much of the voting public is probably unaware of this point and the fact that the industry is supported by taxpayer dollars.

Chapter 14

1. As part of a public health intervention program, social media marketing is used to promote the use of LARC as a responsibility to the earth. Which one of the four A's is the target of this program?
   a. Affordability
   b. Accessibility
   c. **Acceptability**
   d. Availability

   Making something more desirable (i.e., wanted) is very much focused on the principle of acceptability.

2. The fertility rate will always be greater than the birth rate.
   a. **True**
   b. False

   This is because the denominator is much smaller (i.e., only women of reproductive age).

3. Which of the following is least associated with increased urbanization?
   a. Increased pollution of waterways
   b. Increased risk of airborne disease transmission
   c. **Newborn deaths**
   d. Fewer trees to bind carbon

   You learned that **a**, **b**, and **d** are all results of urbanization. Option **c** is completely unrelated.

4. Which one of the following best describes the concept of a demographic transition?
   a. Carbon dioxide levels accelerate global warming.
   b. **The mean age of a population shifts to a much younger average.**
   c. The birth rate exceeds the death rate by a 2:1 ratio.
   d. The fertility rate declines.

   This is usually a result of medical technology extending the lives of the elderly in a population.

5. The Malthus hypothesis implies all of the following except:
   a. **Zoonotic diseases will decimate a large number of people.**
   b. Carrying capacity limits population expansion.
   c. A J-shaped curve involves a rapid die-off of the affected species.
   d. An S-shaped curve is a more optimistic outcome than a J-shaped curve.

   That zoonotic diseases will lead to massive numbers of death is certainly true; however, it was not part of the Malthus hypothesis.

6. Which one of the following public health actions is the least critical to reducing the rate of unintended pregnancy in the United States?

    a. Title X

    b. **Microcredit programs**

    c. LARC

    d. Programs that promote correct condom use

    A key phrase in this question is "in the United States." Thus the action that least applies (because it is used primarily in developing nations) is microcredit.

7. Thinking about all you have learned in this chapter, which form of public health intervention to reduce global overpopulation is the most distal in its goals?

    a. Widespread dissemination of LARC

    b. Teaching young males how to use condoms

    c. Enhancing the provision of low-cost (or free) contraception services for women

    d. **Providing equal education opportunities for girls and young women**

    Distal implies that the influence lies in a superstructure such as economics, education, and so on.

8. Which term represents "bad air" and is thus applicable to explaining the increased risk of respiratory diseases among urban populations?

    a. Right-to-die

    b. IUD

    c. **Miasma**

    d. Zoonotic

    This was a common theory of disease transmission even before the invention of the microscope and the creation of germ theory.

9. Educating girls and young women is vital to controlling overpopulation because this education focuses on teaching knowledge and skills regarding condoms and contraceptive options.

    a. True

    b. **False**

    Education works by giving girls and young women a competitive edge in the global job market. The goal is to increase the number of women who have professional careers.

10. Carrying capacity is exceeded when:

    a. The population birth rate is above 2.0

    b. **Finite resources supporting a population become insufficient**

    c. The S-shaped distribution reaches its peak

    d. The fertility rate exceeds the birth rate

    Always remember that the food and water supplies on earth are finite!

Chapter 15

1. As shown by history, simply creating vaccines and making them available may:

    a. Be ample to create near elimination of the diseases

    b. Be ample to create near eradication of the diseases

    c. **Fail as a public health response due to the unwillingness of people to be vaccinated**

    Remember that even smallpox – a deadly plague – was "marked" by people refusing to take the vaccine.

2. Hemorrhagic fevers lead to death by:
   a. **Causing a loss of blood internally**
   b. Causing the sudden and severe loss of lung function
   c. Creating dangerous swelling of the meninges
   This is because of the destruction occurring in capillary beds.

3. In thinking about the threat of emerging epidemics as a call for the public health system to be prepared, what role is played by case surveillance systems?
   a. These systems quickly determine the causative agent of the disease.
   b. **These system act as a first alarm to trigger a more intensive public health response.**
   c. Case surveillance is a logical conclusion to the public health practice of contact tracing.
   d. All of the above
   Surveillance systems are very much like a fire alarm.

4. Which organization is **not** exclusive to the U.S.-based infrastructure of preparedness for emerging diseases?
   a. The Peace Corp
   b. The CDC
   c. **The WHO**
   d. The Carter Center
   The WHO serves the world in this regard.

5. Which one of the following diseases can be considered eradicated, as opposed to eliminated?
   a. **Smallpox**
   b. Measles
   c. Mumps
   d. Rubella
   Remember that **eradicated** implies a global absence of the disease.

6. Rhonda is a 41-year-old who normally neglects to have an annual flu shot. She also was never vaccinated against COVID-19. Her three children have all attended school and received the entire childhood vaccination series. Which phrase **best** characterizes Rhonda?
   a. Anti-vaxxer
   b. **Not concerned about the threat of disease**
   c. Unwilling to comply with public health guidelines
   Like so many Americans, Rhonda does not make vaccines a priority in her life. But this does not mean she is an anti-vaxxer or somehow unwilling to comply.

7. Vaccines are capable of being the only public health tool in the likely event of an epidemic caused by an emerging disease.
   a. True
   b. **False**
   Remember that a host of other tools must also be used.

8. Emerging diseases also include the prospect of currently known microbes developing antibiotic resistance.
   a. **True**
   b. False
   Gonorrhea is an example from this chapter.

9. As a candidate for president of the United States, Senator X stated, "We must fortify our borders and focus all of our disease prevention efforts on only the citizens of this great nation." What is wrong with this statement?

   a. **It ignores the fundamental principle that the control of emerging infectious diseases must occur at a global level.**

   b. It misses the point that the only way to control emerging infections is to end all travel into the United States.

   This principle is paramount to this chapter!

10. How is it possible that deforestation is a cause of emerging diseases?

   a. It leads to starvation, which then makes people vulnerable to disease.

   b. **It destroys plant and animal species that previously held some microbes in check.**

   c. Deforestation is a direct cause of bacterial-related drug resistance.

   This is a loss of biodiversity.

On 18 July 2022, much of France, Wales, and Britain experienced the most intense heat ever on record. The heat spell was referred to even by government officials as a "heat apocalypse," and reading about it seemed more like science fiction than the daily news. Consider, for example, this passage from *The Washington Post*:

> British authorities declared a national emergency and for the first time issued a 'red extreme' heat warning for large parts of England, as the nation struggled to adapt. In London, workers wrapped the historic Hammersmith Bridge over the river Thames in silver insulation foil to protect the cast-iron spans from cracking. . . . Planes were diverted from at least two airports, amid reports of melting runways and roads. (Noack & Booth, 2022)

As the author of this and nine other public health textbooks, I have always been aware of how quickly material in a textbook becomes outdated. This book was written in 2022. Given the harsh realities of climate change and the endless implications for public health, there is no doubt that new threats to public health will continue to mount and thus challenge the ability of humans and governments to adapt. We must all work for innovative and effective solutions to the health-related problems that occur – even if the problems do not directly impact our lives or the lives of family and friends. The strength and welfare of a nation are as much products of public health as economics, equality, and the exercise of democratic governance.

Public health will become all the more important given the ever-widening health disparities that show no sign of ending. Also, with the earth's ecology permanently altered by climate change, the occurrence of new and emerging diseases is likely to make the COVID-19 pandemic look like a dress rehearsal for more devastating microbes. Perhaps most importantly, as water and food become scarce commodities in parts of the United States, public health will be saddled with the responsibility of finding new ways to provide the basic human necessities for existence and well-being. The full participation of all Americans is required to protect the future of our children (see **Photo E.1**) and ensure that the present times give everyone an equal chance to pursue health and happiness. Thus, the standing lesson from reading this book is that public health is a public responsibility.

As a child, you probably either expected or took for granted that the adults in your world would somehow solve public health problems and create conditions that are safe and healthy. As an adult, however, expecting others to solve the problems that keep us from being safe and healthy is childish thinking. There is no such thing as a "magic bullet" that will cure chronic diseases and avert epidemics – the only magic we have comes from clear, science-based evidence regarding the most effective approaches to improving public health. This book has given you a brief summary of these practices! Now that you are aware of the various actions that can improve public health, the question becomes, "How will you contribute to this public responsibility?"

If you have enjoyed this book and the learning experience, one final point is warranted. Chances are that your career is just starting and this course is part of an undergraduate degree program (perhaps a course you selected as a general education requirement). If you have not

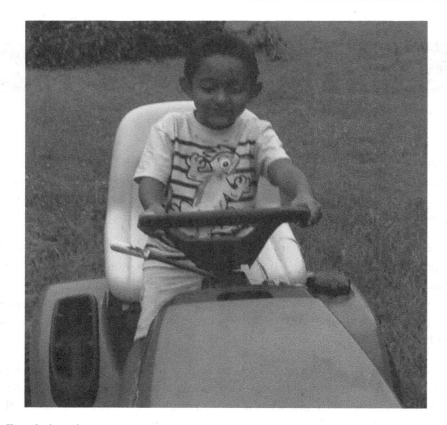

Photo E.1   The author's grandson.

yet fully decided what your career will look like, reflect for a moment on the fact that public health is not a profession per se. As you have learned, all types of professions can involve public health practices: public health architecture, civil engineering (particularly relative to water), solar energy, law, dietary counseling, food programs, urban design, allied health fields, and so on. So, please consider devoting a portion of your ultimate career objective to finding at least one way to make a lasting contribution to improving the health of this nation. And if you decide to devote your career entirely to public health, do not make the mistake of having an "interest area" (i.e., a favorite cause or disease that you want to define your career). Instead, consider that public health practice requires fluidity among its few dedicated professionals – a flexibility that lets these people adapt quickly to the demands imposed by an ever-changing set of challenges to the health and security of the public.

Reference

Noack, R., & Booth, W. (2002). Europeans shocked by "heat apocalypse" as temperature records fall. *Washington Post*, July 18. https://www.washingtonpost.com/world/2022/07/18/britain-europe-heatwave-record-temperatures/